General Surgery

From the publishers of the *Tarascon Pocket Pharmacopoeia*

Jame ~~_~~hambers, MD, MPH

Staff Surgeon
Wilford Hall Medical Center
Lackland Air Force Base, TX

JONES & BARTLETT
L E A R N I N G

World Headquarters
Jones & Bartlett Learning
5 Wall Street
Burlington, MA 01803
978-443-5000
info@jblearning.com
www.jblearning.com

Jones & Bartlett Learning books and products are available through most bookstores and online booksellers. To contact Jones & Bartlett Learning directly, call 800-832-0034, fax 978-443-8000, or visit our website, www.jblearning.com.

Substantial discounts on bulk quantities of Jones & Bartlett Learning publications are available to corporations, professional associations, and other qualified organizations. For details and specific discount information, contact the special sales department at Jones & Bartlett Learning via the above contact information or send an email to specialsales@jblearning.com.

Production Credits

Senior Acquisitions Editor: Nancy Anastasi Duffy
Associate Editor: Laura Burns
Production Assistant: Leia Poritz
Manufacturing and Inventory Control Supervisor: Amy Bacus
Medicine Marketing Manager: Rebecca Rockel

Composition: Exemplarr Worldwide Ltd
Cover Design: Kristin E. Parker
Cover Image: © Image200/Getty Images
Printing and Binding: Malloy, Inc.
Cover Printing: Malloy, Inc.

ISBN: 978-1-4496-3634-0

6048
Printed in the United States of America
15 14 13 12 11   10 9 8 7 6 5 4 3 2 1

DEDICATION

Dedicated to Sylvia, Neil, Brette, my parents, and my brother, Walter. Your love and patience have made everything possible.

Thank you to Drs. Robert McClelland and Gary Purdue for your encouragement and example.

CONTENTS

EDITORIAL BOARD

A NOTE FROM THE AUTHOR

Tarascon Clinical Review Series: General Surgery is intended as a quick reference for the practice of general surgery. It represents a compilation of facts and techniques that I have found useful, and they are referenced where thought to be particularly important. If you find an error or wish to make a suggestion, please let us know (e-mail: editor@tarascon.com).

CHAPTER 1

FLUIDS, ELECTROLYTES, METABOLISM, AND NUTRITION

I. **FLUIDS**
   A. **24 h:** 100 mL/kg for 1st 10 kg (1000 mL), 50 mL/kg for 2nd 10 kg (500 mL), 20 mL/kg thereafter.
   B. **Per h:** 4 mL/kg for 1st 10 kg (40 mL), 2 mL/kg for 2nd 10 kg (20 mL), 1 mL/kg thereafter.

TABLE 1.1. Crystalloid Composition

Crystalloid	Kcal / L	Osm	Na	Cl	K	Ca	Mg	Lactate
NS (0.9%)	0	Iso	154	154	0	0	0	0
D5W	170	Hypo	0	0	0	0	0	0
LR	9	Iso	130	109	4	1.5	0	28
Plasmalyte	21	Iso	140	98	5	0	3	*
D5 ½ NS	170	Hypo	77	77	0	0	0	0

*Plasmalyte uses 27 mEq of acetate and 23 mEq of gluconate as buffers instead of lactate. One advantage of Plasmalyte over RL is its lack of calcium which makes RL incompatible with blood infusions.

   C. **Body fluid composition/rate:**
      1. *Total body water (TBW)*: overall average, 55% body wt is water.
         a. 35% is intracellular, 20% extracellular, 16% interstitial, 4% intravascular.

II. **ELECTROLYTES**
   A. **Sodium:** normal is 140 (135–145).
      1. *Plasma osmolality* = $(2 \times Na) + (Glucose/18) + (Bun/2.8)$.
      2. *Hypernatremia* can result from loss of hypotonic fluids or gain of hypertonic fluids.
         a. Therapy depends on extracellular fluid status.
            i. *Sx of possible metabolic encephalopathy*: altered MS, generalized seizures, and focal neuro deficits.
         b. If pt does not have invasive monitors, consider:
            i. *Recent loss of wt?* (suggests decreased ECV if no edema)
            ii. *Peripheral edema?* (suggests increased ECV if adequate proteinemia)
            iii. *Spot sodium < 10 mEq/L?* (suggests decreased ECV)
         c. *Low ECV* (most common): from loss of hypotonic fluids. Total Na is *decreased* (lost sodium but even more free water), must replace quickly; follow by replacing the free water deficit more slowly.
            i. Crystalloid of choice is isotonic saline, *not* hypotonic.
            ii. Once hypovolemia is corrected, replace the free water deficit:
               • Calculate *normal TBW*.
                  ○ *For hypernatremia*: male TBW → lean body kg × 0.5; female TBW → lean body kg × 0.4. (When not in this circumstance, males are 60% and females 50%.)
               • Calculate *current TBW*: normal TBW × (140/current P_{Na})
               • Calculate *TBW deficit* (L): normal TBW − current TBW
               • Calculate *replacement volume* (L): TBW deficit × (1/1-X) (*Note:* X = Na in replacement fluid / 154)
            iii. *Replace volume*: free water deficit should be replaced over 48–72 h.
         d. *Normal ECV*: from net loss of free water, usu. when hypotonic fluid is replaced w/ isotonic saline 1:1. Slowly replace the free water deficit.

i. Can also occur w/ diabetes insipidus (DI), w/ dilute urine but hypertonic plasma; confirmed if complete fluid restriction does not increase urine osm > 30 mOsm/L w/in hours. Vasopressin (5 U IV) can differentiate between the 2 types.

- *Central DI* (secondary to closed head injury, meningitis, hypoxic encephalopathy): urine osm often < 200; vasopressin increases by 50+% urine osmolality very quickly.
- *Nephrogenic DI* (secondary to hypokalemia, aminoglycosides, amphotericin, iodinated contrast, or polyuric ATN): urine osm usu. 200–500, unaffected by vasopressin.

ii. *Tx for DI*: replace free water only. Calculate TBW deficit, replace over 2–3 d to reduce risk of cerebral edema. If central DI, then generally need to give 5–10 U aqueous vasopressin SC every 6–8 h (monitor Na carefully).

e. *High ECV*: from gain of hypertonic fluids. Seen w/ excessive use of hypertonic saline, sodium bicarbonate, or PO salt. May need furosemide and replace w/ fluids relatively hypotonic to the urine (usu. ~ 75 mEq/L of Na in urine from furosemide diuresis).

3. *Hyponatremia*: therapy depends on volume status, urine sodium, and if sx present. Major risk is potentially irreversible encephalopathy from cerebral edema.

a. *Pseudohyponatremia*:

i. *Hypertriglyceridemia*: mEq/L decrease in plasma sodium = plasma triglycerides (g/L) × 0.002.

ii. *Hyperproteinemia*: mEq/L decrease in plasma sodium = plasma protein − 8 (g/dL) × 0.025.

b. True hyponatremia is, like hypernatremia, classified by ECV status.

i. *Low ECV (hypovolemic)*: from fluid losses that are insufficiently replaced by fluids that are hypotonic relative to the lost fluids. A spot urine sodium may be useful:

Urine Sodium	Site of Sodium Loss
> 20 mEq/L	Renal (diuretics, adrenal insufficiency)
< 20 mEq/L	Extrarenal (diarrhea, vomiting)

- Infuse hypertonic (3%) saline if symptomatic, and normal saline if asymptomatic.

ii. *Normal ECV (isovolemic)*: from gain of up to 5 L of excess water that is not clinically apparent. Spot urine sodium and urine osmolality can be helpful:

U Na	U Osm	Etiology
> 20	> 100	SIADH (plasma tonicity usu. < 290 also)
< 10	< 100	Water intoxication

- Combine furosemide diuresis w/ infusion of hypertonic saline if symptomatic, or w/ normal saline if asymptomatic.

iii. *High ECV (hypervolemic)*: gain water > gain Na. Spot urine sodium can be helpful, although diuretics can confuse the situation.

U Na	Etiology
< 20	Extrarenal (cardiac failure, cirrhosis)
> 20	Renal failure

- Start furosemide diuresis if asymptomatic; combine w/ judicious use of hypertonic saline if sx.

B. **Potassium**: normal is 4 (3.5–4.5).

1. *Hypokalemia*

a. *Etiology*: K^+ → inside cell w/ alkalosis, insulin/anabolism, adrenergic state (can occur w/ beta agonist inhalers), and hypothermia. Most diuretics, steroids, hyperaldosteronism → renal loss of K^+.

    b. *Presentation*: ileus, asthenia. *EKG*: ↑ digitalis effect, flat/inverted T waves, QT prolongation, ST segment depression. Nephrotoxic if chronic.

    c. *Tx*:

        i. Keep above 4 in critically ill pts. Give as KCl (20, 40, 60 mEq) or KPhos (15, 30, 45 mmol).

        ii. Usu. keep administration < 10 mmol/h, although 2× this rate is tolerated.

        iii. *Acidosis*: if prolonged, body will lose lots of K in urine. Watch for hypokalemia if rapidly correct prolonged acidosis.

        iv. *Alkalosis*: although little plasma K, kidney must trade to retain Na (harder to retain HCO_3 to balance or trade H+ in alkalosis, so K is used instead), → urinary loss. Eventually, when K gets too low, kidneys will revert to trading H+ again, resulting in *paradoxical aciduria* (strong sign of total K+ depletion).

          • *Note*: difficult to reverse alkalosis w/out first correcting K+ deficit, as kidneys continue to trade H+ to retain Na+ (or resorb HCO_3 to balance) if not enough K+ to do the job.

          • *Note*: impossible to correct K+ deficit w/ KCl alone if Mg++ is deficient. First replace the Mg++ (important to replace Mg++ for hypocalcemic pts as well).

  2. *Hyperkalemia*

    a. K+ released w/ acidosis, starvation/catabolism, and cell death.

    b. Manifests as paralysis, loss of deep tendon reflexes. *EKG*: peaked T waves (esp. in precordial leads), ↑ PR interval +/− widened QRS. Arrhythmias, ultimately VFib. Increases action of digitalis (tx w/ 2 g IV $MgSO_4$ – NOT Ca++, +/− digitalis Ab).

    c. *Tx*:

        i. *Ca chloride*, 500–1000 mg IVP (5–10 cc of 10% solution).

          • Protects heart from dysrhythmias.

          • Effects in 1–3 min, lasting 30–60 min.

        ii. 1 ampule D_{50} (50 cc) + 10 U regular *insulin* IVP.

          • Effects in 30 min, lasting 4–6 h.

        iii. Nebulized *albuterol*, 10–20 mg nebulized over 15 min.

          • Effects in 15 min, lasting 15–90 min.

        iv. *$NaHCO_3$* 1 mEq/kg IVP.

          • Effects in 5–10 min, lasting 1–2 h.

        v. Consider *furosemide*, 40–80 mg IVP.

        vi. Consider *Kayexalate*, 20–50 g PO in (50 cc) or PR (retention enema) in (200 cc) 20% sorbitol.

          • Effects in 1–2 h, lasting 4–6 h.

        vii. If above fails, consult for *dialysis*.

C. Cl: normal is 100 (99–109).

  1. *Hyperchloremia*

    a. W/ inpts, usu. due to excess IV NS → non-gap metabolic *acidosis*. *Tx*: change IVF (i.e., Na acetate).

  2. *Hypochloremia*

    a. May be from excess GI losses (i.e., gastric outlet obstruction) or volume contraction. Freq. assoc. w/ *alkalosis*. Spot urine Cl− may help determine if alkalosis will be chloride-responsive.

        i. *Chloride-resistant alkalosis*: ↑ U Cl− (> 25 mEq/L), usu. from K+ depletion a/o excess mineralocorticoid activity; assoc. w/ volume expansion. Pts usu. euchloremic.

D. Calcium (*total* 8.0–10.2 mg/dL or 2.2–2.5 mmol/L; *ionized* 2.5–5.0 mg/dL or 0.8–1.6 mmol/L).

  1. ~ 50% bound to plasma proteins (80% is albumin). Ionized fraction is physiologically active. Hypoproteinemia decreases total Ca++, but does not affect the ionized fraction.

  2. *Hypocalcemia* (50–65% of ICU admissions)

    a. *Etiology*: alkalosis, blood transfusions, cardiopulmonary bypass, drugs (aminoglycosides, cimetidine, heparin, theophylline), fat embolism, magnesium depletion, pancreatitis, renal insufficiency, sepsis.

      i. Corrected serum Ca^{++} mg/dL = serum Ca^{++} mg/dL $(0.8 \times [4.0 - \text{albumin g/dL}])$.

   b. *Clinical effects*

      i. *Neuromuscular excitability*: hyperreflexia, seizures, tetany. Chvostek sign is nonspecific (25% in normal adults), Trousseau sign insensitive (30% false-negative).

   c. *Cardiovascular*

      i. Hypotension, decreased CO, ventricular ectopy (ionized Ca < 0.65 mmol/L assoc. w/ VTach and refractory hypotension).

   d. *Tx*:

      i. IV Ca only indicated for symptomatic hypocalcemia or ionized level < 0.65 mmol/L.

      ii. 10% Ca chloride or 10% Ca gluconate. Ca chloride has 3× the elemental Ca (27 mg/mL vs 9 mg/mL), but is also much more osmolar (2000 vs 680 mOsm/L).

      iii. Because of high osmolarity, give either form through central vein if possible; if not, use Ca gluconate through peripheral vein.

      iv. Bolus 200 g elemental Ca (in 100 mL NS over 10 min); as levels will fall again after 30 min, f/u w/ an infusion of 1–2 mg/kg/h elemental Ca for at least 6 h.

      v. Maintain w/ dosage of 2–4 g/d in adults orally w/ calcium carbonate or calcium gluconate tabs.

      vi. Treat any assoc. Mg^{++} depletion as well as hypomagnesemia that impairs PTH release and end-organ responsiveness.

3. *Hypercalcemia*

   a. 90% from malignancy or hyperparathyroidism. Occ. from prolonged immobility, thyrotoxicosis, or drugs (lithium, thiazide diuretics).

   b. Clinical effects (usu. if serum Ca > 12 mg/dL or ionized Ca > 3.0 mmol/L).

      i. *Gastrointestinal*: N/V, constipation, ileus, pancreatitis

      ii. *Cardiovascular*: hypovolemia, hypotension, shortened QT interval

      iii. *Renal*: polyuria, urolithiasis

      iv. *Neuro*: confusion, depressed consciousness, coma

   c. *Tx*: (if symptomatic or serum Ca > 14 mg/dL or ionized Ca > 3.5 mmol/L)

      i. *Saline infusion*: first step as hypercalcemia leads to an osmotic diuresis.

      ii. *Furosemide*: give w/ saline as 40–80 mg IV q 2 h to achieve 100–200 mL/min, which MUST be replaced w/ NS.

      iii. *Bisphosphonates*: more potent than calcitonin, but delayed onset. Pamidronate is agent of choice, given as 90-mg IV infusion over 24 h; peak effect in 4–5 d; can also be repeated in 4–5 d.

      iv. *Dialysis*: for pts w/ renal failure.

E. **Magnesium**

1. *Range*:

   a. *Total* (1.4–2.0 mEq/L or 0.7–1.0 mmol/L)

   b. *Ionized* (0.8–1.1 mEq/L or 0.4–0.6 mmol/L)

   c. *Urinary* (5–15 mEq/24 h or 2.5–7.4 mmol/24 h)

2. Helps maintain cell gradient and calcium movement in smooth muscle. < 1% in the plasma (50% in bone)—can have total body depletion w/ normal plasma levels. In these cases, urine Mg will be abnormally low, however. 55% is in the ionized, active form; most assays only report total Mg, though.

3. *Hypomagnesemia*: up to 65% ICU pts.

   a. Caused by furosemide (most common), aminoglycosides, amphotericin, digitalis, cisplatin, cyclosporine, secretory diarrhea, chronic alcoholism, diabetes mellitus, acute MI.

   b. *Findings*: *hypokalemia* (40%; often need to fix Mg^{++} before K^+ can be fixed), *hypophosphatemia* (30%; often *causes* Mg depletion), *hyponatremia* (27%), *hypocalcemia* (22%; again may need to fix Mg^{++} before Ca^{++}), *thiamin deficiency*.

      i. *Cardiac*: ischemia, arrhythmias, digitalis toxicity. Mg infusion can often stop digitalis toxicity and refractory arrhythmias even in absence of hypomagnesemia.

ii. *Neurologic*: altered mentation, generalized seizures, tremors, and hyperreflexia. Reactive CNS syndrome presents w/ ataxia, slurred speech, metabolic acidosis, excessive salivation, diffuse muscle spasms, seizures, and obtundation.

c. *Tx*: if sx (+) or severe deficiency, IV route preferred. If renal insufficiency, reduce doses by ½, monitor.

   i. *Mild*, asymptomatic cases.
   - Assume deficit of 1–2 mEq/kg.
   - Assume 50% replacement lost in urine; need to replace twice the deficit.
   - Replace 1 mEq/kg the 1st 24 h, then 0.5 mEq/kg/d and over the next 3–5 d.
   - If serum Mg > 1 mEq/L, can use oral Mg.

   ii. *Moderate* cases (serum Mg < 1, or other electrolyte problems).
   - Add 6 g $MgSO_4$ (48 mEq Mg) to 250–500 mL of NS, infused over 3 h.
   - Follow w/ 5 g $MgSO_4$ (40 mEq Mg) in 250–500 mL NS, infused over 6 h.
   - Continue w/ 5 g $MgSO_4$ every 12 h by continuous infusion for the next 5 d.

   iii. *Life-threatening* cases (seizures or serious arrhythmias).
   - Infuse 2 g $MgSO_4$ (16 mEq Mg) IV over 2 min.
   - Follow w/ 5 g $MgSO_4$ (40 mEq Mg) in 250–500 NS infused over 6 h.
   - Continue w/ 5 g $MgSO_4$ every 12 h by continuous infusion for the next 5 d.

   iv. *Parenteral*: each gram of $MgSO_4$ has 8 mEq (4 mmol) of elemental Mg. Dilute w/ NS, not LR.
   - $MgSO_4$ 20%, 200 mg/mL (1.6 mEq/L).
   - $MgSO_4$ 10%, 100 mg/mL (0.8 mEq/L).

4. *Hypermagnesemia*

   a. Rare in absence of renal impairment (creatinine clearance < 30); massive hemolysis ↑ risk.

      i. DKA, adrenal insufficiency, hyperparathyroidism, Li^+ excess can also ↑ levels.

   b. *Manifestation*: clinically, antagonize calcium's effects. Serum Mg > 4 mEq/L may cause hyporeflexia; > 5.0 prolongs AV conduction; > 10 → complete heart block; > 13 → cardiac arrest.

   c. *Tx*:

      i. *Severe* → hemodialysis.

      ii. Calcium gluconate, 1 g IV over 2–3 min for temporary control of cardiac effects.

      iii. If renal function is not impaired, aggressive IVF w/ furosemide can be useful.

F. **Phosphorus** (2.5 mg/dL or 0.8 mmol/L to 5.0 mg/dL or 1.6 mmol/L)

   1. Inorganic state is predominantly intracellular; utilized in glycolysis and high-energy molecule formation.

   2. *Hyperphosphatemia*

      a. *Etiology*: usu. from renal insufficiency or massive cell necrosis (crush injury, tumor lysis, etc.). Less often from DKA.

      b. *Manifestation*: may deposit calcium-phosphate complexes in soft tissue a/o calciphylaxis, typically when product of calcium and phosphorus levels exceeds 60–70.

      c. *Tx*:

         i. *Severe* → consider hemodialysis.

         ii. *Mild/moderate*: aluminum-containing compounds (i.e., antacids, carafate, etc.), or, if pt is hypocalcific, calcium acetate tablets (PhosLo), given as 2 tablets three times per day (each tablet is 667 mg w/ 8.45 mg calcium).

   3. *Hypophosphatemia*

      a. *Etiology*:

         i. Intracellular shift (usual cause), ↑ renal excretion, or ↓ gut absorption.

         ii. *Glucose loading "refeeding syndrome"*: glucose transported w/ P into cells, clinically significant in malnourished pts starting parenteral or enteral feeds; effect starts 1st d, begins to plateau after 7–10 d. Also seen w/ respiratory alkalosis, which raises intracellular pH, stimulating glycolysis.

      iii. Al-containing substances (sucralfate, Amphogel) bind inorganic P, preventing upper GI absorption.

      iv. Hyperglycemia-induced osmotic diuresis → excessive renal losses of P, aggravated w/ insulin as it drives glucose (and thus phosphorus) into cells.

      v. Beta agonists (i.e., bronchodilators) can also increase intracellular movement of P, though rarely significantly. Sepsis is assoc. w/ hypophosphatemia; mechanism not established.

  b. *Manifestation*:

      i. *Severe depletion can*:
- ↓ myocardial contractility.
- ↓ RBC deformability (leading to hemolytic anemia).
- ↓ 2,3-DPG (shifts oxyhemoglobin dissociation curve left; ↓ O_2 off-loading to tissues)
- ↓ glycolytic pathway and production of ATP.

  c. *Tx*:

      i. *IV replacement* if < 1.0 mg/dL or 0.3 mmol/L, or if cardiac dysfunction, respiratory failure, generalized weakness, or impaired tissue oxygenation.

      ii. *Oral replacement*: Neutra-Phos or K-Phos, 1200–1500 mg PO_4 q d. Higher doses may cause diarrhea.

III. METABOLISM

A. Tissue and fuel consumption

1. In absence of stress/starvation, tissues utilize glucose for energy.
2. During stress/starvation, fat/ketones become primary source of energy.
3. *Obligate glucose consumers*: RBC, WBC, adrenal medulla, peripheral nerves.
4. *Facultative glucose consumer*: brain (usu. uses glucose, but can adapt to use ketones during starvation).
5. No pt should go w/out nutrition > 7 d. Gut is preferred route to avoid immunologic, metabolic, and infectious complications.
6. Feeding after prolonged starvation may result in "refeeding syndrome" w/ intacellular hunger for K^+, Mg^{++}, and PO_4^{---} resulting in low serum levels of these molecules. Gradual reintroduction of feeds may prevent this complication.

IV. NUTRITION

A. Calories

1. *Generally*: 30 kcal/kg/d. Most need about 2000–2500 kcal/d.
2. *Alternately*, can use Harris-Benedict equation to determine basal metabolic rate:
   a. *Male*: 66 + (13.7 × wt in kg) + (5 × ht in cm) – (6.8 × age in yr)
   b. *Female* = 65.5 + (9.6 × wt in kg) + (1.7 × ht in cm) – (4.7 × age in yr)
3. *Add*: 10% for head injury, 30% for polytrauma, 75% for sepsis, 150% for extensive burns.
4. Calculate above kcals from carbohydrate or fats (up to 30% of total); do not include protein calories in this total.

B. Protein: in general need 0.66–1.2 g/kg/d minimum.

1. 1 g protein = 4 kcal. However, plan for caloric needs to come from sugar or fat, as proteins use up some energy in metabolism.
2. Protein is 16% nitrogen (or, conversely, 1 g N_2 = 6.25 g protein).
   a. Most pts need about 150 g nonprotein kcal per g nitrogen (150:1).
   b. Pts in renal failure may need a ratio of 400:1, while severely stressed pts may need up to 80:1.
3. Calculate nitrogen balance to determine if adequate protein needs are being met: + value means anabolic; – value means catabolic. N balance = (N_{in} – N_{out}) = ([prot/6.25] – [24 h urine N = 4 g]).
4. *Deficiency*
   a. *Albumin*: goal < 3.5 – single best prognostic nutritional marker. Half-life 21 d.
      i. < 3.0 = 23.7% 30 d mortality.

    ii. $< 2.5 = 43\%$ mortality.

    iii. $< 2.1 = 62\%$ mortality.

  b. *Transferrin*: half-life 9 d. < 200 abnormal. Influenced by body iron levels.

  c. *Prealbumin*: half-life 3 d. < 15 abnormal.

  d. *Lymphocyte count* < 1500 mm^3.

  e. *Hypersensitivity skin test*: presence or absence of anergy has not consistently been shown to be useful as a preoperative marker.

C. Fats

1. 1 g fat = 9 kcal.

2. May be given as 2–5% daily calories (safflower or soybean oil) or ~ 40 g of emulsion weekly.

3. Infuse no faster than 0.1 g/kg/h to avoid hepatic dysfunction.

4. Avoid lipid emulsion if serum triglycerides exceed 400 mg/dL. Levels > 800 mg/dL may induce pancreatitis. Excess lipid infusion may also worsen ALI/ARDS.

D. Carbohydrates

1. Usu. 1 g carbohydrates = 4 kcal, but parenteral dextrose is 3.4 kcal.

E. Vitamin and mineral deficiency

1. *Vitamins*

  a. *Water soluble*

    i. *B$_1$ (thiamin)*:

- "Beriberi" usu. from alcoholism (ethanol inhibits movement of thiamin from enterocyte into portal circulation) in United States; sx (anorexia, paresthesias, irritability, a/o muscle cramps) may be precipitated by beginning pts w/ marginal levels on IV dextrose solutions.

    ◦ *"Wet" form*: cardiovascular sx (peripheral vasodilation, high-output heart failure, dyspnea, peripheral/pulmonary edema).

    ◦ *"Dry" form*: nervous sx (paresthesias, hyporeflexia, pain, Wernicke-Korsakoff syndrome: nystagmus/ophthalmoplegia, ataxia, confusion, amnesia, etc.).

- *Tx*: 100 mg thiamin daily.

    ii. *B$_2$ (riboflavin)*: angular stomatitis, glossitis, cheilosis, asthenia, anemia.

    iii. *Niacin (nicotinic acid)*: pellagra (dermatitis—dry, hyperpigmented, scaly; diarrhea; dementia) may develop after initial sx of anorexia, asthenia, and glossitis.

    iv. *B$_6$ (pyridoxine)*:

- Assoc. w/ INH, penicillamine, OCPs, and alcoholism.

- *Sx*: glossitis, sore mouth, cheilosis, asthenia, peripheral neuropathy, microcytic anemia.

    v. *B$_{12}$ (cyanocobalamin)*:

- Seen after gastric or ileal resection. Require parenteral B$_{12}$. Microcytic anemia if gastric resection, as stomach and duodenum have crucial role in iron absorption.

    vi. *C (ascorbic acid)*:

- Poverty, cancer, smoking, CRF risk factors for clinically significant deficiency (scurvy).

- Early sx include fatigue and asthenia, but may progress to anemia a/o bleeding manifest as petechiae/purpura, hemarthroses, bleeding gums. Late cases demonstrate edema, neuropathy, and intracerebral hemorrhage.

  b. *Fat soluble*

    i. *A*: 5000 µg/d recommended.

- *Early*: night blindness, dry conjunctive (xerosis), white conjunctival patches (Bitot's spots).

- *Late*: keratomalacia, endophthalmitis, blindness.

    ii. *D*: osteomalacia, rickets.

- *Tx orally w/ 50,000 U/wk × 8 wk*: IV replacement risks paradoxically include osteomalacia, although standard TPN dose of 200 U tolerated well.

        iii. *E*: areflexia, gait disturbances, diminished proprioception/vibration sense, ophthalmoplegia.

        iv. *K*: prolongation of PT commonly seen. Addressed with 10 mg vitamin K per wk.

        v. *Essential fatty acids* (deficiency uncommon in obese pts): dry, flaky skin, red papules, alopecia.

2. *Minerals*

    a. *Iron*: microcytic anemia.

       i. Initiallly iron and ferritin ↓ and transferrin level ↑; later microcytic, hypochromic anemia as well.

       ii. Usual daily dose is 15 mg PO or 1–2 mg parenterally.

         • Replacement during active infection or inflammatory state may contribute to immuno-suppression or facilitate bacterial proliferation.

    b. *Copper*: microcytic anemia.

    c. *Zinc*:

       i. Catabolism, diarrhea/malabsorption increases risk; serum levels may be normal in the face of significant depletion.

       ii. Rash, cutaneous anergy, *altered taste/smell*, impaired wound healing, hyperpigmentation of skin creases, neuritis, poor night vision, photophobia, etc., all reported.

       iii. 6 mg/d given if normal GI function; up to 20 mg/d required if malabsorption/diarrhea.

    d. *Calcium*: see section IID. above.

    e. *Magnesium*: see section IIE. above.

    f. *Selenium*: deficiency rare. Proximal muscle weakness, cardiomyopathy, hypopigmentation, and RBC macrocytosis possible.

    g. *Chromium*: refractory hyperglycemia. Up to 150 mcg/d may be required for deficient pts.

F. RQ ratio: reflects amount of carbon dioxide produced per unit of oxygen consumed. 1 = carb; 0.7 = fat; 0.85 = protein.

G. Effects of starvation:

1. *Early (1st wk)*: up to 300 g of protein lost from skeletal muscle; hepatic glycogenolysis also provides a relatively small amount of glucose for energy (exhausted within 24 h). Fat conversion to free fatty acids and ketones represents the largest amount of available energy stores.

2. *Late (> 1 wk)*: proteolysis diminishes as lipolysis assumes even greater role for energy provision.

H. Absorbtion:

1. Where and how is water/food digested and absorbed?

    a. *Water*: small bowel absorbs 10–12 L/d, leaving ~ 500 cc to be absorbed in colon.

    b. *Sodium*: primarily absorbed via active transcellular mechanisms (i.e., N^+-K^+ ATPase pump) in proximal small bowel. Passive absorption less significant.

    c. *Carbohydrates*: salivary amylase begins digestion, which finishes in small bowel (pancreatic amylase, etc.) w/ absorption of 3 specific hexoses along brush border (glucose—Na^+ dependent and Na^+ independent; galactose—Na^+ dependent; and fructose—facilitated transport).

    d. *Proteins*: digestion begun in stomach (pepsin), finished in small bowel by peptidases (require activation of pancreatic trypsinogen to trypsin by enterokinase from brush border). Direct absorption of both amino acids and oligopeptides possible through wide variety of uptake mechanisms.

    e. *Fats*:

       i. Triglycerides (glycerol w/ 3 fatty acid chains) constitute bulk of dietary fat.

       ii. Digestion begins in stomach (acid hydrolysis, gastric lipase), but absorption extremely limited.

       iii. Emulsification in duodenum w/ bile salts and phospholipids facilitates exposure to pancre-atic lipase, which is responsible for brush border membrane absorption.

        • *Micelles* contain free fatty acids, monoglycerides, and cholesterol in small spheres w/ hydrophobic core; interior contents absorbed at brush border into enterocytes, leaving bile salts in gut lumen.

- Alternately, short-chain and medium-chain fatty acids cross brush border directly by simple diffusion. Long-chain fatty acids require specific uptake mechanism.

   iv. Inside enterocyte, fatty acids re-esterified back into triglycerides. These new triglycerides combine w/ apoprotein, cholesterol, and phospolipid to form *chylomicron* (fat-soluble vitamins included).

- Chylomicrons absorbed into lacteals, ultimately draining into thoracic duct and systemic venous system.
- Medium-chain and polyunsaturated fatty acids absorbed directly into portal circulation.

  f. *Vitamins*:

    i. *Water soluble*:

- *Vitamin C*: absorbed in small bowel via Na^+-dependent active transport mechanism.
- *Vitamin B_{12}*: absorption potentially inhibited at several steps.
  - Bound to R protein in stomach; requires hydrolysis by pancreatic enzymes in duodenum.
  - Intrinsic factor (from gastric parietal cells) protects from enzymatic destruction and serves as cofactor for absorption in terminal ileum.

    ii. *Other water soluble* (thiamine, riboflavin, biotin, pantothenic acid): absorbed via Na^+-dependent mechanisms in small bowel.

    iii. *Fat soluble* (A [retinol], D, E [tocopherols], K): absorbed in small bowel via passive diffusion; enter lymph in chylomicrons.

- *Vitamin D*:
  - D_3 *(cholecalciferol)*: results from UV-mediated activation of 7-dehydrocholesterol in skin and subsequently undergoes up to 2 hydroxylations:
    - *Liver* (first): to 25-hydroxycholecalciferol.
    - *Kidney* (second): to 1,25-dihydroxycholecalciferol.
  - D_2 *(ergocalciferol)*: most common form in foods.
- *Vitamin K*:
  - K_1 *(phytomenadione)*:
    - Obtained from dietary sources:
      - *High concentration*: alfalfa, spinach, Brussels sprouts, kale, broccoli, lettuce, soybeans, cabbage, beef liver, wheat bran, parsley.
      - *Medium concentration*: bacon, wheat germ, cheese, butter, avocado, pork liver.
    - Absorbed in small bowel via carrier-dependent, bile salt-facilitated process.
  - K_2 *(prenyl menaquinones)*: elaborated by colonic bacteria, passively absorbed.

  g. *Minerals*

    i. *Calcium*: absorbed predominantly via active transport in duodenum, also through passive diffusion in rest of small intestine. Vitamin D enhances primarily the latter.

    ii. *Magnesium*: absorbed mostly in the ileum through passive diffusion and carrier-mediated processes.

    iii. *Iron*: primarily absorbed through divalent cation transporter in proximal duodenum (has affinity for broad range of divalent cations). In the gut, ferric (Fe^{+++}) iron must be reduced to ferrous (Fe^{++}) form by ferrireductase or ascorbic acid (vitamin C) for absorption.

CHAPTER 2

HEMATOLOGY

I. BLOOD COMPONENT THERAPY

A. Components/products:
1. *Whole blood*: rarely given.
2. *PRBCs*: 300 cc. Each unit should increase Hgb and Hct by 1 and 3, respectively.
3. *Platelets*: 50 cc. 6–10 U given at a time. Each unit should raise plt count 5000–10,000.
4. *Fresh frozen plasma*: 250 cc. Adequate source of coagulation proteins, esp. II, V, VII, IX, XI.
5. *Cryoprecipitate*: contains factor VIII, von Willebrand factor, and fibrinogen.
6. *Prothrombin complex concentrate* (PCC): contains (vitamin K-dependent) factors II, VII, IX, X; useful for reversing warfarin.
7. *Recombinant factor VIIa* (NovoSeven): use in hemophilia A or B w/ inhibitors to FVIII or FIX.

B. Caveats and complications of transfusion
1. *Immunologic*
   a. *Acute hemolytic reaction*: $1/_{12,000}$–25,000; from ABO incompatibility. Presents w/ fever, chills, hemoglobinuria, possibly hypotension and ARF. Tx supportive, directed at preventing ATN w/ IVF.
   b. *Delayed hemolytic reaction*: up to 2 wk posttransfusion; tx w/ supportive care.
   c. *Acute febrile nonhemolytic allergic reaction*: most common transfusion reaction; tx w/ cessation of transfusion, antipyretics.
   d. *Immunosuppression*: assoc. w/ nosocomial infections and increased levels of inflammatory cytokines.
   e. *Transfusion-related acute lung injury* (TRALI): P:F ratio < 300 and bilateral infiltrates on CXR.
2. *Transmission of infectious agents*
   a. *Virus*:
      i. CMV most common.
      ii. HIV, hepatitis C $1/_2$–2.6 million.
      iii. Hepatitis B $1/_{600,000}$.
   b. *Bacterial*: risk ~ $1/_{40,000}$ (some report $1/_{2000}$ plt transfusions).
   c. *Protozoan*: Babesia microti, Trypanosoma cruzi rarely reported.
3. *Metabolic*
   a. *Hyperkalemia*—a risk esp. in older units.
   b. *Hypocalcemia*—from citrate binding.

II. HEMOSTASIS

A. Steps in hemostasis:
1. *Injury to vessel wall* → primary vasoconstriction → formation of platelet plug → clot stabilization → clot dissolution platelet plug.
   a. Adhesion of platelets to subendothelial collagen mediated by von Willebrand factor.
   b. Platelet aggregation.
   c. Activated platelets then bind to fibrinogen via glycoprotein IIa–IIIb complex; stabilization of clot.
2. *Extrinsic pathway*
   a. Begins w/ activation of factor VII (FVII) by tissue factor in exposed endothelium.
3. *Intrinsic pathway*
   a. Begins w/ activation of FXII (Hageman factor), high-molecular wt kinogen (HMWK), and prekallikrein (PK), which in turn activate FXI, which activates FIX.
4. *Common pathway*

     a. Ends in FX activation = prothrombin to thrombin.

B. Assays for hemostasis

  1. *Protime (PT)*

    a. Measures extrinsic (FVII) and common (FX, FV, FII) pathways.

    b. *Prolonged w/:*

      i. Isolated factor deficiency, vitamin K deficiency, hepatic insufficiency.

  2. *PTT*

    a. Measures intrinsic (PK, HMWK, FXII, FXI, FIX, FVIII) and common (FX, FV, FII) pathways.

    b. *Prolonged w/:*

      i. Isolated factor deficiency, heparin use, lupus anticoagulant, hematic insufficiency.

C. Specific disorders of hemostasis (hypocoagulable state) → BLEEDING

  1. *von Willebrand dz*

    a. Most common hereditary bleeding diathesis.

    b. Deficiency or dysfunction of von Willebrand factor.

    c. Manifests as primarily a platelet dysfunction problem.

    d. *Tx*: DDAVP or cryoprecipitate.

  2. *Hemophilia A* (FVIII deficiency)

    a. Second most common hereditary bleeding diathesis. Sex-linked inheritance (same for hemophilia B).

    b. Goal is to replace to 100% level of FVIII.

    c. Mild cases may be treated w/ DDAVP.

  3. *Hemophilia B*, "Christmas disease" (FIX deficiency)

    a. Do not replace > 50% of FIX—assoc. w/ thromboses.

  4. *Lupus*

    a. Occasionally assoc. w/ decreased prothrombin, and occasionally FVII from antibody.

    b. *Tx*: high-dose corticosteroids, component replacement as necessary.

  5. *Platelet functional disorders*

    a. Uremia: inhibits vWF, GP 1b, GP IIb–IIIa.

    b. *Tx*: dialysis, DDAVP, estrogen, recombinant factor VII.

  6. *Vitamin K deficiency*

    a. Usu. from abx that decrease gut bacteria that generate vitamin K, or in TPN-dependent pts. Hepatic insufficiency will often increase PT before PTT as FVII has shortest half-life.

    b. If need to correct immediately, FFP is given.

  7. *Factor X deficiency*

    a. Amyloidosis, multiple myeloma.

D. Hypercoagulable states → *clotting*

  1. *Inherited disorders*:

    a. Factor V Leiden mutation (most common inherited cause): resistance to activated protein C.

    b. Antithrombin deficiency (treat w/ heparin and FFP).

    c. Protein C, protein S deficiencies (prone to warfarin-induced skin necrosis).

    d. Hyperhomocysteinemia (treat w/ folate supplementation).

  2. *Acquired disorders*:

    a. Cancer, pregnancy

    b. Surgery, trauma

    c. Heparin-induced thrombocytopenia

      i. Usu. occurs within 3 wk of heparin administration; can result in arterial "white clots."

      ii. Due to antibodies to platelet factor 4.

      iii. *Tx*: d/c heparin, begin argatroban, lepirudin, or bivalirudin.

    d. Anticardiolipin antibody

e. Lupus anticoagulant (actually a *pro*-coagulant antibody)

III. ANTICOAGULATION

TABLE 2.1. Summary of 2004 ACCP DVT Prophylaxis Recommendations

Risk Level	DVT % Calf / Proximal	PE % Clinical / Fatal	Rec. Prophylaxis
Low • Minor surg • < 40 yo • No risk factors*	2 / 0.4	0.2 / < 0.01	Early mobilization alone
Moderate • Minor surg • 40–60 yo w/out risk factors • Risk factors	10–20 / 2–4	1–2 / 0.1–0.4	LDUH (bid), LMWH (< 3400 U/d), GCS, or IPC
High • > 60 yo • 40–60 w/ risk factors	20–40 / 4–8	2–4 / 0.4–1.0	LDUH (tid), LMWH (> 3400 U/d), or IPC
Highest • Multiple risk factors • Hip/knee arthroplasty • HFS • Maj trauma / SCI	40–80 / 10–20	4–10 / 0.2–5	LMWH (> 3400 U/d), fondaparinux, oral VKA (INR 2–3), or IPC/GCS + LDUH/LMWH

* Risk factors (other than age > 40): prior VTE, cancer, molecular hypercoagulability. LDUH (low-dose unfractionated heparin), LMWH (low-molecular wt heparin), GCS (graded compression stockings), IPC (intermittent pneumatic compression devices), VKA (vitamin K antagonist – i.e., Coumadin).
**Bid = two times per day; tid = three times per day

A. **Indication:** refer to Table 2.1 above.

B. **Mechanical**

1. Sequential compression devices (SCDs) more effective than foot pumps. Work principally by compressing veins (pt should ambulate as soon as possible postop), preventing stasis. No proven system fibrinolytic benefit from SCDs.

C. **Pharmacologic**

1. *Heparin*

   a. Potentiates antithrombin III, which inhibits thrombin and factor Xa.

   b. Unfractionated or fractionated.

   c. Reversed by protamine, usu. given as 1 mg protamine IV (over 10 min) per 100 mg of unfractionated heparin (or per 1 mg enoxaparin).

      i. *Side effect of protamine*: possible immunologically mediated hypotension (give in ICU setting).

   d. HIT is possible side effect of use. Discontinue all heparin products and anticoagulate.

      i. Alternate anticoagulants for pts w/ HIT:

      • *Hirudin derivatives* (Lepirudin): analog of leech salivary anticoagulant, renal clearance. Dosage = 0.1 mg/kg/h w/ goal to achieve PTT 2× normal.

      • *Argatroban*: hepatic clearance, same cost as low-dose hirudin. Half-life 4 h vs hirudin's 24 h (neither has an effective reversal agent). Follow w/ aPTT.

2. *Warfarin* (Coumadin)

   a. Inhibits gamma-carboxylation of vitamin K-dependent coagulation factors (II, VII, IX, X).

   b. Can cause paradoxical hypercoagulable state when first administered (for several days) as half-lives of protein C and protein S (vitamin K-dependent anticoagulant factors) are shorter than procoagulant factors. Thus, heparin should be used as a "bridge" for the first several days.

   c. Reversed by vitamin K (10 U IV/IM/PO) or 2–4 U FFP.

    d. *INR goals*: DVT 2–3; AFib 2–3; post-MI 2.5–3.5; postprosthetic valve placement 2–3.

3. *Clopidogrel* (Plavix)

    a. Inhibitor of ADP-induced platelet aggregation by inhibitory binding of GP IIb/IIIa complex receptor.

4. *Pentoxifylline* (Trental)

    a. Inhibits platelet activation and adhesion.

5. *Cilostazol* (Pletal)

    a. A phosphodiesterase III inhibitor.

6. *Acetylsalicylic acid* (aspirin)

    a. Irreversibly blocks prostacyclin synthetase (cyclooxygenase inhibitor), preventing platelet aggregation.

CHAPTER 3

ANESTHESIA

TABLE 3.1. Common Sedative and Analgesics

Drug	Comments	Dose	Onset and Half-life
Midazolam (Versed)	BZD sedative, excellent retrograde amnesia	IV bolus: 1–5 mg over 2 min q 2–4 h prn IV infusion: 1–20 mg/h (usu. 3 mg/h) Infusion increase: bolus 5 mg, then increase rate by 1 mg/h	2–5 min and 1–4 h (up to 48 h in renal insufficiency)
Lorazepam (Ativan)	BZD sedative, longer acting	PO: 0.5–4 mg q 2–4 h prn IV bolus: 2–4 mg (0.05 mg/kg) over 2–5min IV infusion: 1–20 mg/h (usu. 3 mg/h) Infusion increase: bolus 4 mg, then increase rate by 1 mg/h	5–20 min and 12.9 h (elderly 15.9 h– accumulates w/ time)
Morphine	Opioid analgesic	IV bolus: 1–10 mg prn q 3–4 h prn IV infusion: 1–20 mg/h, titrate by 1 mg/h	3–4 h duration
Fentanyl	Synthetic opioid w/ faster onset, shorter duration than MSO4. Less BP and resp depression. High doses w/ chest wall tightness.	IV bolus: 25–200 mcg q 1 h prn IV infusion: 25–200 mcg/h, titrate by 25 mcg/h	1–2 h duration
Meperidine (Demerol)	Metaboline normeperidine associated with neuropsychiatric side effects	1–1.8 mg/kg (75–150 mg) up to 150 mg IM/SC/PO or slow IV q 3–4 h	
Dilaudid	Potent narcotic	0.5–2.0 mg IM/SC or slow IV q 4–6 h	
Propofol	Anesthetic sedative. Watch for hypotension, apnea, Stop if triglycerides > 300–400. Fat overload. Rapid tolerance to effect. Avoid if allergic to egg, soybean oil, or glycerol; given in 10% Intralipid. Useful bronchodilator.	5 mcg/kg/min, increasing by 5 q 5–10 min. Average: 25–35 mcg/kg/min Anesthetic dose: 50–100 mcg/kg/min	Onset: 9–51 sec Duration: 3–10 min Half-life: 40 min
Haloperidol (Haldol)	For delirium of refractory agitation. Watch for neuroleptic malignant syndrome. Torsades: avoid QTc > 500 msec.	IV bolus: 1–10 mg IV q 1 h prn	*ensure no QTc > 40 msec or increase by 25+%

I. **LOCAL**

    A. **Maximum doses of common local anesthetics:**

        1. *Lidocaine* 1% (10 mg/cc): max dose 5 mg/kg w/out epi; 7 mg/kg w/ epi.

            a. *Onset* 10 min; duration 1–3 h.

            b. *Toxicity*: includes dizziness, circumoral paresthesias, a metallic taste, a/o visual changes, which may culminate in disorientation, seizures (tx w/ benzodiazepines), or even cardiovascular collapse.

        2. *Bupivacaine* (Marcaine): max dose 2 mg/kg w/out epi; 3 mg/kg w/ epi.

            a. *Toxicity*: similar to that of lidocaine, although the cardiovascular effects tend to be more significant and persistent.

TABLE 3.2. Common Paralytic Agents

	Succinylcholine (Anectine)	Pancuronium (Pavulon)	Rocuronium (Zemuron)	Cisatracurium (Nimbex)
Type	Depolarizing	Nondepolarizing	Nondepolarizing	Nondepolarizing
Dose (mg/kg)	1–2 (avg. dose 100 mg)	0.1	0.6–1.0	0.1–2.0
Time to onset	30 sec	90 sec	75 sec	90 sec
Duration	5 min	60–180+ min	30–70 min	35–80 min
Chronotrope effect		† HR (vagolytic effect)	† HR w/ high dose only	None
Miscellaneous	• Can raise K⁺ by 0.5 mEg/L • Avoid if rhabdo., burn, long immobilization, etc. • Potential to cause *malignant hyperthermia*	• Prolonged effect w/ renal > hepatic failure	• Prolonged effect w/ hepatic > renal failure	• No *histamine* release (advantage over other paralytics • can cause ↓ BP, ↑ HR). • Not affected w/ hepatic or renal failure

II. PARALYTICS (NEUROMUSCULAR BLOCKERS)

    A. Train of four: if overdose on paralytics, can lead to polyneuropathy.

III. REVERSAL AGENTS

    A. Narcan 0.4–2.0 mg IV/IM/SC/ET q 2–3 min prn; adult postop reversal 0.1–0.2 mg.

    B. Flumazenil Sed. reversal: 0.2 mg IV over 15 sec, then 0.2 mg q 1 min up to 1 mg. OD reversal: 0.2 mg IV over 30 sec, then 0.3–0.5 mg q 30 sec up to 3 mg.

IV. MALIGNANT HYPERTHERMIA

    A. Life-threatening disorder secondary to defect in calcium metabolism in sarcoplasmic reticulum. Occurs in 1:50,000 adults and more frequently in children. 30% mortality.

    B. Assoc. w/ inhalational anesthetics, amide-class local anesthetics, and succinylcholine.

    C. Dx: fever, tachycardia, cyanosis, a/o rigidity, increased end-tidal CO_2, hyperkalemia, hypercalcemia, and metabolic acidosis.

    D. Tx:

        1. Stop responsible agent and actively cool the pt.

        2. Hyperventilate w/ 100% oxygen.

        3. Dantrolene (2–10 mg/kg IVP), repeat as needed.

        4. Aggressively tx hyperkalemia (see Chapter 1).

V. END-TIDAL CO_2 MONITORING

    A. Abrupt decrease

        1. Plugging or disconnection of tubing.

        2. Venous air/gas (i.e., CO_2) embolism (laparoscopy, GI endoscopy, liver resection).

            a. *Tx*: release pneumoperitoneum; place in Trendelenburg, left side down; hyperventilate w/ 100% oxygen, consider right atrial air aspiration through central line.

        3. Tension PTX.

        4. MI.

        5. Excess pneumoperitoneum or intraabdominal HTN → decreased venous return.

    B. Increase

        1. Insufficient minute/alveolar ventilation.

CHAPTER 4

SURGICAL INTENSIVE CARE UNIT

I. AIRWAY AND BREATHING (VENTILATION)

A. Airway

1. *Intubation criteria*
   a. *Inadequate, unprotected, or threatened airway*: i.e., GCS < 9, vomiting, inhalation injury, etc.
   b. RR > 35 (or significantly increasing work of breathing).
   c. $PaCO_2$ > 50 mm Hg.
   d. Respiratory acidosis w/ pH < 7.25.
   e. PaO_2 < 60 mm Hg.
   f. SaO_2 < 85%.
   g. PaO_2/FiO_2 < 250.
2. *Rapid sequence intubation* (see Chapter 3).
3. *Equipment*
   a. MacIntosh blade is curved, placed in vallecula to lift epiglottis.
   b. Miller blade is straight, placed over/across the epiglottis.
   c. Most adults require a #3 (less commonly #4) blade of either MacIntosh or Miller.
      i. Premature infants, #0 Miller; other infants, #1 Miller; children, #2 Miller.
   d. *Tube size*: adult males 7.5–8.0; adult females 7.0–7.5.
      i. *Children*: ETT width same as 5th fingernail, or use size = (4 + age yr)/4.
   e. In (most) adult males, place tube at 23 cm (incisors or angle of mouth); only go to 21 cm in females. CXR should show tip 2–5 cm above carina in all cases.
      i. Children depth = (age yr/2) + 12.
   f. For tracheostomy, most adults should get a #8 Shiley tracheostomy tube or a 6-0 ETT.

B. Breathing

1. *Pulmonary physiology*
   a. *Peak and plateau pressures*: peak pressure is a function of resistance to inflowing air as well as elastic recoil of lungs (P_{peak} ~ resistance × elasticity). Plateau pressure, however, is proportional only to elasticity of lungs and chest wall (air has already flowed into the lungs → $P_{plateau}$ ~ elasticity). Resultingly, airway resistance ~ $P_{peak} - P_{plateau}$. Remember that peak pressure (normal < 50 cm) correlates w/ luminal obstruction, whereas plateau pressure (normal < 35) corresponds w/ chest/lung compliance.
   b. *Pulmonary gas exchange and oxygen delivery*:
      i. Oxygen delivery = cardiac output (L/min) × CaO_2 × 10:
         • Normal = 0.9 – 1.1 L/min *or* 520 – 600 mL/min/m^2.
         • Arterial O_2 content (CaO_2): (1.34 × Hgb × SaO_2) + (0.003 × PaO_2).
            ◦ Normal PaO_2 ~ 90 mm Hg; normal PvO_2 ~ 40 mm Hg.
      ii. A-a PO_2 gradient (PO_2 difference between alveolar gas and alveolar blood):
         • Affected by age, altitude/barometric pressure, and FiO_2.
         • In general, A-a gradient ~ 2.5 + 0.21 × age. Upper limits of normal by age, on room air (i.e., 20 yo → 17, but 80 yo → 38).
         • Gradient increases ~ 6 mm Hg for every 10% increase in FiO_2.
         • In a healthy young person w/ FiO_2 1.0, A-a gradient should be 25–65, and PaO_2 600 mm Hg.
      iii. *Evaluating hypoxemia*:

- *Hypoventilation* (excess narcotic, weakness, etc.): A-a PO_2 normal, PvO_2 normal.
- *V/Q mismatch* (pneumonia, ARDS, PE, pulmonary edema): A-aPO_2 ↑, PvO_2 normal.
  - Shunt (V/Q < 1) results in no increase in PaO_2 w/ supplemental oxygen.
- DO_2/VO_2 imbalance (low cardiac output, anemia, hypermetabolic state): A-aPO_2 ↑, PvO_2 ↓.

2. *Mechanical ventilation*
   a. *General principles*
      i. *Effect of positive-pressure ventilation*: decreases venous return to heart and thus right ventricular filling (decreases preload); augments left ventricular systolic function (effectively decreases afterload, increases stroke volume). Overall effect is to generally increase cardiac output in normovolemic pts while decreasing cardiac output in volume-depleted pts.
      ii. *Volutrauma*: recent studies suggest that excessive *volume* is more injurious to alveoli than increased pressure, and may be responsible for releasing inflammatory cytokines.
      iii. *PEEP*: functions to increase functional reserve volume and recruit alveoli or diminish atelectasis. Improves P:F ratio. Effects on cardiac output are the same as for positive-pressure ventilation (see entry 2ai. above). Another maneuver to increase oxygenation is inverting the I:E ratio. Potential risk is breath-stacking or auto-PEEP, which can raise pCO_2; it is also uncomfortable for the pt and requires heavy sedation.
   b. *Ventilation modes*
      i. *Assist control*: a form of volume-cycled ventilation where the ventilator delivers a complete cycle when triggered by pt inspiration; will also give breaths if rate of breathing is below a set threshold. Main risks w/ this mode are auto-PEEP a/o respirator alkalosis in pts w/ relatively unimpaired respiratory drive.
      ii. *IMV/SIMV*: delivers a ventilatory cycle if pt does not meet minimum threshold spontaneous breathing rate. Spontaneous breaths may or may not be supported w/ pressure support, depending on settings. In SIMV, the intermittent ventilation breaths are synchronized w/ the spontaneous breaths.
      iii. *Pressure-regulated volume control*: similar to volume control ventilation, but adjusts flow rate to avoid exceeding a programmed peak pressure; useful in decreased lung compliance (i.e., ARDS).
      iv. *Bilevel ventilation* (functionally same concept as *airway pressure release ventilation [APRV]*): essentially a mode of inverse I:E ratio IMV utilized to reduce PIP while maintaining mean airway pressure. Ventilator cycles between 2 different levels of CPAP. Higher level facilitates oxygenation while lower level provides improved ventilation. Hypercapnia is accepted to achieve oxygenation goals.
      v. *Pressure support*: all breaths are initiated by pt and pressure is delivered to augment the breath w/out specifying a particular volume. Generally one can titrate the pressure so that the pt autoregulates minute volume w/ a respiratory rate of 12–20.
      vi. *CPAP* (continuous positive airway pressure): when referring to non-intubated pts, acts as PEEP, and is administered through tightly sealed face or nasal masks. Most often used for pts w/ obstructive sleep apnea.
      vii. *High-frequency percussive ventilation*: uses small tidal volumes w/ rates of 3–8 Hz (adults). Sets baseline pressure control rate, upon which the oscillatory breaths are superimposed. Also known as volumetric diffusive respiration (VDR), which was initially described as a means to "internally percuss" the lungs. Most frequently used in inhalation injury.
   c. *Initial ventilatory settings*
      i. If paralyzed or no respiratory drive → A/C: FiO_2 1.0, RR 12, PEEP 5, Vt 6 cc/kg (~ 500).
      ii. If have respiratory drive → SIMV: similar settings as above.
      iii. Vt should almost never be > 8 cc/kg, and 4 cc/kg is usu. desirable to avoid stretch injury physiology.
      iv. *Oxygenation*: PaO_2 increases/decreases *pari passu* w/ FiO_2 and PEEP.
         - As described above, one may also increase oxygenation w/ increased I:E ratios, adopting a strategy of permissive hypercapnea; respiratory acidosis (even w/ $PaCO_2$ > 100) is better tolerated than hypoxia. See entry 2cvi. below for more information.
      v. *Ventilation*: $PaCO_2$ changes inversely w/ minute ventilation, which is the product of Vt and respiratory rate.

vi. Mechanical ventilation for pts w/ ALI/ARDS [reference in part from *N Engl J Med* 1998;338(6):347–354, *N Engl J Med* 2000;342(18):1301–1308]:

- ALI = acute onset PaO_2:FiO_2 < 300 w/ bilateral infiltrates and no evidence of hydrostatic pulmonary edema (i.e., PAWP ≤ 18 mm Hg).

- ARDS = acute onset PaO_2:FiO_2 < 200 w/ bilateral infiltrates and no evidence of hydrostatic pulmonary edema (i.e., PAWP ≤ 18 mm Hg).

- Work toward a volume of (not exceeding) 6 mL/kg of predicted body wt in conjunction w/ the goal of maintaining end inspiratory plateau pressures ≤ 30 cm H_2O.

- Permissive hypercapnia can be tolerated in pts w/ ALI/ARDS if required to minimize plateau pressures and tidal volumes. The use of hypercarbia is limited in pts w/ preexisting metabolic acidosis and is contraindicated in pts w/ increased intracranial pressure. Sodium bicarbonate infusion may be considered in select pts to facilitate use of permissive hypercapnia (only if pH < 7.15).

d. *Extubation criteria*

i. Gold standard in past has been 2 h of CPAP. With this in mind, many hospitals are going to standard protocol of daily CPAP/SBT trials.

ii. *Consider extubation if tolerates 2 h SBT and*:

- FiO_2 < 0.5
- PEEP < 8 cm H_2O
- RR < 30
- Minute ventilation (VE) < 12 L/min
- pH 7.35–7.47
- PaO_2 > 65
- $PaCO_2$ 33–49
- Condition that led to intubation improved and hemodynamically stable, off pressor/inotrope drips
- Able to obey commands, initiate breaths, clear secretions
- Cuff leak present
- ICP < 20
- RSBI < 105
  - Most accurate method has been to calculate rapid shallow breathing index (RSBI) = resp rate/vol (in liters). < 105 should be able to extubate. < 60 definitely worth a trial.
- Inspiratory force more negative than 25 cm H_2O.

iii. 10–15% reintubation rate acceptable.

e. *Indications for tracheostomy*

i. Upper respiratory tract obstruction (in emergency, use cricothryroidotomy or jet insufflation)

ii. Mental status unable to maintain long-term airway

iii. Anticipated need for mechanical ventilation > 3 wk

iv. Inadequate strength or vital capacity

v. Uncontrolled secretions

II. CIRCULATION (SHOCK, RESUSCITATION, AND CRITICAL CARE MAINTENANCE)

A. Inflammatory response states

1. *SIRS* (systemic inflammatory response syndrome):

   a. *Dx requires 2 of the following 4 criteria*:

   i. *Temperature*: ≤ 36°C or ≤ 38°C

   ii. *Heart rate*: ≤ 90 bpm

   iii. Respiration: ≤ 20 breaths/min *or* $PaCO_2$ < 32 mm Hg

   iv. *WBC*: ≤ 12,000 or ≤ 4000 cells/mm^3 or > 10% bands

2. *Sepsis*: SIRS secondary to identified infectious source.

3. *Severe sepsis*: sepsis assoc. w/ at least one organ system dysfunction.
4. *Septic shock*: refractory hypotension/hypoperfusion despite fluid optimization and vasopressors.
5. *MODS*: multiple organ dysfunction syndrome.

B. Shock
  1. *Types*
     a. *Hypovolemic* (e.g., hemorrhage)
     b. *Distributive* (e.g., neurogenic—different than "spinal shock," which denotes spinal arreflexia after trauma, septic)
     c. *Cardiogenic* (e.g., MI)
     d. *Obstructive* (e.g., cardiac tamponade, tension pneumothorax)

C. Resuscitation
  1. Give crystalloids, PRBCs until CVP 15 and hct of 30. If still unstable (HR > 120, SBP < 90, BD > 6), possible cardiac problems → insert PA catheter, consider echo.
  2. Give fluids until PCWP 15.
     a. If still unstable, bolus 500 cc of crystalloid, until CI (goal 3.8) decreases by 0.3. Consider the PCWP just before the decrease in CI to be optimal PCWP.
  3. If CI < 3.8 after reaching "optimal" PCWP or PCWP of 25, consider inotrope support (i.e., dobutamine, milrinone).
  4. If hypotension (MAP < 60) persists w/ CI < 3.8, consider inotrope w/ vasopressor activity (dopamine, levophed, epinephrine).
  5. If hypotension still present w/ CI > 3.8, consider pressor (levophed, phenylephrine).
  6. *Serum markers for resuscitation*:
     a. *Base deficit*: > 6 worrisome.
     b. *Lactate*: > 2 abnormal, but > 4 is clinically significant.

D. Central venous, PA catheters, and arterial catheters
  1. *Central lines*: U/S guidance rapidly becoming considered standard of care.
  2. *Arterial lines*: Document Allen's test before proceeding.
  3. *Pulmonary artery catheters and shock states*:
     a. May be used to help guide fluid management in pts who are difficult to assess.
        i. No proven mortality benefit from the use of PA-catheters in critically ill pts, however.
     b. *Heart failure patterns*
        i. *Right heart failure*: high CVP, low CI, high PVRI
        ii. *Left heart failure*: high PCWP, low CI, high SVRI
     c. *Hypotension patterns*
        i. *Hypovolemic*: low CVP, low CI, high SVRI
        ii. *Cardiogenic*: high CVP, low CI, high SVRI

TABLE 4.1. Hemodynamic Parameters for Normal and Shock States

Shock Type	CVP	PA	PCWP	CI	SVR
Normal	0–6	25/6–12	6–12	> 2.5	700–1300
Hypovolemic	0–2	15–20/0–2	2–6	< 2.0	> 1500
Cardiogenic	> 8	50/35	> 25	< 2.0	> 1500
Septic	0–2	15–20/0–6	< 6	> 2.5	< 1500
Major PE	8–12	50/12–15	< 12	< 2.0	> 1500
Tamponade	12–16	25/12–16	12–16	< 2.0	> 1500
Neurogenic	0–2	15–20/0–2	6–12	> 2.5	< 700

　　　　iii. *Vasogenic*: low CVP, high CI, low SVRI

　　d. *Valvular/wall patterns*

　　　　i. *Tamponade* (equal diastolic pressures): CVP = PADP = PAWP

　　　　ii. *Mitral stenosis* (increased "a" wave): PAWP = LAP > LVEDP

　　　　iii. *Mitral regurgitation* (increased "v" wave): PAWP = LAP > LVEDP

　　　　iv. *Aortic regurgitation*: LVEDP > LAP = PAWP

III. ADDITIONAL NOTES FOR MANAGEMENT OF SPECIFIC TYPES OF SHOCK

A. **Hypovolemic**

　　1. Aside from fluid administration and mechanical control of bleeding (surgery), consider possible need for blood replacement products and adjunctive maneuvers a/o medications to aid hemostasis (see Chapter 2).

B. **Septic:** outlined are key *portions* of recommendations from the Surviving Sepsis Campaign. [*Crit Care Med* 2004;32(3), Surviving Sepsis Campaign guidelines for management of severe sepsis and septic shock.]

　　1. *Initial resuscitation*

　　　　a. Hyperlactasemia suggests hypoperfusion even if not hypotensive. Goals for 1st 6 h of resuscitation include (higher if on ventilator, or intraabdominal hypertension):

　　　　　　i. *CVP*: 8–12 mm Hg

　　　　　　ii. *MAP* ≥ 65 mm Hg

　　　　　　iii. *UOP* ≥ 0.5 cc/kg/h

　　　　　　iv. *Central venous (superior vena cava) or mixed* SvO_2 ≥ 70%

　　2. *Dx*

　　　　a. Obtain cultures of appropriate body fluids/sites before beginning abx.

　　3. *Antibiotic therapy*

　　　　a. Start IV abx w/in 1 h of severe sepsis dx, after cx have been obtained. In severe sepsis or septic shock, broad empiric coverage warranted until can be directed by cx results. 7–10 d is typically appropriate and should be guided by clinical response.

　　4. *Source control*

　　　　a. Identify and remove infectious foci (lines [probably most common source], necrotic tissue, etc.) ASAP.

　　5. *Fluid therapy*

　　　　a. Boluses (500–1000 cc crystalloid or 300–500 cc colloid over 30 min) may be repeatedly given if BP, UOP suggest benefit w/out untoward effects of hypervolemia.

　　6. *Vasopressors*

　　　　a. Begin vasopressors when appropriate fluid challenges fail to meet goals.

　　　　b. Norepinephrine or dopamine is the first-choice vasopressor agent to correct hypotension in septic shock. Norepinephrine primarily vasoconstrictor; dopamine useful if compromised systolic function but causes more tachycardia.

　　　　c. Consider vasopressin if refractory to fluids, high-dose vasopressors; administered at 0.01–0.04 U/min. Discourage use if cardiac dysfunction, particularly if CI is ≤ 2.5.

　　　　d. Place arterial catheter as soon as practical to help guide pressor titration.

　　7. *Inotropic therapy*

　　　　a. If low CI despite adequate fluid resuscitation, consider use of dobutamine. Once able to monitor cardiac output in addition to blood pressure, a vasopressor such as norepinephrine and an inotrope such as dobutamine may be used separately to target specific levels of mean arterial pressure and cardiac output [*Crit Care Med* 2004;32(3).].

　　8. *Steroids*

　　　　a. Hydrocortisone 200–300 mg/d, for 7 d in 3 or 4 divided doses or by continuous infusion, recommended in pts w/ septic shock who, despite adequate fluid replacement, require vasopressor therapy to maintain adequate blood pressure.

　　　　b. Relative adrenal insufficiency defined as post-ACTH cortisol increase > 9 mcg/dL. Some would use 250-mcg ACTH stimulation test to identify responders (> 9 mcg/dL increase in cortisol 30–60 min post ACTH administration) and discontinue therapy in these pts.

    c. Do not wait for ACTH stimulation results to administer corticosteroids.

    d. Consider administering a dose of dexamethasone until ACTH stimulation test performed because dexamethasone, unlike hydrocortisone, does not interfere w/ the cortisol assay.

9. *Blood product administration*

    a. In absence of hypoperfusion/lactic acidosis, CAD, hemorrhage, or coronary artery dz, RBC transfusion should be limited to hgb < 7.0 g/dL (< 70 g/L) to target a hgb of 7.0–9.0 g/dL.

C. Cardiogenic

1. Generally requires PA catheter monitoring and appropriate fluid and inotrope/pressor management, as described in Chapter 5.

D. Neurogenic

1. Generally limited w/ spinal cord injury above level of T5.

2. Loss of sympathetic tone results in hypotension w/ relatively warm extremities (similar to septic shock), but w/ relative bradycardia. Manage w/ fluids and appropriate alpha agonist (i.e., phenylephrine, norepinephrine, etc.).

3. "Spinal shock" is a different entity, referring to usu. transient arreflexia after blunt spinal trauma.

IV. ABG INTERPRETATION AND ACID-BASE PROBLEMS

A. ABG normal values

1. *Normal pH*: 7.35–7.45

2. *pCO_2*: resp alkalosis < 35–45 < resp acidosis

3. *$HCO3$*: met acidosis < 22–26 < met alkalosis

B. ABG interpretation

1. *First step*: Is the pH high, low, or normal?

2. *Second step*: Is the pCO_2 high, low, or normal?

3. *Third step*: Is the degree of compensation (CO_2 or HCO_3) expected, more, or less?

pH < 7.35

    a. If pCO_2 low or normal, then primary **met acidosis**.

        i. *Check anion gap*: AG = Na − (Cl + HCO_3) → normal < 12 (*Note*: hypoalbuminemia can falsely lower AG).

        • If AG > 12, then gain of acid is responsible (generally a *medical* problem except for lactic acidosis in trauma, bowel infarction, etc.).

           ° *"MUD PILERS"*: methanol, uremia, DKA/starvation, paraldehyde, isopropyl alcohol/ INH, lactic acidosis, ethanol/ethylene glycol, rhabdomyolysis, salicylates.

           ° *DKA tx*: start insulin drip at 0.1 U reg insulin/kg/h; continue insulin until gap is gone, then add dextrose once glucose < 250. To correct Na+, add 1.6 to Na+ level for every 100 mg/dL the glucose is over 100 mg/dL.

           ° mmol/L HCO_3 = (base deficit × kg body wt) (0.3).

        • If AG < 12 (normal), then loss of HCO_3 is responsible (often a surgical issue, such as fistulas, surgical drains, etc.)

           ° *Check urine pH and urine anion gap*: UAG = Na + K − Cl.

           ° UAG = −10 to +10.

           ° UAG < −10 = extrarenal non-AG metacidosis.

           ° UAG > +10 = renal non-AG metacidosis.

           ° In general, urine pH > 6 suggests renal cause, urine pH > 6 suggests GI cause.

           ° *If urine pH < 5.5 and UAG is negative* (often surgical issue): etiology: diarrhea, surgical drains, fistulas, ureterosigmoidostomy/ileal bladder/ileal ureter, cholestyramine. If none of these exist and pt is hypokalemic, consider Type 2 RTA.

           ° *If urine pH < 5.5 and UAG is positive, w/ hyperkalemia*: Type 4 RTA (hyperaldosteronism—hyperkalemia prevents ammoniagenesis, which lowers H+ excretion). Tx hyperkalemia w/ kayexylate or diuretics.

           ° *Other causes of normal AG w/ hyper- or normokalemia*: early renal failure, other renal dz (amyloidosis, hydronephrosis, sickle cell nephropathy), acidifying agents (ammonium chloride, calcium chloride, arginine), sulfur toxicity.

- *If urine pH > 5.5 and UAG is positive, pt usu. hypokalemic*: Type I RTA ("distal": no distal H^+ excretion). Tx w/ 1–2 mEq/kg/d of bicarb.
- *But*: w/ variable urine pH and UAG that is negative, but w/ hypokalemia (may be confused w/ first scenario listed—r/o if no diarrhea, surgical drains, fistulas, etc.): Type 2 RTA ("proximal": low Tm for HCO_3^-?). Tx w/ 10–20 mEq/kg/d of bicarb.
- *Other causes of normal AG w/ hypokalemia*: mineralocorticoid deficiency (angiotensin deficiency/liver failure, ACEi, renin deficiency, aging, extracellular volume expansion, lead, beta blockers, prostaglandin inhibitors, methyldopa, acetazolamide, mafenamide, post-hypocapnia).

   ii. Check difference between measured and expected pCO_2 to identify a superimposed respiratory d/o.
- *Met acidosis*: change pCO_2 = change $HCO_3 \times 1.3$.
  - pCO_2 too high, concurrent resp acidosis.
  - pCO_2 too low, concurrent resp alkalosis.

b. If pCO_2 high, then primary **resp acidosis**.
   i. Pneumonia, narcotic OD, COPD, neuropathy/myopathy.
   ii. Check change in pH to determine acute vs chronic and if superimposed metabolic d/o is present.
- *Acute resp acidosis*: change HCO_3 to change pCO_2 should be 1:10.
  - HCO_3 too high, concurrent met alkalosis.
  - HCO_3 too low, concurrent met acidosis.
- *Chronic resp acidosis*: change HCO_3 to change pCO_2 should be 3:10.
  - HCO_3 too high, concurrent met alkalosis.
  - HCO_3 too low, concurrent met acidosis.

pH > 7.45

c. If pCO_2 high or normal, then primary **met alkalosis**.
   i. Check measured vs expected $PaCO_2$ to see if assoc. resp d/o present. Change pCO_2 = change $HCO_3 \times 0.7$.
- PCO_2 too high, concurrent resp acidosis.
- PCO_2 too low, concurrent resp alkalosis.

   ii. *Check urine chloride*:
- Urine Cl < 20 mEq/L *(chloride responsive)*.
  - *NGT suctioning, vomiting, diuretics, excess LR, TPN, blood transfusions* (usu. > 8), colonic villous adenoma, correction of chronic resp acidosis (conversely, in primary metabolic alkalosis, body will decrease rate to retain acid, which may make vent weaning difficult), CF pt sweating, *volume contraction* (renin-aldosterone retains Na, balanced electrically w/ Cl and HCO_3 retention. H^+, K^+ lost in urine in exchange. Cl preferentially follows H, K, thus HCO_3 is retained comparably more. Must tx by volume expansion w/ emphasis on Na, K, and Cl replacement. Chronic high-dose steroid use results in the same effect).
- Urine Cl > 20 mEq/L *(chloride resistant)*.
  - *Normotensive*: hypokalemia, hypercalcemia, hypomagnesemia, hypoparathyroidism, refeeding carbs after fasting, milk-alkali syndrome, Bartter syndrome.
  - *Hypertensive*: hyperreninism (renal artery stenosis, primary hyperaldosteronism, Cushing syndrome, congenital adrenal hyperplasia, pseudohyperparathyroidism).

d. If pCO_2 low, then a primary **resp alkalosis**.
   i. Check change in pH to see if d/o is acute vs chronic, or if superimposed metabolic d/o is present.
   ii. PE, pregnancy, anxiety, endotoxemia, altitude, fever.
- If altitude, consider acetazolamide.
- If on vent, change from CMV or SIMV, consider rate. Change from CMV to SIMV (neuro picture concern for apnea) or PSV.

   iii. *Acute resp alkalosis*: change HCO$_3$ to change pCO$_2$ should be 2:10.
- HCO$_3$ too high, concurrent met alkalosis.
- HCO$_3$ too low, concurrent met acidosis.

   iv. *Chronic resp alkalosis*: change HCO$_3$ to change PCO$_2$ should be 4:10.
- HCO$_3$ too high, concurrent met alkalosis.
- HCO$_3$ too low, concurrent met acidosis.

pH normal
e. If pCO$_2$ high, mixed resp acidosis, met alkalosis.
f. If pCO$_2$ low, mixed resp alkalosis, met acidosis.
g. If pCO$_2$ normal, a mixed d/o may still exist.
- Check anion gap if elevated or normal.

h. Mixed d/o also exists if PaCO$_2$ is abnormal, but pH is unchanged or normal, or if pH is abnormal and the PaCO$_2$ is unchanged or normal.

CHAPTER 5

CARDIAC AND EKG

I. **CARDIAC**
   A. Anatomy and Physiology
      1. *3 main arteries*: left main (left anterior descending artery w/ septal perforators and diagonals + circumflex w/ obtuse marginals); right main w/ acute marginal; and posterior descending.
      2. $CO = HR \times SV$.
   B. Disease Processes
      1. *Coronary artery disease*
         a. *CABG indications*:
            i. Significant 3-vessel (LAD, circumflex, right main) dz w/ LV dysfunction.
            ii. Significant 3-vessel dz, good LV function, and 1+ important proximal stenoses.
            iii. Significant 2- to 3-vessel dz w/ severe angina, regardless of LV function.
            iv. Left main stenosis > 50%, even if asymptomatic.
            v. 2-vessel dz w/ severe proximal LAD stenosis or LV dysfunction.
         b. *Bypass conduits*: vein grafts 10-yr patency 50–60%, usu. affected by atherosclerosis. IMA grafts more resistant to atherosclerosis w/ 90% 10-yr patency. Radial artery more spastic than IMA; patency > vein grafts but < than IMA.
      2. *Valvular heart disease*
         a. *Mitral valve*
            i. *Stenosis*:
               - Sx (i.e., evidence of pulmonary hypertension, endocarditis, systemic embolization)
               - Valve area < 1 cm^2
                 - ACE inhibitor tx of choice
         b. *Aortic valve*
            i. *Stenosis*:
               - *Sx*: angina, syncope, CHF
               - Pressure gradient transvalvular velocity > 4 m/sec
               - Transvalvular gradient 50 mm Hg or valve area < 1 cm^2
         c. *Endocarditis*: generally 4–6 wk of abx is adequate tx.
      3. *Heart failure*
         a. *Right heart failure*
            i. Fluid cannot be driven forward to lungs, backs up in IVC, leads to JVD, hepatic congestion, LE edema.
            ii. CVP >15 mm Hg and CVP ≥ PCWP.
            iii. Echocardiogram can be useful showing plump IVC.
            iv. If PCWP < 15 mm Hg, give volume until PCWP or CVP increases by 5 *or* either one reaches 20 mm Hg.
            v. If PCWP > 15 or RVEDV is 140 or higher, give dobutamine at 5 mcg/kg/min.
         b. *Left heart failure*
            i. Fluid cannot be driven forward, leads to pulmonary congestion.
            ii. Fluids/preload → if low PCWP, infuse volume.
      4. *Infarction*
         a. *Progression*: T peaking, T inverting, ST segment elevation, Q wave
         b. *Labs*: LDH, troponin, CPK-MB—begins rising in 4–6 h (troponin earliest)
         c. **M**orphine, **O**xygen, **N**itrates, **A**spirin (MONA)!
         d. *Postinfarction complications*:

       i. VSD

      ii. Papillary muscle rupture

     iii. Ventricular aneurysm

     iv. Free wall rupture

     v. CHF w/out VSD

II. EKG ANALYSIS

A. EKG basics

1. *Rate*: 300, 150, 100, 75, 60, 50, etc.
2. *Rhythm*: regular, irregular, irregularly irregular, etc.

B. EKG waves and segments

1. *P wave*
   a. *Amplitude*: > 2.5 mm in II suggests RAE.
   b. *Duration*: > 0.12 sec in II suggests LAE.
   c. *Relationship to QRS*: present before all QRS. Progressive distance between QRS then dropped QRS = Mobitz I (Wenckebach). Fixed interval and fixed ratio of dropped QRSs = Mobitz II. No relation between P and QRS = 3rd-degree (complete AV) block.
2. *PR segment*
   a. *Short*: < 0.12 sec may be WPW or LGL.
   b. *Long*: > 0.20 is 1st-degree AV block.
3. *Q wave*
   a. Significant if > 0.04 sec duration and amplitude > ⅓ QRS complex.
4. *QRS complex*
   a. Prolonged (> 0.12) suggestive of BBB.
   b. *RBBB*: Look for "rabbit ears" (R') in V_1 a/o V_2.
   c. *LBBB*: Look for notched appearance in V_5 a/o V_6.
5. *R and S amplitude*
   a. *Left ventricular hypertrophy*: $RV_1 > SV_1$ and $RV_6 < SV_6$.
   b. *Right ventricular hypertrophy*: $RV_{5 \, or \, 6} + SV_{1 \, or \, 2} > 35$ mm *or* AVL > 12 mm.
6. *ST segment*
   a. *Elevation*: suggests infarction or pericarditis if in all leads.
   b. *Depression*: suggests subendocardial ischemia, or if present in precordial leads w/ elevated R waves indicates strain pattern. *Note:* an upsloping depressed ST segment usu. not worrisome, but horizontal or downsloping ST segments are.
7. *T wave*
   a. *Peaked*: hyperkalemia or early ischemia.
   b. *Flat*: hypokalemia.
   c. *Inverted*: later ischemia.
   d. Generally positive when net QRS positive, negative when net QRS negative.
8. *U wave*
   a. Hypothermia

TABLE 5.1. Localizing Region of Ischemia

Region	Leads	Coronary Artery
Anterior	V1–4	LAD
Lateral	I, AVL, V5–6	LCx
Inferior	II, III, AVF	R
Posterior		R

TABLE 5.2.   Inotropic and Vasoactive Medications

Drug Type and Name(s)	Dose	Indications	Caveats / Miscellaneous
Inotropes			
Dopamine	5–20 mcg/kg/min	•Hypotensive heart failure	•Dopamine, then beta, then alpha •Can lead to myocardial ischemia, tissue hypoxia / necrosis and decreased UOP w/ high doses •Assoc. tachyarrhythmias
Dobutamine (Dobutrex)	5–20 mcg/kg/min	•Normotensive heart failure	•Like intermediate dopamine, see increased HR & SV, but get decreased SVR (opp. of intermed-high dose dopamine) •Assoc. tachyarrythmias, myocardial ischemia, hypotension
Milrinone (Primacor)	50 mcg/kg over 10 min, then 0.375–0.75 mcg/kg/min	•Normotensive heart failure	•Increased SV, but decreased SVR like dobutamine, but little effect on HR. •Rare tachyarrhythmia; mycocardial ischemia, hypotension
Epinephrine	1–10 mcg/min; 1 mg q 3–5 min for resuscitation	•Cardiac arrest •Anaphylaxis •Post-CABG	•Tachyarrythmias, myocardial ischemia, tissue hypoxia / necrosis, hyperglycemia
Norepinephrine (Levophed)	0.5–1 mcg/min may require up to 8–30 mcg/min	•Septic shock, cardiogenic shock, PE	•Increased SVR and SV •Can lead to myocardial ischemia, tissue hypoxia / necrosis, hyperglycemia, oliguria
Vasoconstrictors			
Phenylephrine (Neo-Synephrine)	100–180 mcg/min, then 40-60 mcg/min	•Neurogentic shock, septic shock,anesthesia-induced hypotension	•Myocardial ischemia, tissue hypoxia/necrosis
Norepinephrine (Levophed)	0.5–1 mcg/min may require up to 8–30 mcg/min	•Septic shock, cardiogenic shock, PE	•Increased SVR and SV •Can lead to myocardial ischemia, tissue hypoxia / necrosis, hyperglycemia, oliguria
Vasopressin (Pitressin)	0.01–0.04 U/min;40 U once for resuscitation	•Septic shock, cardiac arrest	•Increases SVR •Myocardial ischemia, tissue hypoxia/necrosis, hyponatremia
Vasodilators			
Hydralazine	5–20 mg q 20–30 min	•Hypertension	•Arteriolar dilator, not good for MI, ischemia, or aortic dissection •Onset 10–30 min •Duration 2–4 h
Nitroglycerine	5–100 mcg/min	•Hypertension	•Venous > arteriolar dilator •Onset 2–5 min •Duration 5–10 min •Good for cardiac ischemia, but poss. unpredictable BP response

Drug Type and Name(s)	Dose	Indications	Caveats / Miscellaneous
Nitroprusside	0.25–10.0 mcg/kg/min	•Hypertension	•Arteriolar > venous dilator •Fast onset (seconds) •Duration = 3 min •Cyanide toxicity w/ prolonged use
Calcium Channel Blockers			
Diltiazim	Load 20 mg, drip	•Afib/Aflutter rate control	
Nicardipine	Begin at 5 mg/h	•Hypertension	•Increase 2.5 mg/h q 5 min up to max of 15 mg/h
Beta Blockers			
Esmolol (Brevibloc)	250–500 mcg/kg/min for 1 min, then 50–300 mcg/kg/min	•Afib/Aflutter rate control •Hypertension	•Pure beta blocker •Onset < 5 min •Duration 10–20 min (half-life 9 min) •Good for aortic dissection or postop hypertension
Metoprolol	5 mg IV push		
Labetalol (Normodyne)	20 mg, then 20–80 mg q 10 min or 2 mg/min Max 300 mg	•Hypertension	•Alpha and beta blocker •Onset 5–10 min •Duration 3–6 h •Not indicated if bronchospasm, 1st-degree heart block, cardiogenic shock, or severe bradycardia
Glycoside			
Digoxin		•CHF •Afib/Aflutter rate control & conversion	
Pde-Inhibitor			
Amiodarone	Load: 150 mg over 10 min, can repeat once, then 1 mg/min over 6 h. (If Vfib 300 mg) Maintenance: 0.5 mg/min	•Afib/Aflutter rate control & conversion •Ventricular arrythmias	•Hypotension, bradycardia, phlebitis, prolongs PR/QRS/QT •Pulmonary fibrosis, hypothyroidism

III. HYPOTENSION AND CARDIAC PHARMACOPOEIA (ALL DOSAGES INTRAVENOUS)

A. Congenital disease

1. *Fetal/perinatal circulation*

   a. 2 umbilical arteries (blood to placenta, relatively unoxygenated), 1 umbilical vein (blood from placenta, relatively well oxygenated).

   b. *Ductus arteriosus*: from left pulmonary artery to descending aorta; blood thus bypasses lungs in utero.

   c. *Ductus venosus*: from portal vein to IVC; shunts blood from liver in utero.

2. *Cyanotic*

   a. Right → left shunt.

   b. Cyanosis may result in polycythemia, endocarditis, hypertrophic osteoarthropathy, and CVA.

   c. CXR and echocardiogram good starters for evaluation.

    d. *Examples*:

      i. *Simple defects*
- Pulmonic stenosis w/ right → left shunt

      ii. *Complex lesions*
- Tetrology of Fallot
  - *Comprised of*: overriding of aorta; pulmonary stenosis, VSD, right ventricular hypertrophy
- Transposition of the great arteries
- Truncus arteriosis
- Tricuspid atresia
- Total anomalous pulmonary venous return

3. *Noncyanotic*

    a. Left → right shunt.

    b. Increased pulmonary congestion leading to Eisenmenger syndrome from prolonged pulmonary HTN.

    c. *Examples*:

      i. *Septal defects*
- *ASD (ostium secundum)*: isolated ASDs represent the most common congenital heart anomaly. 80% spontaneously close in infancy.
- *VSD*: more frequently symptomatic (failure to thrive, tachypnea, cardiomegaly) in infancy than ASDs. Repair usu. advocated if sx or by 1 yo.
- *AV canal defect* (endocardial cushion defect, includes ostium primum ASDs): frequently assoc. w/ trisomy 21.

      ii. *Patent ductus arteriosus*
- Ductus arteriosus comes from confluence of left and main pulmonary artery, and empties into arch just beyond left subclavian artery origin. Patency (increased incidence w/ prematurity) beyond 3 mo postpartum requires intervention to interrupt left → right shunt w/ resultant left heart overload as well as potential endocarditis, obstructive pulmonary vasculopathy, a/o aneurysm development.
- *Presentation*: failure to thrive, pulmonary congestion common in neonates; machinery murmur.
- *Dx*: Echocardiography.
- *Tx*:
  - *Medical*:
    - *Indomethacin*: inhibits prostaglandin synthesis; first-line tx for neonates to close PDA.
  - *Surgical*:
    - Percutaneous catheter closure appropriate after neonate period or if significant pulmonary HTN.
    - Open ligation/clipping via left posterolateral thoracotomy appropriate in poor candidates for catheter closure.

      iii. *Coarctation*: most commonly seen in males and in up to 30% of pts w/ Turner syndrome; results in relative HTN in proximal aorta and upper extremities. CXR classically shows notched ribs from enlarged intercostal arteries. Untreated, can cause CHF, hemorrhagic CVA, endocarditis, a/o rupture of aorta. Resection and grafting is traditional tx.

CHAPTER 6

THORACIC AND ESOPHAGUS

I. **THORACIC**
  A. **Anatomy and Physiology**
    1. *Anatomy*
      a. Right lung 55% volume (3 lobes), left lung 45% volume (2 lobes).
      b. Azygous vein on right side, empties into SVC. Thoracic duct begins on right, crosses to left (at approx T6) to empty to left subclavian at confluence w/ internal jugular vein.
      c. Phrenic n. anterior (to hilum) but vagus n. posterior (to hilum).
      d. *Pneumocytes*: type I (> 95%) involved in gas exchange; type II (< 5%) produce surfactant.
    2. *Physiology*
      a. *Functional adequacy for resection*:
        i. Need postop $FEV_1 > 0.8$ (or $\geq 40\%$ predicted value).
          • Can assay relative contribution of FEV_1 from planned resection portion w/ V/Q scan preop.
        ii. Need predicted postop FVC > 1.5 L.
        iii. Need preop (room air) $pCO_2 \leq 45$ or $pO_2 \geq 50$.
        iv. Need preop VO_2 max ≥ 10 cc/min/kg.
        v. Desired DLCO $\geq 11–12$ cc/min/mm Hg CO ($\geq 50\%$ predicted value).
      b. *Ventilation volumes* (also see Chapter 4, section I. on ventilation).
        i. *FVC* (forced vital capacity): if decreased, suggests restrictive dz. FVC < 2 L (or < 50%) concerning for postop complications. Vital capacity refers to volume of air in maximal expiration after maximal inspiration.
        ii. *FEV_1* (forced expiratory volume in 1 sec): if decreased, suggests obstructive dz. FEV1 < 0.8 L concerning for postop complications.
        iii. *FEV_1/FVC*: low number suggests obstructive dz.
        vi. *MVV* (maximal voluntary ventilation): < 50% predicts moderate postop risk.
        v. *FRV* (functional residual volume/capacity): amount of air left in lungs after normal expiration. This volume is increased w/ PEEP, stemming from alveolar recruitment.
        vi. *TV* (tidal volume): volume of air in normal expiration after normal inspiration.
        vii. *TLC* (total lung capacity): total maximum volume of lungs (i.e., measured at maximum inspiration, and including residual volume).
  B. **Pathology**
    1. *Abnormal lesions*
      a. *Malignant*
      b. *Solitary pulmonary nodule*
        i. Asymptomatic mass, well-circumscribed, < 3 cm diameter.
        ii. *Excisional bx indicated unless*:
          • No radiographic change in 2 yr.
          • Calcification pattern c/w hamartoma.
          • Clear evidence of infectious process (i.e., tuberculosis).
          • Prohibitive operative risk ($\rightarrow$ FNA).
          • Strong clinical suspicion for small cell carcinoma ($\rightarrow$ FNA).
        iii. *If hx of previous cancer, ddx changes*:
          • *Prior h/o sarcoma or melanoma*: lesion most likely a met.
          • *Prior h/o GI or GU cancer*: lesion equal chance of met or lung primary.
          • *Prior h/o head/neck or breast CA*: lesion more likely lung primary.

c. *Pulmonary sequestrations*: aberrant lung tissue not connected to bronchial tree, receiving systemic (not pulmonary) arterial blood flow (usu. thoracic aorta). Tx = resection.

   i. *Intralobar*: within a lobe, more likely to drain into pulmonary vein, more commonly diagnosed in adults.

   ii. *Extralobar*: outside a lobe, more likely to drain into systemic vein, more commonly identified in children.

d. *Cystic adenoid malformation*: see Chapter 18.

e. *Bronchogenic cysts*: most common mediastinal cysts; no connection w/ bronchial system; tx = resect.

f. *Thymoma*

   i. 50% malignant, 50% symptomatic, 50% have myasthenia gravis.
   - Conversely, only 10% of pts w/ myasthenia gravis (Ab to acetylcholine receptors) have a thymoma.
     - *Myasthenia gravis sx*: weakness, ptosis, diplopia.
     - *Myasthenia gravis tx*: anticholinesterase meds, plasmapheresis, steroids. 80% of all cases improve w/ thymectomy, even if no evident thymoma present.

   ii. All thymomas should be resected.

g. *Mediastinal masses* (neurogenic most common overall)

   i. *Anterior* (most common site)
   - Thymoma (most common)
   - Thyroid mass (much less commonly, parathyroid)
   - Teratoma/germ-cell tumor
   - Lymphoma (see Chapter 10)

   ii. *Middle* (heart, trachea, etc.)
   - Cysts (bronchogenic, pericardial, enteric)
   - Lymphoma

   iii. *Posterior* (esophagus, descending aorta, etc.)
   - Neurogenic tumors
   - Enteric cysts
   - Lymphoma

2. *Infectious pathology*

a. *Empyema*

   i. Infected pleural fluid, most often secondary to pneumonia, but may result from trauma or systemic infection as well. Uncomplicated, can lead to invasion of chest wall (empyema necessitatis), bronchopleural fistula, spread to pericardium, rib osteomyelitis, a/o general sepsis: *3 phases*:
   - *Exudative*: thin fluid, low cell count.
     - *Tx*: IV abx and (almost always) large-bore chest tube.
   - *Fibrinopurulent*: fibrinous deposition on pleura, abundant PMNs, may begin to loculate.
     - *Tx*: IV abx and open vs video-assisted decortication. VATS contraindicated if evidence of stage III dz (thickened rind/peel, contracted hemothorax, possibility of abscess or malignancy).
   - *Organizing/chronic*: thick exudate, heavy sedimentation. Empyema wall organizes w/ fibroplast proliferation and angiogenesis. Lung will not spontaneously reexpand after simple evacuation.
     - *Tx*: IV abx and open decortication.
       - Empyema tube(s) placed through partially resected rib bed may be appropriate if extensive amounts of thick pus/loculations.
       - Eloesser flap refers to marsupialization of a thoracostomy to drain the empyema, achieved by suturing skin to parietal pleura to create a controlled drainage sinus.
       - Clagett technique refers to open drainage, pleural cavity irrigation w/ abx (short or long term), and subsequent closure of chest wall w/ tube left in place to continue abx irrigation. Most often done for fistulas resulting from empyema.

b. *Abscess*

   i. Usu. from aspiration (followed by pneumonia, lung cancer, septic emboli, etc.), located in superior segment RLL > posterior segment RUL > superior segment LLL > elsewhere. Consider in ddx bronchiectasis and carcinoma. Aspiration abscesses most often involve anaerobes whereas pneumonic cases are usu. from *S. aureus*.

   ii. *Dx*: CXR and bronchoscopy. Latter can get washings for cx and cytology, removal of FB (if present), and drainage.

   iii. *Tx*:
- Initially tx w/ abx (8 wk standard, some advocate 16 wk) and bronchoscopic drainage—95% effective.
- Percutaneous drainage may be attempted as adjunctive therapy.
- Surgery reserved for failure of medical management, significant hemorrhage, possibility of malignancy. Resection is preferred over pneumonostomy/pneumonotomy. For poor surgical candidates, a Mondaldi catheter/tube may be placed for drainage, but requires presence of pleural adhesions for adequate seal.

c. *Fungal*

   i. *Aspergillosis*: opportunistic; voriconazole often DOC. Surgery for refractory cases.

   ii. *Coccidioidomycosis and histoplasmosis*: antifungals if persistent or mod to severe sx.

d. *Other*

   i. *M. tuberculosis*: surgery rarely indicated.

   ii. *Nocardia*: can present as multiple abscesses, may invade chest wall, producing draining sinuses. Tx of choice: TMP-SMX or linezolid.

   iii. *Actinomyces*: potential to erode into chest wall, w/ abscesses and draining sinuses w/ sulfur granules. PCN is drug class of choice.

3. *Other*

a. *Pneumothorax*: see Chapter 7 for injury-related.

   i. *Spontaneous*: 20% recur after 1st event, 60% after 2nd, 80% after 3rd.
- More common on right.
- Initial tx w/ chest tube, w/ surgery indicated for recurrence, large apical blebs (see on CT), air leak > 7 d, failure to reexpand, or in high-risk professions (divers, pilots).
- *Surgery*: usu. VATS mechanical pleurodesis +/– resection of blebs.

b. *Hemothorax* (see Chapter 7)

c. *Chylothorax*: milky-white character w/ increased lymphocytes and triacylglycerols; fat stained by Sudan red; defined by pleural fluid w/ > 110 mg/dL triglycerides.

   i. Lesion *above* T5–6 → left side chylothorax.

   ii. Lesion *below* T5–6 → right side chylothorax.

   iii. Conservative tx if < 700–1000 cc/d; up to 4 wk chest tube, low-fat diet or TPN, octreotide.
- Failure of conservative management → ligate thoracic duct on right, low in mediastinum for isolated lesion. If due to malignant dz, try pleurodesis (mechanical or chemical/talc); lower success rate.

d. *Pleural effusion*:

   i. *Etiology*: most common reason for bilateral effusion is CHF. Divide into transudative and exudative w/ Light's criteria below (need 1 criterion to call exudates; need all 3 to call transudate).
- *Transudate*: CHF, infection/empyema, cirrhosis, Meigs syndrome.

TABLE 6.1. Pleural Fluid Analysis

	Transudate	Exudate
Pleural fluid protein : serum protein	< 0.5	> 0.5
Pleural fluid LDH : serum LDH	< 0.6	> 0.6
Absolute pleural fluid LDH	< $2/3$ upper limit of normal for serum	> $2/3$ upper limit of normal for serum

- *Exudate*: malignancy, catamenial hemothorax, chylothorax.

ii. *Management*:
  - Medical management of systemic issues (i.e., CHF, cirrhosis).
  - Thoracentesis (diagnostic and therapeutic).
  - Chest tube or Pleur-X catheter.
  - *Pleurodesis*:
    - *Chemical*: tetracycline, talc, bleomycin, and others have been used.
    - *Mechanical*: sponge pad or other abrasive means is effective.

e. *Chest tubes*:

i. *Indications*: pneumothorax, hemothorax, chylothorax; subcutaneous emphysema in trauma pt. PTX seen on chest CT but not CXR (occult PTX) usu. does *not* need intervention.

ii. If placed for traumatic reason, should cover w/ 1st-generation cephalosporin for no longer than 24 h (per Eastern Association for the Surgery of Trauma guidelines at www.east.org).

iii. See Chapter 7 for management of retained hemothorax or massive air leak w/ subcutaneous emphysema in trauma setting.

iv. Place initially on suction (usu. 20 cm water wall suction) for 24 h. Change to water seal after that. If CXR 6 h after the change to water seal demonstrates no ptx, and pt has no air leak or significant drainage (> 200 cc/24 h), consider removing chest tube. Repeat CXR 6 h after d/c CT.

v. If placed for pleural effusion, limit drainage to no more than 1 L/d to avoid reexpansion pulmonary edema.

vi. Chest tube drainage system (Pleur-evac by Teleflex): has 3 reservoirs, evolved from older 3-bottle system. Facing the Pleur-evac, from right to left, the chambers are (note, the order of the first and second reservoirs are reversed in the old bottle system):
  - *First reservoir* collects the draining fluid (collection chamber).
  - *Second reservoir* is the air trap. Fluid here allows air to egress from pleural space, but not return. Fill to 2 cm of water level through the suction tube (large tube at top left of box).
  - *Third reservoir* is the suction control chamber, which acts to regulate the amount of pressure from wall suction. Wall suction above the level set here will suck air through a vent; bubbles in this setting do NOT indicate an air leak. Fill w/ water (usu. 20 cm) through the atmospheric vent (rubber flap at top left of box).

vii. Check for air leak in the air leak meter located between the suction control chamber and the collection chamber. Small air leaks may also be suggested by holding a U of tubing up and observing the column of fluid. If it is of symmetric height, that is normal, but if the column is displaced away from the pt (i.e., the level is higher on the distal arm), then an air leak may be present (called the meniscus sign).

f. *Thoracic emergencies*

i. *Hemoptysis*
  - *Etiologies*: bronchiectasis, neoplasm, embolism (including septic), PA rupture.
  - *Tx*: depends on etiology.
    - In general, first maneuver is turned to side w/ bleeding side down if known, give 100% O_2 and check coags, CBC, T&C, etc.
    - In OR, perform rigid bronchoscopy and suction.
    - If from left bronchus, place #8 Fogarty catheter in bronchus and inflate, then intubate trachea.
    - If from right bronchus (too short for Fogarty), replace rigid w/ flexible bronchoscope, then intubate left bronchus over scope w/ ETT.
    - Consider a-gram and selective bronchial artery embolization, but if deteriorates, will need thoracotomy and resection.

ii. *Pulmonary embolism* (PE)
  - Primary risk factor is iliac DVT; more peripheral DVTs—unknown risk increase. If patent foramen ovale, risk for paradoxical embolism.
  - *Presentation*:

- Range from asymptomatic to w/ dyspnea; chest pain; hypoxemia; normal, low, or high $PaCO_2$; or hemodynamically instability.
- Most common EKG finding: sinus tachycardia. Right heart strain pattern, RBBB, anterior T wave inversion less common. $S_1Q_3T_3$ frequently mentioned, rarely seen.
- CXR: normal or demonstrate Hampton's hump (focal consolidation at costophrenic angle or lateral pleural edge), Westermark's sign (diminished peripheral pulmonary vasculature markings), or Palla's sign (enlarged right descending pulmonary artery).

- *Dx*:
  - CT angiogram of chest most common imaging modality.
  - V/Q scan largely supplanted by chest CT, although, if obtained, a "high-probability" study (decreased perfusion w/ normal ventilation) should prompt intervention.
  - D-dimers may be elevated due to a number of conditions (including recent surgery), but a normal D-dimer suggests dx other than PE.

- *Tx*:
  - *Immediate*: supplemental oxygen, and airway maintenance.
  - In pts w/out contraindications to heparinization, begin IV unfractionated heparin w/ bolus of 80 U/kg (5000–10,000 U) followed by drip of 18 U/kg/h (no greater than 1600 U/h), titrating to keep PTT 1.5–2.5× > control. Some institutions are allowing therapy w/ low-molecular wt heparin instead; no titration needed.
  - Long-term anticoagulation w/ warfarin should be bridged w/ concomitant heparin/warfarin for 3–5 d, followed by warfarin alone w/ INR of ~ 2 (to avoid paradoxical thrombosis or warfarin-induced skin necrosis), continuing for 3–6 mo. Consider low-molecular wt heparin.
  - IVC (level ~ L3) filter reserved for pts w/ known DVT and contraindications to heparinization.
    - Provides no therapeutic benefit for established PE, but 95% effective at preventing further emboli.
  - Life-threatening hemodynamic instability may warrant more extreme measures such as catheter-based thrombolytics or embolectomy (venous/suction or open method).

iii. *Air embolism*
- Can occur from venous trauma, improper technique in managing central lines, or laparoscopic surgery.
- *Classic sx*: hypotension, bradycardia, or "mill wheel" murmur. Poss. cardiac arrest or convulsions.
- *Dx*: suggested by hx and physical, definitive dx w/ esophageal echocardiogram.
- *Tx*:
  - Do not delay intervention waiting for definitive dx (i.e., echocardiogram).
  - Usu. should put pt head-down, left side down. Attempt to aspirate air via central line from heart.
  - If due to pulmonary trauma, place in Trendelenburg, occlude hilum of affected lung, aspirate air from left ventricular apex/aorta, and perform open cardiac massage.
    - *Alternate recommendations*:
      - If suspect air still in right side of system, place head-up, right side up; attempt to aspirate w/ central venous catheter from right atrium.
      - If suspect left-sided emboli (often present w/ cardiac arrest), address w/ thoracotomy after placing pt in Trendelenburg to trap air in left ventricle.
  - Neuro deficits may be successfully treated w/ hyperbaric oxygen therapy.

iv. *Fat embolism*
- Sx in up to 2% of pts w/ long bone fx, 10% of pts w/ unstable pelvic fx, usu. w/in 48 h.
- Triad of confusion, dyspnea, and petechiae (esp. of upper trunk and subconjunctiva) considered classic. Fever, seizures, coma, right-sided heart failure, dysrhythmia, and other sx may occur.
- *Dx*: clinical. Thrombocytopenia often reported. Fat in urine is neither sensitive nor specific for dx.

- *Tx*: aggressive hemodynamic and ventilatory support are the only interventions of proven benefit. Early fx stabilization helps avoid the syndrome.

v. *Sudden change in end-tidal CO_2.*
  - *Increase*: malignant hypothermia (see Chapter 3).
  - *Decrease*: PE, airway disconnection, right main stem intubation.

II. ESOPHAGUS AND DIAPHRAGM

A. Esophageal Anatomy and Physiology

1. *Length*: male 40 cm, females 37 cm. Comprised of inner layer of circular muscle and outer layer of longitudinal muscle. No serosa. Upper $1/3$ is striated, w/ progressively more smooth muscle distally.

2. *3 points of narrowing*: cricopharyngeus (most narrow), aortic arch/left main stem bronchus, GE junction/diaphragmatic hiatus.

3. Thoracic duct is dorsal to esophagus, crossing from right → left in upper $1/3$ of chest, entering neck posterior to left SC vein. Vagus nerve lies on both sides, and forms 2 plexi—right vagus → posterior, left vagus → anterior.

B. Benign Pathology

1. *Congenital*
   a. Tracheoesophageal fistula
      i (Gross classification) Type C "common type:" 87%, proximal atresia w/ distal fistula.
      ii Type A (isolated atresia) and Type B ("H"), each 5–7%.
      iii 50% of cases w/ other VACTERL (vertebral, anorectal, cardiac, tracheoesophageal, renal, limb) defects.
      iv *Acquired TEF* occurs rarely, usu. from ET tube cuff erosion.
      v *Tx*:
         - Place feeding gastrostomy tube (and low-pressure ET tube cuff distal to fistula if still requiring ventilatory support).
         - Divide fistula through cervical approach and close esophagus in 2 layers.
         - Resect involved portion of trachea and primarily close (generally possible w/ up to 5-cm gap), and interpose pedicled muscle flap between esophagus and trachea.

2. *Mechanical/trauma*:
   a. *Esophageal perforation*: most often iatrogenic. Thoracic > cervical > abdominal.
      i. *Dx*: initial test should be Gastrografin (*not* barium—has particulate matter that binds to bacteria) swallow. If nondiagnostic, then consider barium study.
      ii. *Tx*: if pt not septic *and* Gastrografin drains back into esophagus from cavity, can treat w/ careful observation, NPO, and abx × 7–10 d.
         - Perforation at thoracic inlet or midesophagus w/ leakage → right thoracotomy drainage +/– patch.
         - Perforation in lower esophagus w/ leakage into abdomen → left thoracotomy a/o celiotomy drainage and patch/repair.
         - If presents > 24 h, debride lesion, and drain internally w/ T tube or Malecot tube; drain externally w/ mediastinal/chest tubes.
         - May resume feeding if repeat esophagogram after tx demonstrates healing.
      iii. *Caustic injury*:
         - *Acid*: coagulative necrosis limits penetration.
         - *Alkali*: liquefactive necrosis frequently causes full-thickness injury.
         - *Acutely*: maintain airway. CXR, AXR.
            ○ *If suspect perforation*: see section 2a. above on esophageal perforation.
            ○ *If do not suspect perforation*:
               ■ Esophagoscopy to grade injury. If ulceration or necrosis (2nd or 3rd degree), admit to ICU, make NPO, give IVF, abx, PPI. Steroids may be given to prevent strictures, but may also mask signs of perforation. Gastrografin swallow at 24 h.
                  ▪ Feeding gastrostomy and retrograde passage of string for subsequent dilatation is commonly recommended. Otherwise, for 2nd- or 3rd-degree burns,

endoscopic stent placement (for 3–4 wk) can help maintain patency. A final option is TPN or feeds via Dobhoff tube.

■ Maintain pt NPO until can swallow saliva w/out pain. EGD at 3 wk, 3 mo, and 6 mo.

— Stricture typically occurs 1–2 mo post-injury. Generally begin tx w/ dilatations w/ completion of re-epithelialization.

— TE fistula, hiatal hernia, achalasia, and carcinoma are less common long-term sequelae.

■ Alternately, some authors advocate exploratory celiotomy for 2nd- or 3rd-degree injury, w/ esophagogastrectomy, cervical esophagostomy, and feeding jejunostomy.

b. *Boerhaave syndrome*

i. Refers to tear in distal esophagus from vigorous retching/emesis, usu. resulting in longitudinal *left* posterolateral tear several cm cephalad to GE junction.

ii. *Mackler triad*: h/o vomiting, abrupt-onset lower thoracic pain, SC emphysema in base of neck.

c. *Mallory-Weiss tear*: tear in GE junction from mechanism similar to Boerhaave (above). Generally self-limited, although endoscopic management (heater probe, epinephrine injection, etc.) often useful adjunct. Surgery rarely needed to oversew lesion.

d. *Foreign body ingestion*:

i. *Tends to get caught in 3 locations*: cricopharyngeus, aortic arch/left main stem bronchus, diaphragmatic hiatus. Rigid esophagoscopy indicated for removal.

ii. If passes into stomach, almost always passes spontaneously, and can be managed expectantly following serial x-rays and clinical exam. Some advocate early celiotomy for batteries, however, given risk of caustic injury.

3. *Diverticula*

a. *False* (Pulsion)

i. *Zenker's (cricopharyngeal)*:

• Due to hypertonic/uncoordinated cricopharyngeus, mucosa bulges most often on left posterolateral side behind SCM.

• Classic sx dysphagia, regurgitation of undigested food, halitosis. Dx w/ barium swallow, not endoscopy (perforation risk).

• *Tx*: myotomy of cricopharyngeus and (if large) diverticulectomy, via left cervical incision between carotid sheath and trachea. High-risk pts may be managed w/ diverticulopexy +/– cricopharyngeal myotomy.

ii. *Epiphrenic*: r/o GERD (endoscopy), achalasia (BE, manometry). Tx w/ diverticulectomy via left thoracotomy or VATS stapling. If LES pressure elevated, consider myotomy.

b. *True*

i. *Traction*: usu. small and in midthorax. Result from adjacent inflammatory process (usu. LN, often from TB), which draws wall out. Generally asymptomatic, not requiring tx.

4. *Strictures*

a. *Plummer-Vinson syndrome*: cervical dysphagia in setting of chronic iron-deficiency anemia, usu. from *upper* esophageal web. 10% → SCCA in hypopharynx or esophagus. *Tx*: iron supplementation, prn esophageal dilatation.

b. *Schatzki ring*: a *lower* esophageal web or ring, found at the squamocolumnar junction, and almost invariably in conjunction w/ a hiatal hernia. Often responds to dilatation and rx for GERD.

5. *Motility disorders*

a. *Achalasia*: sine qua non = increased resting pressure of lower esophageal sphincter.

i. *Dx*: GI swallow—see "beak-like" tapering in distal esophagus. F/u w/ upper endoscopy (look for esophagitis, CA, Bx [decreased/absent ganglion cells in Auerbach's plexus]) and manometry (*need*: usu. aperistalsis; incomplete EGS relaxation; high resting pressure [usu. > 30 mm Hg]).

ii. *Standard*: esophagus has little to no peristalsis.

iii. *Vigorous*: esophagus has normal or exaggerated peristalsis.

vi. *Tx*:

• *Medical*: Calcium channel blockers, nitrate, endoscopic botulinum toxin.

- *Surgical*: Heller myotomy: perform laparoscopically or through left chest, extending from lower pulmonary vein to 1–2 cm onto stomach. If pt has reflux, do a Dor or loose Nissen (abdominal approach) or partial wrap such as Belsey-Mark IV (thoracic approach).
- *Other*: dilation: contraindicated in children or vigorous achalasia. Reasonable initial results in up to $3/4$ of pts, but often transient in effect.

b. *Nutcracker esophagus*

c. *Diffuse esophageal spasm*: may mimic cardiac chest pain. Barium swallow → "corkscrew" appearance. Manometry → tertiary, nonpropulsive contractions and normal LES pressure. *Medical tx*: tx life stressors, NTG or isosorbide, calcium channel blockers. *Surgical tx* = extended myotomy of thoracic esophagus through right chest, rare.

6. *Gastroesophageal reflux* (including Barrett esophagus)

   a. *Dx*: suggested by sx such as heartburn, regurgitation, chest pain, etc. Gold standard for confirmation is 24-h pH probe (i.e., pH < 4 for > 7% of the time definite evidence of dz). MUSE score used to classify extent: **M**etaplasia, **U**lcer, **S**tricture, **E**rosions. Each component scored 0–3 pts.

   b. *Tx*:

      i. *Medical*: lifestyle modification (elevate HOB 6–10" w/ blocks, lose wt, cease smoking, reduce EtOH, avoid late evening meals, limit chocolate/fat/peppermint/caffeine/acid) and H_2 blockers/PPI.

      ii. *Surgical*
         - *Indications for partial fundoplication*: poor esophageal motility; severe aerophagia; previous gastrectomy or other reason to have insufficient fundus for loose total fundoplication; planned Heller myotomy for achalasia.
         - *Specific repairs*:
            - *Nissen fundoplication*: 360-degree fundal wrap (the only nonpartial wrap)
            - *Dor fundoplication*: 150- to 200-degree anterior wrap
            - *Belsey-Mark IV*: transthoracic 270-degree anterior wrap
            - *Hill repair*: 90-degree lesser curve plication and pexy to medial arcuate ligament
            - *Toupet fundoplication*: 270-degree posterior wrap
            - *Watson*: 120-degree anterolateral wrap
            - *Collis gastroplasty*: tubularization of distal stomach for foreshortened esophagus

   c. *Barrett esophagus*

      i. Premalignant condition, most frequently found in white males, found 10–15% of pts w/ symptomatic GERD. 9–45% of pts w/ Barrett have concurrent esophageal adenocarcinoma.

      ii. *Dx*: endoscopic bx → squamous epithelium replaced by columnar ("intestinal") epithelium.

      iii. *Tx*: endoscopic surveillance at least every 2 yr results in slightly lower stage dz at dx of cancer.
         - Antireflux surgery/fundoplication reserved for GERD refractory to medical management.
         - *Low-grade* dysplasia → options include ablation w/ laser, photodynamic tx, etc.
         - *High-grade* dysplasia → esophagectomy (nearly indistinguishable from carcinoma in situ, and $1/3$ of pts w/ high-grade dyplasia have carcinoma somewhere in the esophagus).

7. *Hiatal hernias*:

   a. *Type I* (sliding): esophagus slides up through hiatus into thorax.

   b. *Type II* (paraesophageal): esophagus stays intraabdominal, but fundus of stomach slides through defect lateral to left phrenoesophageal ligament into thorax.

      i. Risk is incarceration a/o volvulus of stomach. Manage by laparoscopy or celiotomy, reduction of hernia, repair of crural defect, and gastropexy via Stamm gastrostomy tube or Nissen fundoplication. After reduction and repair, almost half of pts develop GERD sx postop, adding to rationale for fundoplication. Poor operative candidates may be managed w/ endoscopic reduction and PEG placement w/ fixation to stomach in 2 places.

   c. *Type III* (paraesophageal): coexistence of type I and type II hiatal hernias.

   d. *Type IV*: viscera or intestine herniated into thorax.

8. *Varices*: see Chapter 14.

CHAPTER 7

TRAUMA

I. RESUSCITATION PRIORITIES

A. Airway

1. *Chin lift or jaw thrust initially w/ c-spine control.*

   a. *Nasopharyngeal airway* can be used if pt spontaneously breathing and w/out if midface trauma. 7.0 ETT for men, 6.0 ETT for women.

      i. Pass through nose, listening for air movement, then pass through vocal cords as pt inspires.

   b. *Oral airway* appropriate for unconscious or altered mental status unable to protect airway. First ensure no airway protection.

      i. Preoxygenate before RSI (etomidate 0.2 mg/kg IV + succinylcholine 1 mg/kg—often give 20 and 100, respectively). Do not use succinylcholine if risk of hyperkalemia (renal failure, CVA, or other debilitating neuro d/o > 48 h old, burns > 48 h old). 8.0 ETT for men, 7.0 for women.

   c. Consider cricothyroidotomy if unable to place ETT. 5.5–6.0 ETT (men), or #5–6 Shiley tracheostomy tube (men). Slightly smaller size usu. appropriate for women.

   d. Needle/jet insufflation may be a useful temporizing measure (up to 45 min) in children (cricothyroidotomy contraindicated in children).

   e. ETT contraindicated if suspect laryngeal fx (feel crepitus or see on laryngoscopy); *tracheostomy*, not cricothyroidotomy, indicated in this instance.

   f. Combitube used by some EMT in the field. Consists of dual-lumen tube w/ 2 balloons.

   g. Placement of NGT usu. indicated to prevent aspiration, but is controversial and contraindicated if suspect esophagus or penetrating cervical vascular injury.

B. Breathing

1. Check if can talk, cyanotic, respiratory rate, volume, chest symmetry, JVD distension, tracheal deviation. Auscultate and percuss; also palpate for subcutaneous emphysema and bony stability.

2. *THINK and RULE OUT—if present, TREAT IMMEDIATELY*:

   a. *Open pneumothorax*

      i. Cover w/ occlusive dressing; place chest tube at separate site.

      ii. Historically, small lesions treated by taping dressing on 3 sides to create flutter valve.
         - United States military experience in Iraq suggests no need for flutter valve (just place dressing).

   b. *Hemothorax*

      i. Ipsilateral decreased breath sounds and decreased percussive resonance.

      ii. Drain w/ chest tube.

      iii. Pleural space can hold up to 3 L of blood each hemithorax.

      iv. Immediate output of 1500 cc *or* 4+ consecutive hours of > 200 cc/h *or* 800 cc/4 h indication for thoracotomy.

   c. *Tension pneumothorax*

      i. Hypotension, tracheal deviation, distended neck veins, ipsilateral decreased breath sounds, and increased percussive resonance.

      ii. First decompress w/ 14-g needle in midclavicular line, 2nd intercostal space.

      iii. F/u w/ chest tube.

   d. *Pericardial tamponade*

      i. Like tension PTX, hypotension, distended neck veins. Distant heart sounds.

      ii. Pericardial window preferred over pericardiocentesis.

   e. *Flail chest*

      i. 2 or more fxs in 2 or more adjacent ribs; paradoxical chest movement w/ respiration is pathognomonic.

ii. Problems include decreased respitory excursion from pain and underlying pulmonary occlusion.

iii. Treat rib pain w/ rib blocks or epidural anesthesia.

iv. Treat contusion by carefully titrating fluids, supplemental oxygen, intubate as necessary.

C. Circulation

1. *Establish 2 large-bore IVs; give fluid bolus*:

   a. *Adults*: 1–2 L

   b. *Children*: 20 cc/kg

   c. Evaluate response via BP, HR, mental status, capillary refill, urinary output.

2. *Estimations of blood loss.*

   a. *Degrees*

   b. *Orthostatics* (not generally noted in a trauma pt)

      i. Check vitals in supine position, then sit pt up w/ legs hanging for 5 min. Pulse increase of > 20 bpm or decrease in SBP > 10 mm Hg suggests 20+% blood loss.

3. *Trauma CPR and ED thoracotomy* (*Note*: resuscitative thoracotomies occur in OR and have expanded indications).

   a. *Key issues*

      i. *Electrical activity?* If none, pronounce dead.

      ii. *Blunt mechanism w/ electrical activity.*

      - If unable to resuscitate via ACLS/ATLS, pronounce dead.
      - If resuscitated, proceed as usual.

      iii. *Penetrating mechanism w/ electrical activity*

      - Resuscitate w/ ACLS/ATLS; possible resuscitate thoracotomy.
      - If unable to resuscitate, pronounce dead.
      - If able to resuscitate, proceed, consult CVTS.

II. DISABILITY

A. Glasgow Coma Scale: like vital signs, reassess frequently.

1. *Eyes*

   a. 4—open spontaneously

   b. 3—open to voice

   c. 2—open to pain

   d. 1—do not open

2. *Verbal*

   a. 5—oriented

   b. 4—confused

   c. 3—inappropriate words

   d. 2—unintelligible words

   e. 1—no speech

3. *Motor* (the most important component)

   a. 6—obeys commands

   b. 5—localizes pain

   c. 4—withdraws from pain

   d. 3—decorticate posturing (abn flexion)

   e. 2—decerebrate posturing (abn extension)

   f. 1—unresponsive

III. EXPOSURE: undress pt and evaluate entire body, but provide coverage and warmth as soon as possible.

IV. SECONDARY SURVEY: complete physical exam, FAST exam; may introduce radiological exams and DPL.

V. HEAD, NECK, AND SPINAL CORD

A. Head (see Chapter 22, section IC. on Trauma)

1. *Get head CT if loss of consciousness or focal neurologic deficits.*
2. *Increased cerebral pressure may be reduced by:*
   a. Elevating head of bed
   b. Mannitol (0.25–1.0 g/kg IV)
   c. Intubation w/ mild hyperventilation (keep pCO_2 around 35)
   d. Barbituates
3. *Epidural hematoma:* accociated w/ parietal bone fx, infrequently see "lucid interval." Lenticular shape on noncontrast CT.
4. *Subdural hematoma:* assoc. w/ dural tears. Crescent shape on CT.
5. For intracranial hemorrhage after blunt head trauma, load pt w/ fosphenytoin (Cerebyx) as 1 g IV, followed by phenytoin (Dilantin) as approximately 100 mg PO three times per day. More precisely, can load phenytoin equivalent as 10–20 mg/kg depending on severity of risk, followed by 5–6 mg/kg phenytoin IV or PO q d, holding TF for 2 h before and after dosing.
6. *Diffuse axonal injury* (DAI).

B. Spinal cord

1. *Blunt injury may be treated w/ IV methylprednisolone:*
   a. Bolus w/ 30 mg/kg over 15 min.
   b. Follow w/ 5.4 mg/kg/h given over the next 23 h.
2. *Neck:*
   a. *C-spine* (see Chapter 19)
   b. *Indications for CTA a/o angiogram:*
      i. Neurologic sx not explained by head CT.
      ii. Seat belt mark across neck.
      iii. Bruit in young person.
      iv. Fx involving foraminal canal.
      v. Severe cervical hyperextension/hyperflexion.
      vi. Near-hanging or strangulation.
      vii. C-spine fx of vertebral body, pedicle, or transverse process.
      viii. Basilar skull fx involving carotid canal or petrous bone.
      ix. GCS ≤ 8 w/out CT or MRI findings in brain to explain.
      x. LeFort II or III fx.
   c. *Incision*
      i. *If unable to localize preop* → anterior sternocleidomastoid.
      ii. *For innominate or proximal right subclavian* → median sternotomy +/– supraclavicular.
      iii. *For proximal left subclavian* → left thoracotomy +/– supraclavicular.

C. Neck

1. *Penetrating neck injury*
   a. Remember that *airway* control is paramount—stridor, hoarseness, hemoptysis, tracheal deviation, a/o expanding hematoma may herald loss of airway. Emergent intubation, cricothyroidotomy, or even emergent tracheostomy (if laryngeal injury) may be required.
   b. If suspect possible esophageal injury or possible cervical vascular injury, do not place NGT as may worsen perforation or dislodge clot, either directly or by stimulating retching.
   c. Regardless of location in neck, pts w/ airway problems, expanding hematoma, or other evidence of active bleeding should go straight to the OR.
   d. Less overtly injured pts have traditionally had their injury management defined by zones:
      i. *Zone I* (thoracic inlet to cricoid cartilage)
         • CT angiogram (arteriogram a/o esophagram/esophagoscopy if CTA abnormal); +/– tracheobronchoscopy.

    ii. *Zone II* (cricoid cartilage to angle of mandible)
- *Surgical exploration* or CTA (possible arteriogram a/o esophagram/esophagoscopy if CTA abnormal); pharyngoscopy/laryngoscopy (not tracheobronchoscopy).

    iii. *Zone III* (angle of mandible to skull base)
- CT angiogram (arteriogram if CTA abnormal); pharyngoscopy (no tracheobronchoscopy or esophagoscopy).

  e. If injury identified in any of 4 cervical vessels, must evaluate all vessels *as well as* intracranial circulation.

  f. *Penetrating cervical vascular injury*:
- i. Neck exploration through incisions over anterior SCM. Venous ligation tolerated well if not B jugular. Vertebral art. injury usu. best managed by embolization.

  g. *Penetrating cervical esophageal injury*:
- i. Typically approach retracting carotid sheath laterally (going medial to carotid; left-sided approach easier if no concerns on the right neck). To fully expose, must divide omohyoid, middle thyroid vein, +/− inferior thyroid artery. If NGT present, palpate to find esophagus.
- ii. *Tx*:
  - Debride then repair in 1 (i.e., PDS) or 2 layers.
  - Interpose healthy muscle flap between suture line and other neck structures or suture lines.
  - Drain uncontrolled leaks if esophagus is inaccessible. Fistula should close w/ time. Lateral esophagostomy is other option for large defects.

2. *Blunt neck injury*
  a. *Suspect cerebrovascular lesion if*: severe cervical hyperextension/rotation or hyperflexion; near-hanging or strangulation; basilar skull fx involving carotid canal or petrous bone fx; C-spine fx involving vertebral body, pedicle, or transverse process; GCS ≤ 8 w/out evident cerebral lesion on CT or DAI; LeFort II or III fx; lateralizing neuro deficit w/out CT findings to explain; cerebral infarct on head CT; massive epistaxis; anisocoria/Horner syndrome; seat belt sign above clavicle; cervical bruit or thrill. [Biffl WL, Moore EE, Offner PJ, Burch JM, *World J Surg*, 2001;25:1036–43.]

  b. *Any of the above findings should prompt*:
- i. Standard 3-view plain films of cervical spine.
- ii. CT angiogram of head/neck (as good as 4-vessel angiogram for dx).

  c. *Management of carotid/vertebral injuries* [by grading sytem of Biffl et al., *J Trauma*, 1999;47(5):845–58.]
- i. *Grade I*: luminal irregularity or dissection w/ < 25% luminal narrowing; hemodynamically insignificant.
  - Consider systemic fractionated or unfractionated heparin a/o ASA/antiplatelet tx.
- ii. *Grade II*: dissection or intramural hematoma w/ > 25% luminal narrowing, intraluminal thrombus, or raised intimal flap. May progress to pseudoaneurysms/thrombotic occlusions.
  - Systemically anticoagulate and repeat angiography.
- iii. *Grade III*: pseudoaneurysm—risk of thrombosis a/o rupture.
  - Repair if accessible (open or endovascular).
- iv. *Grade IV*: occlusion; very high stroke rate.
  - Systemically heparinize.
- v. *Grade V*: transaction w/ free extravasation; rare, usu. lethal.

VI. THORAX

A. Lungs
1. CXR can detect as little as 200 cc in hemithorax.
2. 85% problems corrected w/ chest tube.
3. All pts w/ pneumothoraces must have chest tube before beginning mechanical ventilation.
4. Subcutaneous air or sx of tension pneumothorax in an unstable trauma pt merits a chest tube *before* CXR.

a. Chest tubes placed for trauma should receive 1 dose 1st-generation IV cephalosporin.

b. Retained hemothorax traditionally treated w/ second chest tube to prevent empyema and fibrothorax, but early VATS often result in earlier discharge from hospital. [Meyer DM, Jessen ME, Wait MA, Estrera AS, Early evacuation of traumatic retained hemothoraces using thoracoscopy: a prospective, randomized trial, *Ann Thorac Surg* 1997;64:1396–401.]

5. *Indications for thoracotomy*:

    a. Immediate output of 1500 cc from chest tube.

    b. > 2 h of > 200 cc blood from chest tube.

    c. Hemopericardium/tamponade.

    d. Expanding hematoma at thoracic outlet.

    e. Exsanguinating hemorrhage from supraclavicular penetrating wound.

    f. Radiographic evidence of thoracic great vessel injury.

6. *Emergency Department Thoracotomy (EDT)* [Cothren CC, Moore EE, *World J Emerg Surg* 2006;1:4, Powell DW, Moore EE, *J Am Coll Surg* 2004;1999:211–5.]

    a. *Indications*:

      i. *Cardiac arrest*:

        • Witnessed penetrating trauma w/ < 15 min prehospital CPR.

        • Witnessed blunt trauma w/ < 5 min prehospital CPR.

      ii. *Persistent severe hypotension (SBP ≤ 60) secondary to*:

        • Pericardial tamponade.

        • Hemorrhage (thoracic, abdominal, extremity).

        • Air embolism.

    b. *Contraindications*:

      i. Penetrating trauma w/ > 15 min CPR and no signs of life (papillary reflexes, spontaneous respiration, or motor activity).

      ii. Blunt trauma w/ > 5 min of CPR and no signs of life or asytole.

    c. *Goals (6)*:

      i. (1) Decompress pericardial tamponade; (2) control cardiac bleeding; (3) control intrathoracic bleeding; (4) temporarily occlude descending thoracic aorta; (5) perform open cardiac massage/defibrillation; (6) evacuate massive air embolism.

      ii. *Other*: overall survival < 1.4%. Better for penetrating trauma (particularly stab wound to heart w/ pericardial tamponade) than blunt trauma.

    d. *Incisions*

      i. *Left anterolateral thoracotomy*: most thoracic great vessel injuries and proximal left subclavian artery injury.

      ii. *Left posterolateral thoracotomy*: descending aorta, proximal left carotid artery.

      iii. *Median sternotomy*: thoracic vena cava, ascending aorta and arch, innominate artery, intrathoracic left carotid artery, proximal right subclavian artery, pulmonary arteries/veins.

      iv. *MS + neck extension*: thoracic outlet injury.

      v. *Right posterolateral*: azygous vein, distal right pulmonary vein, thoracic esophagus.

7. *Tracheobronchial injury*

    a. Suggested by hemoptysis, mediastinal emphysema, and persistent air leak.

    b. First maneuver should generally be bronchoscopy to confirm and localize (usu. w/in 2 cm of carina).

    c. Double-lumen ETT may be indicated in some cases.

B. Cardiac

1. *Tamponade*

    a. If stable w/ (+) pericardial effusion/tamponade, most begin w/ pericardial window, then extend to median sternotomy if (+). If pt unstable, begin w/ emergent left lateral thoracotomy, dividing pericardium anterior to phrenic nerve, which may be visible or obscured by assoc. overlying fatty tissue.

2. *Laceration*

   a. If partial thickness, repair w/ staples or pledgeted sutures.

   b. If full thickness, first occlude hole to prevent exsanguination. May use finger initially, then consider other such as Foley catheter. Repair w/ pledgeted sutures, taking care not to entrap/ occlude coronary arteries; if near one, can repair w/ horizontal mattress stitches passed under the vessel.

C. Non-Cardiac

1. *Great vessels*

   a. Findings assoc. w/ aortic rupture or other significant injury:

      i. Widened mediastinum most accurate (> 8 cm).

      ii. Fx of scapula or first 2 ribs (controversial).

      iii. Loss of pulmonary window a/o aortic knob.

2. *Mediastinal traversing injury*

   a. If unstable, immediate chest tube, followed by CXR, OR.

   b. If indication for extrathoracic surgery, need to evaluate cardiothoracic system, the thoracic aorta, and aerodigestive tract. Can be accomplished via celiotomy for other indication; pericardial window; esophagoscopy; bronchoscopy; aortography (postop).

   c. If no indication for any surgery, can w/u via CXR w/ chest tube as indicated; arteriography; esophagography; echocardiography.

3. *Blunt aortic injury*

   a. *CXR risk factors*: widened mediastinum (> 8 cm), indistinct aortic knob, indistinct AP window, indistinct descending aorta, apical cap, deviation of NGT/trachea to right, depression of left main stem bronchus, fx of ribs 1 a/o 2, or scapula.

   b. *Once pt stabilized, obtain spiral CT of thorax to further screen.*

      i. *If normal, no further w/u necessary.*

      ii. *Abnormal*:

      • *Ascending aortic injury*: CVTS consult for immediate operative intervention.

      • *Descending arotic injury*: CVTS consult, SICU admission for aggressive BP control (esmolol, labetalol). Consider endovascular exclusion of the injury.

      • Anterior mediastinal hematoma → no further w/u or tx necessary.

      • Peri-aortic hematoma/pseudoaneursym/intimal flap → CVTS consult to determine need for aortography.

   c. *Aortography*

      i. *If normal, no further w/u necessary.*

      ii. *Abnormal*:

      • If operative candidate, should go to OR.

      • If not operative candidate (traumatic CHI, etc.), need aggressive medical control of rate-pressure product. Maintain SBP below 100–110 mm Hg, ideally w/ short-acting beta blocker such as esmolol, which is also a negative inotrope. Additional control may be gained w/ nitroprusside if beta blocker ineffective. Obviously, in pts w/ CHI, there will be conflicting goals for BP, which will require close cooperation of specialty services and ICU team.

4. *Blunt cardiac injury*

   a. *If suspect*, get EKG.

   b. *If unstable*, get emergent echocardiography, admission to ICU, invasive monitoring, and aggressive resuscitation.

   c. *If stable* w/ normal EKG, no further w/u. If stable w/ abnormal EKG → telemetry monitoring × 24 h. Tx arrhythmias if symptomatic.

5. *Pneumothorax/hemothorax*

a. If pt unstable w/ clinical indications of PTX/HTX, perform emergent tube thoracostomy before CXR.

b. If stable, mechanism is blunt, and CXR is normal, no further w/u necessary.

c. If stable, mechanism is penetrating, and CXR is normal, repeat CXR in 6 h for latent PTX.

   i. Occult PTX (PTX seen on CT but not on CXR) does not need decompression.

d. Hemothorax or PTX (non-occult) require chest tube.

e. Persistent PTX requires placement of additional tube directed at PTX.

f. If still have PTX or persistent air leak, need bronchoscopy to evaluate for tracheobronchial injury. CVTS consult.

   i. Airway injury requires thoracotomy.

g. Persistent HTX should be managed w/ right angle tube in posterior sulcus or VATS/thoracotomy.

h. Chest tubes placed outside of OR are indication for 24 h of abx (i.e., 1st-degree cephalosporin).

6. *Thoracoabdominal injury*

7. *Trauma CPR*

   a. If no electrical activity, pronounce pt dead.

   b. If blunt mechanism and electrical activity, perform ACLS/ATLS until dead or to OR/ICU.

   c. If penetrating mechanism and electrical activity, perform ACLS/ATLS. If aortic cross-clamp and pericardiotomy successful (ED thoracotomy), take to OR and consult CVTS.

8. *Rib fx/pulmonary contusion*: ensure adequate analgesia, including possible thoracic epidural. ICU monitoring necessary if respiratory embarrassment.

9. *Esophageal injury* (not from transthoracic trauma): see Chapter 6.

VII. ABDOMEN

A. General principles

1. *Penetrating abdominal trauma* (count numbers of holes—should be even if missile not in body)

   a. *GSW to abdomen or trauma to abdomen w/ pneumoperitoneum*:

      i. All go to OR.

   b. *Stab wounds to abdomen*:

      i. $1/3$ of stab wounds to abdomen do not penetrate peritoneum; another $1/3$ cause no significant harm.

      - *To OR if*: peritonitis, bowel evisceration (omental evisceration only → admit for serial exams), or evidence of intraabdominal bleeding.

      - *Otherwise, locally explore*:
        - "Positive" = tract penetrates posterior fascia or peritoneum.
        - "Positive" or equivocal cases get DPL unless ex lap indicated.
          - *Positive DPL criteria*:
            - Aspiration of 10 cc gross blood
            - > 100,000 RBC/mm^3
            - > 500 WBC/mm^3
            - Bile or vegetable matter

2. *Blunt abdominal trauma*

   a. *To OR if*: evisceration, peritonitis, or (+) FAST and hemodynamic instability.

      i. Only items needed before OR are CXR, pelvis film, and T&C.

   b. If no immediate indication for OR, all get at least examination, FAST, CXR, and pelvic x-ray.

3. *Damage control celiotomy*

   a. *Indication to get out of operation and to ICU for resuscitation ("the lethal triad/triangle")*:

      i. *Hypothermia* (< 34°C)

      - *Passive rewarming*: BAER hugger, warm blankets, etc.

- *Active rewarming* (preferred): warmed IV fluids, CAVR, warmed bladder/NGT lavage, warmed DPL fluid, warmed fluid lavage of thorax through chest tubes; warming of pt's blood and reintroducing it to body via pump (Gentilello technique).

ii. *Acidosis* (< 7.2) or other evidence of profound shock (e.g., BD < −7, lactate > 5, etc.)

iii. *Coagulopathy*

b. *Steps*:

    i. *Control hemorrhage!* If involves liver, *pack*.

    ii. *Control enteral spillage*: staple off bowel, leave in discontinuity, or occlude w/ clamps.

    iii. *Control GU injury*: ligate ureters, etc.

    iv. *Temporary closure of the abdomen* (i.e., close skin w/ nylons or towel clips, or VAC, etc.).

    v. *Planned return to OR in ~ 24 h*, after resuscitation in the ICU.

4. *Stab wounds to back and flank*

  a. Peritoneal sx, shock, or evisceration → OR.

  b. Otherwise, locally explore wound to determine direction (for flank), and depth/end of tract.

    i. If clearly ends w/out entry into abdomen, debride wound. *Otherwise*, see below:

      - *Flank wounds*: if tracks toward peritoneal cavity and penetrates fascia → DPL. If tracks toward retroperitoneum → CT (w/ rectal contrast if concern for colorectal injury).

      - *Back wounds* → CT scan (w/ rectal contrast if concern for colorectal injury).

      - (+) DPL or suggestion of injury on CT scan → OR.

5. *Suspected rectal injury*:

  a. Perform proctosigmoidoscopy if blood on rectal exam or if suspect colorectal injury. If abnormal, do retrograde cystourethrogram as well.

B. Abdominal vascular injury

1. 5–10% of blunt trauma celiotomies. 10% of stab wound celiotomies. 10–25% of gunshot wound celiotomies.

2. Open abdomen, pack in all quadrants and then remove lower packs, then LUQ, then RUQ.

3. Hematoma in midline *supramesocolic* area → *left* medial rotation (Mattox maneuver) including colon, kidney, pancreatic tail, gastric fundus.

4. Hematoma/hemorrhage in midline *inframesocolic* area → *right* medial rotation (Cattell-Braasch maneuver) including transverse colon, midgut, w/ proximal infrarenal aortic control inferior to left renal vein.

C. Diaphragm

1. Always warrant primary closure; mesh may be used for extensive defects. F/u w/ chest tube.

2. If hemothorax or gastric/intestinal spillage, irrigate thoracic cavity through chest tube or red rubber catheter placed through defect. Incidence of empyema highest after gastric spillage followed by colonic spillage.

D. Distal esophagus and stomach (as for all penetrating trauma, should generally have even number of holes)

1. *Distal esophagus*: Mobilize GE junction (see section 2. on stomach below).

  a. In damage-control situations, large defects can be managed w/ drain placed into the hole and brought out through skin.

  b. *Definitive repair*:

    i. *Simple defect*: debride, close in 1 layer (i.e., PDS), drain. If possible, bring up antrum to create serosal patch (Thal patch).

    ii. *Destruction of GE junction*: typically has significant assoc. injuries. Staple esophagus and stomach, drain, then come back later for anastamosis.

2. *Stomach*:

  a. *Examine entire stomach*: divide gastrocolic omentum to enter lesser sac and visualize posterior stomach. Mobilize GE junction (take down left triangular ligament of liver, retract left lobe, and open peritoneum).

  b. Most injuries can be managed w/ stapled wedge resection, although more extensive gastrec-tomy may be occasionally necessary.

E. Pancreas

1. *Anatomy/physiology/epidemiology*

   a. *Dx*: essential to have high index of suspicion based upon mechanism of injury and any of the following: worsening abdominal exam; CT scan w/ peri-pancreatic hematoma or parenchymal filling defect. FAST exam and DPL (amylase) not very sensitive as pancreas is retroperitoneal. Consider structures that are commonly injured along w/ pancreas (head/body = biliary tree, duodenum, portal vein, liver right kidney, SMA/SMV, L-1; tail = spleen, proximal jejunum, left kidney). Elevated serum amylase/lipase not specific, but absence of these means likely no significant pancreatic injury (+/–).

   b. *Tx*:

      i. Minor contusion or laceration w/out duct injury (*grade I*): externally drain.

      ii. Major contusion or laceration w/out duct injury (*grade II*): externally drain.

      iii. Distal (left of SMA/SMV) injury w/ duct injury (*grade III*): distal pancreatectomy is generally recommended w/ drainage and oversewing of duct +/– splenectomy. Stapling thought by some to be not as good an option as fishmouth hand-sewn resection.

      iv. Proximal (right of SMA/SMV) inury +/– papilla injury (*grade IV*):

         • *Intraoperative pancreatogram*: can perform duodenotomy and cannulate ampulla, but to avoid additional potential morbidity, recommend performing high-pressure cholangiogram via needle in cystic duct.

         • *Consider*:

            ◦ Resection and external drainage.

            ◦ External drainage and endoscopic ductal stent.

            ◦ Internal drainage using Roux-en-Y limb (rarely used).

         • *Pancreatic head injury*: can usu. be managed w/ ample drainage via closed silastic catheters, but complex, massive damage (grade V; esp. if duodenum also injured) may Whipple in 2 stages (resection and subsequent reconstruction; rarely actually performed—normal/soft pancreatic parenchyma high risk for leak).

F. Small intestine

1. *Duodenum*

   a. *Anatomy/physiology/epidemiology*:

      i. Between L1 and L3, first segment (duodenal bulb) intraperitoneal; the remainder is retroperitoneal. Ampulla of Vater separates 2nd, 3rd segments. SMA divides 3rd, 4th portions.

      ii. 5–10 L/d pass through duodenum.

      iii. Injured in 3–5% abdominal injuries, 75% from penetrating trauma. Blunt injury most often from "handlebar" compression/"blowout" or deceleration.

   b. *Dx*: essential to have high index of suspicion based upon mechanism of injury and any of the following: worsening abdominal exam; KUB w/ retroperitoneal air; (+) FAST; DPL w/ bile; CT w/ right-sided contrast leak or periduodenal hematoma; upper GI contrast study w/ leak or intraluminal filling defect. Consider structures that are commonly injured along w/ duodenum (D1/D2 = stomach, pancreas, biliary tree, liver, kidney, portal vein; D3/D4 = SMA/SMV, proximal jejunum, kidney, L1 vertebral body or transverse processes).

   c. *Tx*:

      i. Nonperforated (*grade I*): may be managed nonoperatively.

      ii. < 50% circumferential laceration (*grade II*): primary repair (transversely/obliquely to avoid stenosis).

      iii. > 50% circumferential laceration (*grade III*):

         • Pyloric exclusion and gastrojejunostomy

         • Duodenal diverticulization

            ◦ Perform antrectomy and gastrojejunostomy IV

      iv. 75% circumferential laceration + CBD/ampulla injury (*grade IV*)

         • Roux-en-Y bypass

      v. *Complex pancreaticoduodenal injury*:

         • Pancreaticoduodenectomy

2. *Jejunum, ileum*: small full-thickness injury is easily managed w/ running 4-0 absorbable suture, followed by 3-0 silk Lembert sutures; close transversely if possible to avoid luminal narrowing. Otherwise, resect area and perform primary anastamosis.

G. Colon

1. 15–39% penetrating abdominal trauma; rare in blunt trauma.
2. Can usu. resect injured area and perform primary anastamosis (if too edematous to staple, then hand-sew).
3. *Indications for diversion instead of primary anastamosis*:
   a. Destructive lesions (> 50% bowel wall or devascularization of bowel segment) *and . . .*
      i. Hemodynamic instability (pre- or intraop SBP < 90), *or . . .*
      ii. Significant comorbidities, *or . . .*
      iii. Significant assoc. injuries (PATI < 25, ISS < 25, Flint grade < 11), *or . . .*
      iv. Peritonitis

H. Rectum

1. Rare (3–5% colon injury), but prone to disaster.
2. 4 traditional linchpins of management (debride, dilute, divert, drain [presacral]) have been challenged recently by authorities. Several studies have questioned the need for presacral drainage.
3. If able to easily identify and repair injury, do so; protect repair/anastomosis (intraperitoneal portion) w/ diverting ostomy. Otherwise, if suspect extraperitoneal rectal injury, perform diverting loop ostomy, and consider presacral drainage.

I. Liver

1. *Injury scale* (similar to spleen scale)
   a. *Hematoma/vascular*
      i. *Grade I*—subcapsular, nonexpanding, < 10% SA
      ii. *Grade II*— subcapsular, nonexpanding, 10–50% SA
      iii. *Grade III*—subcapsular, > 50% or expanding, ruptured subcapsular actively bleeding, intraparenchymal > 2 cm or expanding
      iv. *Grade IV*—ruptured intraparenchymal hematoma actively bleeding
      v. *Grade V*—juxtahepatic venous injuries (i.e., retrohepatic vena cava or major hepatic veins)
      vi. *Grade VI*—hepatic avulsion
   b. *Laceration*
      i. *Grade I*—capsular, nonbleeding, < 1 cm deep
      ii. *Grade II*—capsular, bleeding, 1–3 cm deep, < 10 cm long
      iii. *Grade III*—> 3 cm deep
      iv. *Grade IV*—25–50% lobar disruption
      v. *Grade V*—> 50% lobar disruption
2. Most commonly injured abdominal organ w/ blunt trauma, but vast majority is relatively minor, not requiring operative intervention.
3. Given unique vascular supply, many hepatic injuries can be managed through interventional radiology.
4. Intraoperative maneuvers to obtain hemostasis include first taking down falciform ligament, bimanual compression, Pringle maneuver, taking down triangular and coronary ligaments (contraindicated if massive retrohepatic bleeding), shunt, total hepatic vascular isolation, finger fx and ligation, insertion of red rubber catheter w/ side holes, and overlying Penrose.
5. *Hemobilia*: classically, this manifests as triad of RUQ pain, jaundice, and upper GI bleed occurring ~ 2–3 wk after hepatic trauma. Results from fistula between hepatic arterial supply and biliary system. Confirmatory dx and tx are angiographic.
6. *Bile leak*: manifests as RUQ discomfort, sx of ileus or gastric obstruction, and jaundice. Evaluate w/ U/S or CT. CT-guided drainage w/ ERCP to localize source (and, if more significant than cystic duct leak after cholecystectomy, treat via stenting) is generally sufficient tx.

J. Spleen

1. Most common *significantly* (requiring operative intervention) injured organ in blunt trauma.
2. Rupture may manifest as falling hct and rising WBC.
3. *Injury scale* (similar to liver scale)
   a. *Hematoma/vascular*
      i. *Grade I*—subcapsular, nonexpanding, < 10% surface area
      ii. *Grade II*—subcapsular, nonexpanding 10–50% SA
      iii. *Grade III*—subcapsular, > 50% or expanding, ruptured subcapsular actively bleeding, intraparenchymal > 2 cm or expanding.
      iv. *Grade IV*—ruptured intraparenchymal hematoma actively bleeding
      v. *Grade V*—major bleeding
   b. *Laceration*
      i. *Grade I*—capsular, nonbleeding, < 1 cm deep
      ii. *Grade II*—capsular, bleeding, 1–3 cm deep but not involving trabecular vessels
      iii. *Grade III*—> 3 cm deep or involving trabecular vessel(s)
      iv. *Grade IV*—involves segmental or hilar vessels w/ > 25% splenic devascularization
      v. *Grade V*—shattered/pulpified spleen, hilar disruption, devascularized or avulsed fragments
4. *Indications for operation in pts w/ splenic rupture*:
   a. Need for blood transfusion.
   b. Peritonitis.
   c. Inability to follow exam (i.e., head injury).
   d. Failed embolization of pseudoaneurysm.
5. *Splenorrhaphy vs splenectomy*
   a. *Salvage may be considered if*:
      i. < 500 cc (or $\frac{1}{3}$ pt volume) lost or if pt hemodynamically stable
      ii. No hilar involvement
      iii. No coagulopathy
      iv. Minimal assoc. injuries
   b. *Splenic salvage may be attempted w/*: electrocautery, argon beam laser, hemostatic gel, polyglycolic mesh (to keep multiple shattered segments together), debridement/suture repair, partial splenectomy (stapler or suture w/ pledgets), etc.
   c. Must retain 30–40% of spleen and hilar blood flow architecture to preserve immune function.
6. *Pseudoaneurysm*
   a. Suggested by blush on CT.
   b. Initial management may be attempted by interventional radiology if no other indications for operation.
7. Pediatric (< 2 yo better than < 6 yo better than adult) spleen more elastic; more often can be managed nonoperatively.
8. *Postsplenectomy sequelae*: refer to Chapter 16.

K. Great vessels

1. *Retroperitoneal zone I hematoma* (*Zone I = between renal hila*)
   a. Explore all.
2. *Retroperitoneal zone II hematoma* (*Zone II = lateral to renal hila*)
   a. Explore if penetrating trauma or expanding or pulsatile.
3. *Retroperitoneal zone III hematoma* (*Zone III = pelvis*)
   a. Explore if penetrating trauma or expanding or pulsatile.

L. Abdominal compartment syndrome (watch for decreased UOP):

Grade	cm H$_2$O	mm Hg
I	10–15	7–11 (normal)
II	15–25	11–18 (close watch)
III	25–35	18–26 (+/– decompress)
IV	35	> 26 (nec. decompress)

M. Genitourinary

1. *Initial management*

   a. Most trauma pts require Foley catherization. However, blood at meatus, high-riding prostate, or palpable bladder suggest urethral injury and warrant retrograde urethrogram. Perform by instilling 10 cc of contrast through catheter inside urethral meatus.

   b. Gross hematuria warrants evaluation w/ CT cystogram or retrograde cystogram w/ ~300 cc of contrast in bladder.

   c. Microscopic hematuria warrants imaging only if penetrating injury *or* h/o hypotension (SBP < 90 mm Hg) *or* in pediatric pts.

   d. Unstable pts can be evaluated in OR w/ "one-shot" IVP using 2 mg/kg IV contrast 10 min before plain radiograph.

2. *Specific injuries*

   a. *Kidney*: recent literature suggests vast majority of injuries can be managed nonoperatively. Operative principles of repair include débridement of nonviable tissue, water-tight repair of collecting system, coverage w/ renal capsule or omentum. Nephrectomy indicated in unstable pt w/ expanding or pulsatile perinephric hematoma.

   b. *Ureter*

      i. Most often iatrogenic.

      ii. Management depends on level of injury.

         - *Upper third*:
            ◦ Primary ureteroureterostomy tx of choice.
            ◦ Renal autotransplantation or bowel interposition less-favored options.
         - *Middle third*
            ◦ Primary ureteroureterostomy tx of choice.
         - *Lower third*
            ◦ Bladder reimplantation w/ psoas hitch to decrease anastamotic tension is preferred.
               ▪ Requires division of urachus and contralateral medial ligament, followed by incising the bladder anteriorly to create antireflux anastamosis from within. Avoid injuring genitofemoral nerve when suturing to psoas.
            ◦ Primary ureteroureterostomy acceptable if no loss of length and no pelvic sepsis or urinoma.
            ◦ Boari flap (tubularization of portion of bladder to anastamose to ureter).

      iii. In a damage-control situation, one can ligate the ureter and place a nephrostomy tube using a red rubber catheter.

   c. *Bladder*

      i. 10% of pelvic fx assoc. w/ bladder injury. 80+% of bladder injuries assoc. w/ pelvic fx. 50% extraperitoneal, 30% intraperitoneal, 20% combined.

      ii. *Extraperitoneal*
         - Can be managed w/ catheter drainage alone for 2 wk.

      iii. *Intraperitoneal*
         - Managed w/ 2 layers of running suture (chromic gut preferred, esp. for inner layer, to decrease risk nidus for stone formation) and catheter drainage for 8–10 d.

    d. *Urethra*
        i. 5% of pelvic fx assoc. w/ urethral injury, usu. at junction of prostatic and membranous portions.
        ii. Do not place Foley if suspect injury, unless urethrogram normal.
        iii. Blunt injury managed initially w/ suprapubic cystostomy. Depending on location and nature of injury, urethral voiding and possible urethroplasty schedules vary.

VIII. PELVIS (see Chapter 19)

IX. EXTREMITIES (see Chapter 19 for specific types of fx/dislocation)

A. Mangled extremity severity score (MESS): consider amputation if total score > 7. *Note*, the original article that reported this threshold was retrospective. Prospective data suggest that up to ⅓ of "non-salvageable" limbs may in fact be salvageable w/ reasonable outcome.

TABLE 7.1. Mangled Extremity Severity Score (MESS) [Johansen et al., *J Trauma*, 1990:30(5);568-72.]

Skeletal soft tissue injury	Low energy	1 point
	Medium energy (open fx)	2 points
	High energy (military gsw)	3 points
	Very high energy (gross contamination)	4 points
Limb ischemia (2x if > 6 h isch.)	Near-normal	1 point
	Pulseless, decreased cap. refill	2 points
	Cool, insensate, paralyzed	3 points
Shock	SBP always > 90 mm Hg	0 points
	Transient hypotension	1 point
	Persistent hypotension	2 points
Age (years)	< 30	0 points
	30–50	1 point
	> 50	2 points

B. Gustilo classification for open fx (initially developed for tibia fx):
1. *Gustilo II*: moderate soft-tissue injury and stripping
2. *Gustilo IIIA*: high-energy, but adequate soft tissue despite laceration or undermining
3. *Gustilo IIIB*: extensive soft-tissue injury and periosteal stripping, usu. gross contamination
4. *Gustilo IIIC*: Gustilo B w/ limb ischemia

C. Contraindications for salvage of Gustilo IIIC injury in lower extremity:
1. Preexisting severe comorbidity
2. Severed limb
3. Tibial loss > 8 cm
4. Ischemia > 6 h
5. Severance of posterior tibial nerve in adults, or sciatic nerve in anyone (increasingly controversial)

D. Extremity vascular injury (see Chapter 9 for exposures)
1. *Hard signs of vascular injury* (mandate exploration in OR)
    a. Circulatory deficit
    b. Ischemia
    c. Pulse deficit

    d. Bruit

    e. Expanding or pulsatile hematoma

    f. Arterial bleeding

2. *Soft signs of vascular injury* (generally mandate further w/u such as angiography)

    a. Small or stable hematoma

    b. Adjacent nerve injury

    c. Otherwise unexplained shock

    d. Proximity to major vessel (< 1 cm), bony injury, nerve injury

    e. ABI < 0.9 or difference of > 0.15 from uninjured side

CHAPTER 8

BURNS

I. **INITIAL CARE AND RESUSCITATION** (The following burns should be referred to a designated burn center if possible: 2nd- and 3rd-degree burns > 10% BSA; full-thickness burns > 5% BSA; any burn to face, hands, eyes, ears, or perineum that could result in cosmetic or functional disability; high-voltage electrical injury including lightning, inhalation injury, or assoc. trauma; chemical burns; burns in pts w/ major comorbidities [DM, COPD, etc.]. In addition to steps mentioned below, all significant burns merit NGT and Foley.)

   A. **Airway, breathing, and other important considerations**
      1. Always suspect inhalation injury; give 100% oxygen by mask.
      2. Expose chest to assess breathing.
      3. Consider early intubation, esp. if face/neck burns, or inhalation injury.

   B. **Circulation:** fluid resuscitation (see below for calculation of TBSA)
      1. BP may be difficult to assess in extremities; follow pulse, skin perfusion.
      2. 2 peripheral IVs should be *sutured* at multiple points to the skin; as the pt will become edematous; this helps prevent lines from being dislodged.
      3. While calculating fluid deficits, start RL at 500 cc/h (adult) or 250 cc/h (child > 5 yo).
         a. *Parkland formula* (for adults w/ burn BSA > 20%; peds/elderly BSA > 10%); developed by Dr. Charles Baxter:
            i. 4 cc/kg/24 h—initial guide, follow UOP, other clinical parameters.
            ii. *Note:* the Brooke formula recommends 2 cc/kg/24 h.
         b. *Galveston formula* (designed for children):
            i. 5000 cc/m^2 burn + 2000 cc/TBSA m^2/24 h.
      4. The Parkland, Brooke, and Galveston Formulas *all* use Ringer's lactate for the crystalloid, and *all* administer half the total fluid volume over the first 8 h *post-injury* (*not post-hospital arrival*), w/ the second half total fluid volume distributed over the ensuing 16 h.
      5. *Urine:*
         a. *UOP:* maintain ≥ 30 cc/h (30–50 ideal) (0.5 cc/kg/h) for adults or 1.0 cc/kg/h for children.
         b. *Alkalinization:* high-voltage burns, crush injuries w/ myoglobinuria/hemoglobinuria at risk of ATN. Not necessary to treat microscopic myoglobinuria, just grossly obvious cases. Consider use of mannitol a/o sodium bicarbonate for these pts (i.e., 2 amps sodium bicarbonate and 25 mg mannitol IV prn).
      6. *Other adjuncts:* in the intensive care setting, pediatric pts may benefit from reducing the hypermeta-bolic demands on the heart by tx w/ beta blockade (i.e., propanolol).

   C. **Nutrition and electrolytes**
      1. *Energy expenditure:*
         a. *Nonintubated:* 629 − 11 (age) + 25 (wt in kgs) − 609 (if obese)
         b. *Intubated:* 1925 − 10 (age) + 292 (if trauma) + 5 (wt in kgs) + 281 (if male) + 851 (if > 20% TBSA burn)
      2. Begin nutritional support postburn d 1.
      3. Enteral feeds are preferred to parenteral nutrition.

II. **THERMAL BURNS**

   A. **Initial pt considerations**
      1. Avoid hypothermia, remove all jewelry/constricting items; edema *will* follow major burns.
      2. Perform standard trauma assessment as well as ABG, CXR, carboxyhemoglobin. Examine pulses, consider escharotomies (different incisions than fasciotomies) at bedside w/ IV sedation. Chest wall escharotomy on chest wall may be needed if ventilation impaired.

3. *Accurately estimate burn size and depth.*
   a. *Wallace's rule of nines* (for 2nd-, 3rd-degree burns—in honor of A. B. Wallace, a Scottish plastic surgeon):
      i. *Adult*:
         - Head, 9%
         - Upper extremity, 9%
         - Neck, 1%
         - Anterior trunk, 18%
         - Posterior trunk, 18%
         - Lower extremity, 18%
      ii. *Child*:
         - Head/neck, 18%
         - Upper extremity, 9%
         - Anterior trunk, 18%
         - Posterior trunk, 18%
         - Lower extremity, 14%
      iii. *Note*: pt's palm (fingers included) is roughly 1% of BSA.
4. *Tetanus prophylaxis*: if burn > 10% BSA, give 0.5 cc tetanus toxoid. If tetanus immunization hx > 10 yr ago, or if received less than 3 total doses, or uncertain, also administer 250 U of tetanus immunoglobulin. Both Td and TIG are given IM. In short, treat all burn wounds like dirty wounds.

B. Scald injuries
1. Most common form of burn injury in pts < 5 yo.
2. Unlike other burns, which appear white or black (as well as dry and leathery), w/ full-thickness burns, 3rd-degree scald burns generally appear red (as well as dry and leathery).

C. Infection: leading cause of death in adequately resuscitated pts.
1. Mortality used to be from wound sepsis, but now pneumonia is main risk.
2. Generally do not consider a fever significant in a burn pt unless ≥ 39.5, as all pts will be hypermetabolic.
3. *Topical agents*: indicated immediately after debridement

TABLE 8.1.   Topical Burn Care Agents

Agent	Indications / Advantages	Caveats
Silver sulfadiazine (Silvadene)	Painless, nonstaining. Agent of choice except for face, ears, thick eschars, or skin grafts (causes sloughing).	Poor eschar penetration, mild reversible neutropenia
Silvadene + mycostatin (Silvamyco)	Extended coverage against fungi	" "
Mafenide acetate (Sulfamylon)	Good eschar penetration. Agent of choice for ears, thick eschars	Painful, metabolic alkalosis 20 carbonic anhydrase inhibitor. In some pts, allergy can cause a chondritis mimicking infection of auricle
Silver nitrate	Broad spectrum	Poor eschar penetration, electrolyte abnormalities
Sodium hypochlorite (Dakin's solution)	Broad spectrum	High doses impair wound healing
Neomycin	Useful for uncomplicated facial burns	Minimal
Bacitracin	Gram (+) coverage. Agent of choice for face	Minimal

III. INHALATION INJURY

A. Generally do not cause direct thermal injury below level of vocal cords (exception = steam). Therefore, mechanism is from chemical injury. Majority of house burn fatalities are from anoxia, not thermal injury.

B. Injury may mature up to 48 h postexposure and is generally underappreciated initially.

C. Pulse oximetry not accurate. Obtain ABG and carboxyhemoglobin levels. If have high index of suspicion, treat w/ nonrebreather mask oxygen, and sit pt up at 45° to minimize airway edema.

  1. *CO level of 50–60%* usu. fatal.

  2. *CO level > 5%* abnormal except in smokers (> 10%).

  3. *Tx until < 10%* (nonrebreather mask decreases half-life from 240 min to 40 min).

  4. Suspect cyanide toxicity if persistent metabolic acidosis despite what should be adequate resuscitation.

   a. If have pulmonary artery catheter, may also see increased SvO_2 (*ddx:* sepsis, hepatic failure, AV shunt, nitroprusside toxicity).

   b. *Tx:* amyl nitrite, sodium nitrite, followed by sodium thiosulfate.

D. Bronchoscopy indicated to document dx, but can also be therapeutic (suctioning plugs, etc.). Xenon diffusion scan alterative means of dx.

E. Nebulized heparin (decrease cast formation) and acetylcysteine (loosen secretions, decrease oxygen toxicity) shown in one study to be of benefit along w/ bronchodilators and aggressive pulmonary toilet [Desai, *J Burn Care Rehab*, 1998;19(3): 210-212].

IV. ELECTRICAL BURNS

A. **Low voltage** (< 1000 V)

B. **High voltage** (> 1000 V)

  1. *Neurologic:* neurologic complications can develop early or late after trauma including encephalopathy, hemiplegia, aphasia, and brain stem dysfunction up to 9 mo after injury.

  2. *Cardiac:* arrhythmias, particularly ventricular fibrillation can occur.

  3. *Renal:* myoglobinuria can induce acute tubular necrosis. The earliest sign of impending problems is a distinctive "cranberry" color urine; once dark sediment is noted in the urine, more aggressive tx (beyond keeping UOP at 2 cc/kg/h) may be warranted. Mannitol and sodium bicarbonate may be given in a variety of methods. Some give a one-time dose of 25 mg mannitol and 1 bicarb ampule. Others recommend 25 mg IV of mannitol q 6 h and a 5% continuous bicarb infusion titrated to urine pH.

  4. *Extremity:*

   a. Tetanic convulsions can lead to fxs/dislocations. Consider use of c-collar until injury can be ruled out.

   b. Fasciotomies (not just escharotomies) must be considered in any extremities w/ tense compartments, circumferential injury, rhabdomyolysis, or other evidence of muscle compromise. Unlike flame burns, damage to deep tissues is much greater than suggested by skin pathology, esp. around bone, which serves as a heat sink for electrical current.

  5. *Abdomen*

   a. Intraabdominal injury, including bowel perforation, can occur.

  6. *Other*

   a. Cataracts develop in almost $1/3$ of pts after high-voltage injuries as a long-term complication.

C. **Lightning**

  1. May cause *temporary* (unlike high-voltage electrical injury) paralysis (keraunoparalysis) a/o apnea.

  2. Evaluate for blast effect (burst tympanic membranes).

  3. Can cause arborizing, dendritic burn pattern over skin w/ (often) relatively spared internal tissues.

V. CHEMICAL BURNS

A. **General:** remove clothing, copiously irrigate w/ (minimum 15 L) water. Brush powders away before irrigation.

B. **Acids:** irrigate w/ water. Do not attempt to neutralize; tends to form eschars.

1. *Hydrofluoric/oxalic/phosphoric acids*: chelate calcium and magnesium, causing extensive, extremely painful local tissue destruction and potential arrhythmias. Copious irrigation w/ water followed by immediate application of calcium gluconate gel (2.5%); replacing the gel every 15 min until pain is relieved is appropriate.
2. *Hydrochloric acid*: fumes can cause pneumonitis.
3. *Dichromate salts*: consider aggressive debridement (LD 50 is 50 mg/kg).
4. *Sulfosalicyclic/tannic/trichloroacetic acids*: systemic absorption can lead to hepato/renal toxicity.
5. *Formic acid*: can cause considerable electrolyte abnormalities, metabolic acidosis, renal failure, ARDS, and hemolysis. Hemodialysis may be required for large exposures. Wounds are characteristically greenish, deeper than are initially apparent, and are optimally managed by excision.

C. Bases (lime, bleach, sodium/potassium hydroxide): liquefactive necrosis invades more deeply than acid burns.

1. Irrigate w/ water; may take longer than w/ acids.
2. Cement (calcium oxide) leads to similar injury from hydroxyl ion. Irrigate (water/soap) until effluent has pH < 8.

CHAPTER 9

VASCULAR

I. ANATOMY

A. Supradiaphragmatic

1. Aorta gives off brachiocephalic trunk (innominate a.) to the right.
2. Common carotid is first branch off of both aorta and brachiocephalic trunk (innominate a.). Internal carotid has no extracranial branches. The branches of the external carotid are superior thyroid a., ascending pharyngeal a., lingual a., facial a., occipital a., posterior auricular a., maxillary a., and superficial temporal a. Consider mnemonic: **S**ome **A**stute **L**awyers **F**ind **O**ut **P**ost-**M**ortem **S**tudies.
3. After the common carotid, the innominate becomes the subclavian a. The first branches of the subclavian are the vertebral a.'s, which go cephalad while the interior mammary (int. thoracic) a. heads caudally.

B. Infradiaphragmatic

1. Aorta gives off phrenic arteries bilaterally once through hiatus.
2. Celiac axis is first major branch, giving off left gastric a., splenic a., and common hepatic a.
   a. *Left gastric a.* runs along the superior aspect of the lesser curvature of stomach, collateralizing w/ the right gastric a., which runs along the inferior aspect of the lesser curve.
   b. *Splenic a.* gives off dorsal and great pancreatic a.'s en route to spleen, then . . .
   c. *Common hepatic a.* divides into proper hepatic a. and gastroduodenal a. after giving off the right gastric a., which anastamoses w/ the left gastric a. in the lesser curvature of the stomach.
      i. Common hepatic divides into *right* and *left* hepatic a.'s. Typically the cystic a. comes off the right hepatic a.
      ii. *Gastroduodenal a.* gives off ant. and post. superior pancreaticoduodenal a.'s, which anastamose w/ their inferior counterparts stemming from the superior mesenteric a. (SMA) below. The gastroduodenal a. then turns left to become the right gastroepiploic a., running along the greater curve of the stomach, anastamosing w/ the left gastroepiploic, which has its origin w/ the distal splenic a.
3. *SMA is below celiac axis and yields 4 branches*: (1) inferior pancreaticoduodenal a., (2) ileocolic a., (3) right colic a., and (4) middle colic a. Adrenal a.'s take off the aorta near the SMA bilaterally. Renal a.'s are below the adrenal a.'s.
4. Gonadal a.'s branch off between SMA and IMA.
5. *IMA yields 3 branches*: (1) left colic a., (2) sigmoid a., (3) superior rectal a.
6. Aorta then branches into common iliacs.
7. Common iliacs divide into internal and external iliacs at L4, ~2 cm inferior to umbilicus.
   a. *Internal iliac* (hypogastric a.): can ligate unilaterally w/ impunity on 1 side only. Divides into large anterior (6 branches) and small posterior (3 branches) divisions.
   b. *External iliac*: gives off the inferior epigastric a. and deep circumflex a. before exiting the abdomen. Note, ureter crosses external iliac, just distal to takeoff of internal iliacs (runs parallel to internal iliac a.).

C. Infrainguinal

1. Common femoral emerges from femoral canal (had been ext. iliac), giving off profunda femoris about 5 cm below inguinal ligament, then continuing on as superficial femoral.
2. Superficial femoral a. emerges from adductor canal (Hunter's canal) as the popliteal a., which trifurcates into the anterior tibial a., posterior tibial a. (medial), and peroneal a. (lateral).

II. NONMESENTERIC ARTERIAL DISEASE

A. Carotid

1. Dx: duplex is excellent test for carotid screening.
   a. *Symptomatic (amaurosis fugax, CVA, TIA, etc.) tx guided by NASCET*: decreases 5-yr stroke risk from 26% to 9% w/ CEA if ICA is stenosed by 50% or more. In symptomatic pts, higher degrees of stenosis results in higher risk of stroke (unlike asymptomatic pts).

b. *Asymptomatic tx guided by ACAS*: decreases 5-yr stroke risk from 11% to 5% w/ CEA if ICA is stenosed by 60% or more. Unlike symptomatic pts, those w/out sx do not have significantly higher risk of CVA w/ stenosis once beyond at/beyond 60–70%.

c. *Endarterectomy anatomy*:

   i. *ECA branches*: superior thyroid, lingual, facial, maxillary, superficial temporal, posterior auricular, occipital, and ascending pharyngeal.

   ii. *Nerves*:

   - *Vagus*: 90% posterior to carotid, 10% anterior, most commonly injured nerve (usu. causes hoarseness as gives off superior and recurrent laryngeal nerves).

   - *Hypoglossal*: loops in superior field, damage leads to ipsilateral tongue deviation.

   - *Ansa ("loop") cervicalis*: loops in midfield, can transect w/ impunity as only innervates strap muscles (sternothyroid, sternohyoid, omothyroid, omohyoid) w/ no significant function.

   - *Glossopharyngeal*: found high in superior field, damage results in dysphagia, gives off "Hering's nerve" to innervate carotid sinus.

   - *Facial*: marginal mandibular branch has motor function; damage results in inability to depress ipsilateral lip, may result in accidental lip biting.

d. *Endarterectomy complications*:

   i. *Nerve damage*: see entry 1cii. above.

   ii. *Hyper-/hypotension*: results from denervation (i.e., neurapraxia) or increased stimulation (overlying plaque now gone) of carotid sinus. Treat HTN w/ nitroprusside, hypotension w/ dopamine. Generally self-limited 48–72 h.

   iii. *Hemorrhage*: stroke.

   iv. *CNS hypoperfusion*: stroke.

   v. *Restenosis*:

   - Up to 25–40% affected, only 10% significant flow velocity increase, 1–3% symptomatic over 5 yr.

   - < 2 yr: secondary to intimal hyperplasia, comparatively benign natural hx.

   - > 2 yr: atherosclerotic plaque more common.

   - Operate if symptomatic and > 80% stenosis.

   vi. *Cerebral hyperperfusion syndrome*: can occur up to 2 wk postop. Related to temporary loss of autoregulatory ability of intracranial circulation due to chronic vasodilation in vessels past the stenosis.

   - Risk factors include a contralateral tight stenosis/occlusion, advanced age (> 70), ipsilateral tight stenosis.

   - Manifested by headache, seizure, hemorrhagic stroke.

   - Tx is aggressive blood pressure control titrated to relief of sx.

B. Lower extremity

1. *Acute arterial occlusion*

   a. *6 Ps*: **P**ulselessness, **P**ain, **P**oikilothermia, **P**aralysis, **P**aresthesias, **P**allor.

   b. If see foot drop, nonblanching skin, no capillary refill, no sensation, and no motor, do not revascularize (K^+, rhabdomyolysis can be fatal w/ reperfusion).

   c. Anticoagulate (heparin inhibits propagation of thrombus via potentiation of antithrombin III, inactivating thrombin as well as activated factors IX–XII and plasmin, preventing conversion of fibrinogen to fibrin; it also promotes NO release), then thrombolysis or surgery:

   i. Thrombolytics take several h to work, but may be appropriate if comorbidities, multiple levels of obstruction.

   ii. If do surgery, fix most proximal lesion first. Backbleeding is a poor predictor of success. Get intraop arteriography at completion. Have low threshold for fasciotomy. Watch carefully during reperfusion period for rhabdomyolysis, hyperkalemia, and renal failure.

2. *Chronic arterial occlusion*

   a. *Medical tx, 1st line*: pentoxifylline (Trental), cilostazol (Pletal), clopidogrel (Plavix)—block platelet ADP receptor, preventing fibrinogen binding and decreasing platelet aggregation; aspirin blocks prostacycline synthetase, preventing formation of thromboxane A_2, a potent platelet aggregator.

   b. *Intermittent claudication*: except for smokers and diabetics, most pts improve or remain the same. Risk of limb loss at 5 yr = 5%, 10 yr = 11%. Initial tx is exercise, smoking cessation, and rheologic agents. 10-yr limb loss risk drops to 2% w/ smoking cessation. Pentoxifylline helps claudication distance, but not rest pain. Nocturnal calf cramps common in general population, not assoc. w/ vascular dz.

   c. *Limb threatening*: ulceration, gangrene, ischemic rest pain, metatarsalgia, dependent rubor (specificity increases if latter 3 increase w/ elevation of extremity). Rest pain means pain increases w/ elevation a/o decreases w/ dependency, generally over metatarsal heads; toe pain may mean gout or infection. Arterial ulcers form at distal areas of toes, foot. Venous insufficiency ulcers, in contrast, form at medial malleoli. Neurotrophic ulcers often between toes and over metatarsal heads (pressure points).

   d. 90% have CAD, w/ significant 5- to 10-yr mortality (> 50%). 30% have > 50% internal carotid compromise.

   e. *Dx*: Doppler, ankle-brachial indexes (ABIs) → 1–1.2 normal; 0.4–0.9 claudication; 0.0–0.4 rest pain/limb threat. Correlation poor in diabetics (get false negatives from Ca^{++} causing non-compressible vessels). Lower extremity formal ABIs w/ waveform analysis may be esp. useful w/ diabetics or ABI > 1.2. ABI is ratio of highest systolic pressure in either arm to systolic pressure in pedal vessels. Artificially elevated in diabetics frequently secondary to mural calcinosis in (particularly tibial, pedal) arteries. Toe pressures: 30 mm Hg nondiabetics, 50–55 mg Hg in diabetics should be down to level of transmetatarsal.

      i. In these pts esp., toe pressures are much more reflective of perfusion. 30–45 mm Hg good threshold for revascularization.

      ii. Pulse volume recordings can estimate burden of stenotic dz at various levels in LE.

   f. *Manifestations*: claudication, arterial ulceration/painful/distal/pale, rest pain, dependent rubor, ulceration, gangrene. Differentiate from blue toe syndrome, esp. in asymptomatic pts, nonclaudicators. Typically see tissue loss only w/ multilevel dz; single-level dz more often just causes claudication.

      i. *Outflow dz*: treat w/ either open bypass or endovascular recannulization.
         - Femoropopliteal dz
         - Tibial dz

C. Aneurysms (aneurysm = increase in diameter > 50% normal)

   1. *Aortic*

      a. *Epidemiology*: 3% men, 2.1% women; 13th leading cause of death in United States, most common peripheral arterial aneurysm. Assoc. w/ iliac (41%), femoral and/or popliteal aneurysms (15%), carotid stenosis/ectasia (if see carotid ectasia, do AAA U/S), and arterial ectasia. Normal diameter is 2.0 cm: 5.5 cm is indication for surgery (5.0 in females), as is increase in diameter > 0.5 cm/yr, or symptomatic aneurysms. 50% have CAD; 50% deaths due to CAD (5–15% postop MI).

      b. *Presentation*: infrarenal (90%) >> juxtarenal > suprarenal. Usu. asymptomatic, but may manifest as abdominal, back, or groin pain, or thromboembolic sx. 20–25% present ruptured. If see midabdominal pain and shock, think ruptured AAA! Rupture risk (annual) assoc. w/ LaPlace's law (T = PR); < 5 cm 1%, 5 cm 3–15%, 6–7 cm 10–20%, 7–8 cm 20–40%, > 8 cm 30–50%. Over 5 yr: < 5 cm 20%, 5–7 cm 33%, > 7 cm 95%.

      c. *Dx*: U/S good, CT is better; if unstable, straight to OR.

      d. *Tx*:

         i. *Open repair*: approach either transabdominal or retroperitoneal.
            - *Abdominal approach*: better visualization of right iliac, poor for suprarenal aneurysm, poor visualization of left colon, less chance of retractor damage (spleen), possibly has worse pulmonary complications.

- *Retroperitoneal*: avoid opening abdomen, better for suprarenal and thoracic aortal, cannot visualize colon, difficult access to right iliac.
  - *Complications*:
    - *Ischemic colitis*: if see postop diarrhea (esp. bloody), get sigmoidoscopy; go to OR if necrosis is present. 2–4% of all AAA repair pts.
    - *Spinal ischemia*: 0.1% w/ infrarenal, 5–10% w/ suprarenal.
    - *Aortoenteric fistula*: usu. aortoduodenal and presents w/ upper GI bleed. Need to remove aortic graft and do extraanatomic bypass.

ii. *Endograft*:
- Studies show a perioperative mortality benefit EVAR vs open repair, but 2-yr survival is the same.
- Endograft leak (50% may have some type of leak, 25% w/in 1st yr; vast majority not clinically important).
  - *Type I*: leak at proximal/distal aspect of device (type Ia and Ib, respectively). Often can be repaired w/ endovascular tx; must be repaired at the time of surgery if seen intraop.
  - *Type II* (most common): leakage outside graft but inside native vessel from back-bleeding lumbar arteries, IMA, etc. Can embolize. Requires at least 2 patent vessels (inflow and outflow). Usu. one lumbar and patent IMA.
  - *Type III*: mechanical problem w/ graft (i.e., modular disassociation).
  - *Type IV*: leak from fabric porosity, usu. seals spontaneously.
- Aneurysm enlargement must be looked for on CT compared w/ baseline at time of graft placement (growth in size more important than presence of endoleak). Expect small decrease in size in first 6–12 mo, but no change is not uncommon. Growth in diameter > 0.25 cm in 6 mo warrants concern.

e. *Special circumstances*:
  i. *"Mycotic" aneurysm*: Staph most common pathogen; Salmonella seen less commonly. Pts have abdominal pain, pulsatile mass, and *fever*. CT often reveals eccentric aneurysm that is thickened, w/ surrounding fluid. Tx w/ abx, debridement, and in situ grafting. "Mycotic" does not refer to infectious cause, but rather dates back to early (preantibiotic) days of "malignant endocarditis," which seeded systemic arterial tree w/ infectious emboli causing multiple aneurysms along path, resembling hyphae.
  ii. *Inflammatory AAA*: 5% of cases; ↑ ESR; abdominal pain w/ ureteral obstruction/medial deviation. Get CT scan; use retroperitoneal approach to avoid duodenum. (Also use retroperitoneal approach for pts w/ horseshoe kidneys.)

2. *Visceral*
   a. *Hepatic artery*: 20% of splanchnic aneurysms.
      i. Rupture rate probably ~ 20%. Resection and repair warranted unless prohibitive operative risk.
   b. *Splenic artery*: most common (60%).
      i. Highest risk of rupture in gravid females (75% fetal loss, 50% maternal mortality).
      ii. Ligation or embolization if > 2 cm, symptomatic, or in reproductive-age female.
      iii. Splenectomy usu. not necessary, as short gastrics provide good collateral flow to spleen.

3. *Peripheral*
   a. *True*
      i. *Popliteal*:
         - ½ bilateral.
         - ⅓ assoc. w/ AAA (get abdominal U/S to evaluate aorta, iliac arteries).
         - Risk is thrombosis/embolism, not rupture (40–50% limb loss over 5 yr if no tx).
         - Exclude and bypass if > 2 cm.

    ii. *Femoral*: most common true peripheral aneurysms, but low rupture and thromboembolic risk.

  b. *Pseudoaneursyms*

    i. Femoral most common. Iatrogenic. May be treated w/ local compression for ~ 1 h, but local injection of thrombin greatly accelerates closure (true for most peripheral pseudoaneurysms).

III. VENOUS DISEASE

A. Deep venous thromboembolism (DVT)

  1. *Impact and risk factors*:

    a. *United States incidence* [1]/1000 person/yr w/ mortality approaching 10% per case.

    b. *Virchow's triad*: venous stasis, endothelial injury, hypercoagulable state.

    c. *Risk factors*: trauma (esp. pelvic, spine), recent surgery, age > 65 yo, malignancy, exogenous estrogens, obesity, venous varicosities, family hx of thrombophilia.

    d. *Thrombophilia*

      i. Factor V Leiden (most common thrombophilia in Caucasians)

      ii. Prothrombin 20210 (Factor II mutation)

      iii. Protein C deficiency

      iv. Protein S deficiency

      v. Antithrombin IIII deficiency

      vi. Hyperhomocysteinemia

      vii. Antiphospholipid syndrome

      viii. Lupus anticoagulant

  2. *Presentation and pathology*

    a. < 50% of pts have signs or sx initially.

    b. Most commonly begin in calf. (+) Homan's sign (pain w/ passive dorsiflexion of ankle) suggestive, although (–) test does not r/o DVT.

    c. Early findings may include pain a/o LE circumferential asymmetry. W/ large pelvic DVTs, may progress to *phlegmasia alba dolens*, or even *phlegmasia cerulea dolens*.

    d. *Sequelae*:

      i. ⅓ of calf DVTs embolize or propagate proximally.

      ii. Pulmonary emboli.

      iii. Chronic venous insufficiency.

  3. *Dx*:

    a. Duplex study demonstrating noncompressible vein w/ no flow increase w/ distal compression is most commonly used modality. Pelvic or retroperitoneal DVT may be better assessed w/ magnetic resonance venography.

    b. Normal D-dimer level (marker for fibrin degradation by plasmin) essentially excludes dx; elevated level nonspecific in surgery pts (effects of trauma a/o surgery elevate level).

  4. *Tx*:

    a. *Heparin*

      i. *Unfractionated*:

        • Begin w/ 80 U/kg bolus, then start 18 U/kg/h infusion for goal PTT of 60–80 sec as initiate warfarin (see section 4b. below); titrate as needed.

      ii. *Fractionated (low-molecular-wt) heparin*:

        • Given predictable response, no need to follow lab values.

        • Can use as bridge for warfarin or as stand-alone therapy (*agent of choice during pregnancy*, as warfarin teratogenic).

      iii. *Argatroban or hirudin if heparin-induced thrombocytopenia* (see Chapter 2 for choice of agent and dosing).

b. *Warfarin*:

    i. Goal INR of 2.0–3.0 for 3 mo usu. indicated. Lifetime anticoagulation (or IVC filter, see section 4c. below) likely indicated if recurrent DVTs or known thrombophilia.

c. *IVC filter*: indicated if anticoagulation not appropriate (i.e., CNS hemorrhage) or if develop pulmonary embolism or propagation of iliofemoral thrombus while appropriately anticoagulated. < 5% PE rate. 5% long-term occlusion rate—tx w/ fluid resuscitation.

d. *Other*: for significant pain or impending gangrene from *phlegmasia*, consideration may be given to thrombolysis or surgical thrombectomy followed by long-term anticoagulatoin.

5. *Prophylaxis*:

    a. Ambulation.

    b. Sequential compression devices.

    c. Unfractionated heparin 5000 U SQ three times per day.

    d. *Fractionated low-molecular-wt heparin*:

        i. Directly inhibits factors Xa, IIa.

        ii. More predictable response than unfractionated heparin, but additional cost limits its use to moderate- and high-risk pts.

B. Venous insufficiency (lower extremity):

1. Twice as common in females. Secondary to valvular incompetence.

2. *Anatomy*:

    a. *Saphenofemoral*: reflux present in ~ 70% of pts w/ LE venous insufficiency.

    b. *Saphenopopliteal*: reflux present in ~ 15% of pts w/ LE venous insufficiency.

3. *Dx*:

    a. On physical exam, pt often has swelling over legs/feet, relatively sparing toes (different than lymphedema).

    b. Physical exam adjuncts (now largely supplanted by radiography/ultrasonography).

        i. *Trendelenburg test*: elevate leg to drain veins, then apply pressure (hand or tourniquet) to saphenofemoral junction. Have pt stand and observe filling pattern.

          • Gradual calf filling occurs in normal anatomy w/ competent perforators.

          • Rapid (< 30 sec) calf filling occurs w/ incompetent perforators.

          • After observing calf, release pressure in thigh.

             • Rapid filling of thigh varices signifies saphenofemoral incompetence.

        ii. *Perthes test*: place tourniquet around upper leg, then have pt ambulate.

          • If varicosities disappear, signifies patent deep system w/ competent perforators.

          • If pt has pain w/ ambulation, signifies deep obstruction (pt relies on superficial veins for drainage).

    c. *Duplex U/S*: required for class 2–6 dz.

    d. *Plethysmography*: required (in addition to duplex U/S) for class 4–6 dz.

    e. *Venography*: required if evidence of deep system reflux/incompetence or obstruction.

4. *Tx*:

    a. *Class 1* (telangiectasias, "spider veins:" compression hose, injection sclerotherapy)

    b. *Class 2–6*:

        i. *Superficial incompetence only*:

          • Saphenous vein stripping (or ablation w/ RF or laser).

        ii. *Superficial* and *perforator incompetence*:

          • Saphenous vein stripping *and* subfascial endoscopic perforator surgery (SEPS).

        iii. *Deep reflux a/o obstruction*:

          • Valve reconstruction, transposition, or transplant; *or* PTA + stent; *or* bypass.

5. *Klippel-Trenaunay-Weber syndrome*: classic findings of limb hypertrophy, birthmark (port wine stain, or venous malformation), and varicose veins. In these pts, deep veins are frequently absent

or otherwise anomalous; *saphenous vein stripping should be avoided*. Instead, more conservative measures such as support hose and stab avulsion are preferred.

IV. MESENTERIC ISCHEMIA

A. Arterial

1. *Chronic* (CMI, intestinal angina):

   a. *Etiology*: most from atherosclerosis of mesenteric arteries, although vasculitides or compressive syndromes possible (i.e., median arcuate ligament syndrome from compression of celiac axis by part of diaphragm, esp. during full expiration).

   b. *Presentation*: generally elderly, *female* (3:1 over males) postprandial pain (w/in 10–30 min), develops into food avoidance. Wt loss, other GI complaints (diarrhea/constipation, flatulence, etc.) common. *As w/ acute dz, pain is classically out of proportion to physical findings.*

   c. *Dx*: duplex imaging may be useful for screening. Portal vein blood flow does *not* significantly ↑ w/ eating (abn). Arteriography gold standard, must show stenosis or occlusion of at least 2 of the major mesenteric vessels; 50% of cases involve all 3.

   d. *Tx*: if peritonitis → celiotomy. Attempt at revascularization should be made before resecting bowel if feasible. Prosthetic graft bypass to 1 or 2 vessels (SMA +/– celiac) standard unless contaminated abdomen (would require autogenous—i.e., reversed saphenous bypass vs femoral vein). Celiac a/o SMA endarterectomy also option for short stenoses; antegrade (supraceliac) is generally preferred over retrograde b/c of less atherosclerotic burden cephalad to celiac vessels and less risk of kinking (esp. w/ vein). Conversely, infrarenal aorta is easier to expose, and less potential for hemodynamic instability a/o distal embolization w/ clamping/unclamping. Endovascular stenting increasingly popular, esp. in elderly pts who are poor operative candidates, but patency is poor (50% primary patency at 1 yr; often serves as a bridge to definitive bypass). Divide median arcuate ligament along w/ bypass if this is offending structure (*note*: this is dx of exclusion). Predictors of success include female gender, postprandial pain, wt loss > 20 lb, no psych/drug abuse hx, arteriography w/ celiac axis compression w/ poststenotic dilatation a/o collateral flow.

2. *Acute mesenteric ischemia* (AMI)

   a. *Embolic*: ~ 50% of cases of AMI, majority from cardiac source (w/u CHF, MI, Afib, valve dz). Embolization of atheromatous plaques and iatrogenic insults generally result in smaller emboli that travel more distally, w/ more focal involvement (usu. middle/distal jejunum and ileum) than a proximal SMA lesion.

      i. *Presentation/dx*: abrupt onset acute abdominal pain, out of proportion to physical findings early on, +/– N/V/D. Progresses to frank peritonitis over time, often w/ sx of hypovolemia. Leukocytosis, hyperamylasemia, and later, increased lactate levels may be found. In the absence of perforation or bowel wall pneumatosis, plain films not helpful. U/S is operator- and properly prepared pt-dependent. (i.e. pt should be NPO for at least 8 h prior to U/S to decrease bowel gas). Study of choice is abdominal CT angiogram (nonfilling of mesenteric vessel, bowel edema, and mesenteric stranding).

      ii. *Tx*:

         • Resuscitate, get EKG (check for Afib and MI), get invasive monitoring. Begin systemic anticoagulation and IV abx.

         • If peritonitis or unstable → resuscitate and celiotomy (bypass radiographic w/u—can do on-table angiography if necessary). Prep abdomen and both LE to knees. Make midline incision; assess viability of bowel. If amount of infarcted bowel is incompatible w/ life, close abdomen. Unless bowel is clearly necrotic, revascularize before resect. *Options*:

            ○ *SMA embolectomy*: open the vessel transversely if normal; longitudinally if atherosclerotic and a patch angioplasty is anticipated. Default should be longitudinal arteriotomy if uncertain.

            ○ *SMA bypass*: antegrade vs retrograde aorto-SMA vs retrograde ilio-SMA bypass. Prosthetic OK if no frank bowel necrosis or perforation.

   b. *Thrombotic*: accounts for ~ 25% of AMI. Usu. manifests during low-flow state from preocclusive lesion (see section 1. on CMI above). Presentation and dx are same as for embolic dz (see section 2a. above). Lesion more proximal than w/ embolic dz, usu. near SMA origin. Ischemic area usu. extends from ligament to Treitz to mid-transverse colon.

c. *Nonocclusive*:

   i. *Etiology*: low perfusion despite patent vessels—CHF, hypotension/hypovolemia, digoxin, etc.

   ii. *Dx*: index of suspicion + "pruning" of mesenteric branch vessels typically seen on angiogram.

   iii. *Tx*: reverse etiology (increase perfusion w/ fluids, inotropes, etc., fluoroscopically guided papaverine or tolazoline may assist). Celiotomy if peritonitis. Bowel resection if nonviable.

B. Venous thrombosis: dx w/ abd CT—edematous bowel, venous thrombus. Assoc. w/ prothrombotic diatheses, intraabdominal inflammation (i.e., pancreatitis), postop state, and portal hypertension. Mild sx may be addressed w/ full heparinization alone. If have peritonitis, need celiotomy. Infarcted bowel (look at color, Doppler, Wood's lamp, etc.) should be resected, then reanticoagulate, planning for second-look celiotomy in 24 h. Should w/u predisposing conditions.

C. Vasculitides and vasospastic disorders

1. *Takayasu's*: chronic inflammatory dz primarily of aorta and large arteries, although subclavian, carotid, and renal arteries may also be affected. More common in females, and sometimes referred to as "pulseless dz" due to difficulty in palpating peripheral pulses in some pts. *Tx*: corticosteroids; cyclophosphamide may be used in refractory cases. Surgery rarely indicated for burned-out dz. Stenting and angioplasty → poor results.

2. *Buerger's dz* (thromboangiitis obliterans): poor response to medical and surgical tx. Only effective tx is cessation of smoking. *Dx*: young smokers (usu. male) w/ abnormal pressures and no risk factors for obstructive vasculopathies (hypercoagulable diathesis, etc.), essentially diagnostic w/out arteriogram. May present w/ nonhealing ulcers in fingers/toes. Arteriograms classically show normal vessels down to mid-leg/forearm w/ abrupt occlusions and "corkscrew" appearance of collateral vessels.

3. *Temporal arteritis* (giant cell arteritis): inflammatory disorder primarily of medium and large carotid artery branches. Classically, fever, HA, anemia, and high ESR + tender temporal artery +/− scalp pain and jaw/tongue claudication; severe cases may lead to blindness. Path dx via bx of temporal artery. Tx w/ prednisone usu. successful.

4. *Kawasaki's dz*: inflammatory dz of children; fever, cutaneous/mucosal, and vasculitis of small and medium blood vessels. Incidence is 10× higher in Asians. At risk for coronary aneurysms (~ 20–25%), which generally regress and are reduced in incidence w/ prompt medical tx. Peripheral ischemia reported. Tx 1st w/ ASA and IV IgG; steroids usu. avoided. PTCA, surgery rarely indicated.

5. *Raynaud's dz*: vasospastic disorder triggered by cold exposure or emotional stress. Classically, white (pallor) → blue (cyanosis) → red (rubor) skin. Sometimes assoc. w/ connective tissue dz, occupational stress (i.e., vibration), diabetes mellitus. Tx includes avoidance of cold, tobacco/nicotine, beta antagonists, ergotamines, and oral contraceptives. Calcium channel blockers, Botox injections may be helpful.

6. *Polyarteritis nodosa* (PAN): inflammatory d/o of medium-sized arteries, w/ systemic sx such as fever. Etiology unknown, assoc. w/ hepatitis B. Cyclophosphamide reserved for the remainder, or those w/ evidence of end-organ dz (renal, CNS, cardiac, etc.).

7. *Vascular surgery dilemmas*:

   a. AAA and concomitant intraabdominal malignancy (up to 4% of all AAA). Symptomatic or ruptured AAA trumps concerns w/ malignancy (treat the most life-threatening condition first).

      i. *Colon cancer*
         - If AAA asymptomatic and < 5 cm, resect cancer first, esp. if obstructing, bleeding, or perforated.
         - If AAA asymptomatic but > 5 cm and cancer asymptomatic, repair AAA first.
         - If AAA symptomatic or ruptured, repair first, then resect cancer at subsequent operation.
            - If cancer is obstructing, consider exteriorizing loop of colon after reperitonealizing AAA repair, keep pt on NGT suction, then mature ostomy the following day. Resect cancer at subsequent date.

      ii. *Ovarian mass*
         - See Chapter 20. Again, the principle is tx the process that is most immediately life threatening.

b. *Concomitant cholelithiasis and AAA.*

   i. Repair AAA first. Endovascular or open retroperitoneal approach facilitates subsequent laparoscopic cholecystectomy (compared w/ transperitoneal approach).

c. *Aortoenteric fistula:*

   i. Most commonly occurs from erosion between proximal suture line of AAA graft w/ duodenum/proximal jejunum, although primary cases (unoperated AAAs) have been reported as have other parts of intestine.

   ii. Often presents w/ small "herald" bleed h to wks before massive hemorrhage.

   iii. If suspect dx (and pt not hemodynamically unstable), procure upper endoscopy for confirmation.

      • If endoscopy negative, proceed to CT w/ oral and IV contrast to identify area(s) of possible inflammation. If CT negative, proceed to angiography (w/ lateral views).

   iv. *If dx secured or if pt unstable, proceed to operating room:*

      • Obtain proximal control of supraceliac aorta.

      • Mobilize affected bowel (i.e., Kocher maneuver) as necessary, then separate graft from bowel.

         ○ Maintain direct pressure over aortic defect.

      • Inject heparin in distal aortic segment to prevent stasis thrombosis.

      • Close bowel defect transversely if able.

      • If AAA has not previously been operated upon (rare) and bowel lesion is duodenal, many authors recommend standard graft repair followed by wrapping graft in omentum in absence of extensive local sepsis.

      • More commonly, fistula from aortic graft is encountered, which mandates removal of graft, oversewing aortic stump, and buttressing w/ local soft tissue (i.e., anterior spinal ligament, omentum, etc.).

         ○ Distal flow is achieved via extraanatomic bypass (i.e., axillobifemoral bypass). Aorta can also be reconstructed using femoral vein (NAIS) or cryopreserved aorta/vein, which avoids the issue of preventing aortic stump dehiscence and blowout.

      • *Note:* in hemodynamically stable pts w/ firm dx, one can perform extraanatomic bypass first, and then repair fistula or remove graft 1 to several days later.

CHAPTER 10

ONCOLOGY*

I. GENERAL ONCOLOGY FACTS AND PRINCIPLES

A. **Cancer mortality in United States:** lung >> colorectal >> breast > prostate > pancreas > leukemia

B. **Genetics** (gene → CA)

1. *p53*
   a. Regulates apoptosis by arresting cell cycle before G_1/S transition (facilitates repair vs apoptosis).
      i. Apoptosis mediated through class of proteases called caspases (10+ different types).
   b. Deletion or mutation results in damaged DNA replication.
   c. Likely most common genetic etiology for human neoplasms.
   d. *Li-Fraumeni syndrome:* sarcomas, breast CA, brain tumors, leukemia, adrenal CA, poss. uterine CA.

2. *Birc-5* (Survivin): anti-apoptosis gene (bad for pts w/ cancer, good for pts w/ MI)

3. *C-myc*
   a. Small cell lung CA, neuroblastoma, Burkitt's lymphoma.

4. *K-ras*
   a. Proto-oncogene.
   b. Implicated in 90% pancreatic CA, 50% colon CA, some lung CA.

5. *Ret*
   a. Proto-oncogene.
   b. Assoc. w/ medullary thyroid CA (MEN II syndrome), Hirschsprung's dz.

6. *BRCA I, II*
   a. I = breast CA (50–80%), ovarian CA (40–65%).
   b. II = breast CA (35–80%), ovarian CA (10–20%), male breast CA.

7. *Adenomatous polyposis cancer* (APC)
   a. Tumor suppressor gene on chromosome 5q. Mutation assoc. w/ 80% of colorectal tumors.
   b. *Familial adenomatous polyposis (FAP) syndrome*: 100% get colon cancer if not taken out, almost universally AD.
      i. *Gardner's* (AD): GI polyposis, osteomas, epidermoid cysts, desmoid tumors.
      ii. *Turcot's* (AR): GI polyposis, CNS tumors (medulloblastoma, glioblastoma). Young presentation.

8. *Mismatch repair gene*
   a. *Hereditary nonpolyposis colon cancer* (HNPCC).
      i. *Lynch I, II*: defect in mismatch-repair gene, assoc. w/ microsatellite instability, right-sided colon cancer, and generally more favorable prognosis.
         • *Lynch I*: no assoc. extracolonic malignancies.
         • *Lynch II*: assoc. w/ malignancy in endometrium, ovaries, cholangiocarcinoma, stomach.

9. *Deleted in colorecal cancer (DCC) gene*
   a. Postulated to be tumor suppression gene on chromosome 18q.
   b. Possibly induces apoptosis in normal cells.

10. *COX-2 gene*
    a. Overexpressed in many colorectal tumors.
    b. Use of Cox-2 inhibitors may facilitate appropriate apoptosis and angiogenesis inhibition; reduce polyp burden in FAP pts (see section 7a. above).

11. *Hamartomatous* (no malignant potential) often confused w/ above, although no genetic locus identified

---

*Gynecologic, orthopaedic, genitourinary, neurologic, and head/neck neoplasms discussed in their respective chapters.

    a. *Peutz-Jeghers*: autosomal dominant, assoc. w/ STK11 gene mutation; mucosal hyperpig., mucocut. melanin spots. May develop extracolonic malignancies (GI, panc, breast/ov.).

    b. *Cronkhite-Canada*: GI polyps, nail dystrophy, alopecia, cutaneous hyperpigmentation. Nonfamilial, but up to ⅔ of pts have Japanese ancestry.

    c. *Cowden's*: autosomal dominant, assoc. w/ PTEN gene mutation. GI-tract hamartomas, breast CA, colon CA, uterine CA, lung CA, bladder CA, thyroid CA, circumoral papillomatosis, nodular gingival hyperplasia.

C. Genetics (CA → gene)

    1. *Colon CA*: APC (esp. in FAP), COX-2, K-ras. p53, 18q (all are tumor suppressors except K-ras oncogene).

    2. *Breast CA*: p53, bcl-2, c-myc, her 2 neu, BRCA1/2.

    3. *Pancreas*: K-ras, INK4A, p53, SMAD4/DPC4, BRCA2.

D. Environmental factors

    1. *Diet*: fatty diets lead to increased bile salts in gut, which is assoc. w/ colorectal CA.

E. Common sites of metastasis

    1. *Receiving metastases*:

        a. *Brain*: males—lung, colon, renal most common; females—breast, lung, colon, melanoma most common

        b. *Lung*: breast, sarcoma

        c. *Liver*: GI (esp. colorectal), pancreas

            i. Liver has been shown to increase ICAM-1, VCAM-1, and selectin expression while decreasing iNOS expression during times of (even distant) inflammation, making the hepatic parenchyma more suitable for metastasis implantation and survival.

        d. *Bone*: breast (mixed osteoblastic/clastic), prostate (osteoclastic), follicular thyroid CA

        e. *Ovaries*: stomach, colon

        f. *LN*: breast, papillary thyroid CA, liver, SCCA, melanoma

        g. *Adrenal*: lung, stomach, breast, melanoma, renal, prostate

        h. *Thyroid*: breast, kidney, colon, lung

    2. *Sending metastases*:

        a. *Breast*: lung, bone, liver, brain, thyroid

        b. *Renal*: thryoid

        c. *Colon*: liver, lung, ovaries

        d. *Stomach*: liver

        e. *Melanoma*: liver, lung, GI tract, brain, skin

        f. *Prostate*: bone

        g. *Lung*: liver, adrenal, bone, brain

        h. *Pancreas*: liver

        i. *Sarcoma*: lung (for extremity sarcomas—retroperitoneal sarcomas usu. go to liver); sarcoma usu. does *not* spread via lymphatics

F. Tumor markers (**bold** represents primary usage)

    1. *Carcinoembryonic antigen* (CEA): may be elevated w/ **colorectal** CA, melanoma, lymphoma, breast CA, lung CA, pancreatic CA, gastric CA, cervical CA, bladder CA, renal CA, thyroid CA, hepatic CA, ovarian CA, IBD, pancreatic dz, hepatopathy, and tobacco smoking.

    2. *Alpha-fetoprotein* (AFP): may be elevated w/ **liver** CA or **germ cell** CA. Rarely elevated w/ cirrhosis, hepatitis, ataxia telangiectasia, Wiskott-Aldrich syndrome, and pregnancy.

    3. *CA 125*: may be elevated w/ **ovarian** CA, uterine CA, cervical CA, pancreatic CA, liver CA, colon CA, breast CA, lung CA, GI tract CA, endometriosis, PID, pancreatitis, hepatopathy, pleuritis, menstruation, and pregnancy.

    4. *CA 19-9*: cholangiocarcinoma, pancreatic adenocarcinoma.

    5. *Lactate dehydrogenase* (LDH): extremely nonspecific, but used to follow testicular CA, Ewing's sarcoma, melanoma, NHL. Also elevated w/ CHF, hypothyroidism, anemia, and various lung and liver dz's.

    6. *Prostate-specific antigen* (PSA): elevated w/ **prostate** CA, prostatitis, and BPH.

7. *Prostatic acid phosphatase*: elevated w/ **prostate** CA, testicular CA, leukemia, NHL, cirrhosis, PE, hyperparathyroidism, Gaucher's dz, and Paget's dz.

8. *Human chorionic gonadotropin* (hCG): elevated during pregnancy and may be also be elevated w/ **choriocarcinoma** and cancers of **testis**, ovary, liver, stomach, pancreas, and lung. Marijuana may also elevate levels.

    a. *Neuron-specific enolase* (NSE): may be elevated w/ **neuroblastoma**, **small cell lung** CA, nephroblastoma (Wilm's tumor), melanoma, and cancers of thyroid, kidney, testis, and pancreas.

G. **Paraneoplastic syndromes**

1. *By source*

    a. Lung (*small cell*): ACTH, ADH

    b. Lung (*non-small cell*): PTH-like hormone

2. *By-product/result*

    a. *ACTH*: bronchial carcinoids, small-cell lung carcinoids >> gut/thymic carcinoids, endocrine pancreatic neoplasms, pancreatic cystadenomas, thyroid medullary carcinoma, pheochromocytoma

    b. *CRH*: thyroid medullary CA, prostate CA

    c. *Hypercalcemia*: breast, lung, kidney, multiple myeloma, parathyroid CA, renal cell, SCCA

    d. *SIADH*: small cell CA of lung >> prostate, adrenal, esophagus, pancreas, colon, head/neck, carcinoids, mesotheliomas

    e. *Hypoglycemia*: insulinoma, hepatoma, adrenocortical, mesothelioma, fibrosarcoma, neurofibrosarcoma

    f. *Tumor lysis syndrome* (hyperuricemia, hyperkalemia, hyperphosphatemia, hypocalcemia): lymphoma, leukemia, rarely small cell lung CA, metastatic breast CA, metastatic medulloblastoma

H. **Multiple Endocrine Neoplasm** (MEN); see Table 10.1.

TABLE 10.1   Multiple Endocrine Neoplasia (MEN) Syndromes

	MEN I	MEN IIa	MEN IIb
Acronym	Wermer's Syndrome	Sipple's Syndrome	Sizemore's Syndrome
Associated Tumors	**Parathyroid** (90%) (four-gland hyperplasia) — — — **Pancreas** (80%) (gastrin > insulinoma) **Pituitary Adenoma** (55%) (prolactin >> GH > ACTH)	**Parathyroid** (20–60%) (four-gland hyperplasia) *Medullary Thyroid CA* (100%) *Pheochromocytoma* (20–40%) — — —	— — *Medullary Thyroid CA* (100%) *Pheochromocytoma* (20–40%) Neuromas (lips, tongue, oral mucosa, GI tract) —

II. SPECIFIC CANCERS ORGANIZED BY ORGAN (ALPHABETICALLY)*

A. **Anal**

1. *Risk factors*: immunosuppression, anal receptive intercourse, and (for squamous cell cancers) HPV (subtypes 6, 11, 16, 18) infection.

2. *Subtype by location*:

    a. *Anal canal cancers* (proximal to anal verge): ⅔ of all anal cancers, more common in women. Locally aggressive, w/ ½ locally advanced at dx, ⅓ to ½ w/ mesenteric LN spread.

    b. *Anal margin cancers* (distal to anal verge, including 5-cm radius of perianal skin): more common in homosexual males. Relatively favorable prognosis; rarely metastasize (usu. to superficial inguinal LN—15% of cases overall).

*Staging information from *AJCC Cancer Staging Handbook*, 7th edition, SB Edge, et al., 2010, Springer.

3. *Subtype by histology*:
   a. *SCCA*: 80% of anal cancer. Includes basaloid, mucoepidermoid, and cloacogenic.
   b. *Adenocarcinoma*: exceptionally rare; poor prognosis. Optimal tx likely surgery + chemo + XRT.
   c. *Melanoma*: poor prognosis. Typically tx w/ WLE (1–2) cm if able to spare sphincter mechanism; otherwise APR indicated. See section N. below on skin cancers for more information.

4. *W/u*:
   a. Complete H&P, w/ focus on anal sphincter function. CXR, abdomen/pelvis CT scan, proctoscopy endorectal U/S appropriate. Clinically (+) inguinal LN should be investigated w/ FNA.

5. *Tx*:
   a. *Anal canal cancers*:
      i. Tumors < 5 cm (T1, T2) that do not invade sphincter → WLE.
      ii. All others → Nigro protocol of chemoradiation (*note:* below regimen assoc. w/ high incidents of complications in AIDS pts; alternatives may be appropriate). 85% 5-yr survival.
      - *Day 1*: Mitomycin C IV bolus (or bleomycin or cisplatin).
      - *Days 1–4*: 5-FU continuous IV infusion.
      - *Days 1–35*: XRT 5 d/wk for 45–55 Gy. Boosts to anus a/o inguinal basins allowed.
      - *Days 29–32*: 5-FU continuous IV infusion.
      - *Exceptions*: surgery still indicated for:
         - Salvage for persistence or recurrence after Nigro tx → APR.
         - Significant local sx (rectovesical fistula, perineal sepsis, incontinence, etc.) → APR.
         - Recurrent LN dz after XRT → inguinal LN dissection.
         - Obstructing lesions → temporary fecal diversion.
   b. *Anal margin cancers*:
      i. Tumors < 5 cm (T1, T2) that do not invade sphnincter → WLE (80% 5-yr survival).
      - XRT alone yields similar survival, but w/ higher incidence of complications.
      ii. Tumors > 5 cm (T3) or w/ LN (+):
      - APR w/ inguinal XRT (inguinal LN dissection if residual/recurrent LN).

6. *Premalignant lesions*
   a. Paget's dz (intraepithelial adenocarcinoma).
   b. Bowen's dz (intraepithelial squamous cell carcinoma).

AJCC TNM Classification for Anal Carcinoma

Primary Tumor (T)	Regional Lymph Nodes (N)–Clinical & Pathological	Distant Metastasis (M)
Tis – Carcinoma in situ	N1 – Metastasis in perirectal LN(s)	M1 – Distant metastasis
T1 – < 2 cm in greatest dimension	N2 – Metastasis in unilateral internal iliac and/or inguinal LN(s)	
T2 – > 2 but not > 5 cm in greatest dimension	N3 – Metastasis in perirectal and inguinal lymph nodes and/or bilateral interal iliac and/or inguinal LN(s)	
T3 – > 5 cm in greatest dimension		
T4 – Any size tumor which invades adjacent organ(s)		

c. Both manifest as perianal eczematoid plaque; r/o synchronous invasive colorectal CA w/ endoscopy. Local excision is preferred tx (although topical agents such as 5-FU may be effective), along w/ "anal mapping" bx's of remaining perianal skin (sample 4 quadrants of verge, margin, and dentate line).

AJCC Staging for Anal Carcinoma (2009 Version)

Stage	TNM	Survival (Squamous)	Survival (Nonsquamous)
0	TisN0M0		
I	T1N0M0	71.4	59.1
II	T2N0M0 T3N0M0	63.5	52.9
IIIa	T1N1M0 T2N1M0 T3N1M0 T4N0M0	48.1	37.7
IIIb	T4N1M0 Any T, N2, M0 Any T, N3, M0	43.2	24.4
IV	Any T, Any N, M1	20.9	7.4

B. Breast

1. *Genetics*:

   a. Majority of breast CA are sporadic (90–95%), not familial.

   b. *Risk factors*: early menarche, late menopause, hormone replacement therapy, late childbirth.

   c. *BRCA 1*; chromosome 17q, tumor suppressor gene. Lifetime risk breast CA 50–85%. Risk of ovarian CA 40–65%. Assoc. w/ medullary breast CA.

   d. *BRCA 2*; chromosome 13, autosomal dominant. Lifetime risk breast CA ~ 35–80%. Lifetime risk ovarian CA 10–20%. Increased risk male breast CA.

   e. *Syndromes*: Li-Fraumeni assoc. w/ p53 mutation; sarcoma, brain, leukemia, adrenocortical CA. Cowden syndrome assoc. w/ PTEN; uterus, lung, bladder, thyroid, colon, GI polyps. RBI w/ bilateral retinoblastoma, soft tissue sarcoma.

2. *Screening*: USPTF 2009 recommendations: biennial mammogram starting at age 50; however, ACS and NCCN still recommend annual screening at age 40 (in cases of 1st-degree relatives w/ breast CA, recommend 10 yr before age of cancer dx). Clinical breast exam by physician at least every 3 yr in 20s–30s, then annually therafter. Breast self-exam may be suggested in the 20s, but evidence of significant benefit compared to other screening modalities is lacking.

3. *LCIS*: a marker of increased risk for breast CA, most frequently found in white females; 80–90% premenopausal. Risk of developing cancer = 21% over 17 yr (~ 1%/yr), usu. favorable histology. Of those who develop invasive dz, ⅔ ductal. Can observe as high risk (most common), chemoprevention (tamoxifen), or prophylactic B mastectomy. NSABP Cancer Prevention Trial showed tamoxifen for 5 yr → 56% ↓ risk invasive cancer. F/u: PEx and MMG (or MRI) q 6–12 mo × 5 yr, then annually.

4. *DCIS*: 20–25% of breast CA. Presents as microcalcifications or mass. Prognosis excellent, tx w/ total mastectomy or lumpectomy and radiation.

   a. DCIS w/ widespread dz (2+ quadrants) requires total mastectomy w/out LN dissection. 1–2% (+) LN. For more limited dz and those w/ (–) margins (primary or re-excised), either total mastectomy or breast conserving therapy. If apparent pure DCIS tx'd w/ mastectomy or tail of breast (could compromise future SLNBx), consider doing SLNBx. If < 0.5 cm, unicentric, low-grade of solid, cribriform, or papillary subtype, can do excision + RT; TM w/out LN dissection; or excision alone + observation. Margins > 10 mm are negative; less than 1 mm inadequate.

   b. Long-term survival w/ mastectomy = excision and whole breast irradiation. Whole breast irradiation added to margin-free resection ↓ recurrence, but no ↑ in survival. XRT indicated after local excision for DCIS > 0.5-cm diameter.

c. *Early Breast CA Trial overview*: 5 yr of tamoxifen → 52% ↓ annual recurrence in pts w/ ER (+) or receptor-unknown tumors. NSABP B-24 = tamoxifen of benefit for DCIS after breast conservation tx and XRT (5% absolute ↓ recurrence and 37% relative risk ↓), esp. good for ER (+) dz.

d. *F/u*: PEx q 6 mo for 5 yr and then annually, and annual mammography.

5. *Breast CA Staging and Prognosis*
    a. *Stage I, II breast CA*: partial mastectomy + XRT vs total *and* SLNBx.
        i. *Breast conservation contraindicated if*: pt doesn't want it, (+) margins (if positive after re-excision mastectomy indicated), diffuse malignant calcifications, 1st/2nd-trimester pregnancy, pregnant, widespread dz, inadequate radiation, or hx of prior XRT in the area. Breast-conserving tx relative contraindications: connective tissue dz in skin (lupus, scleroderma), tumor > 5 cm, focally positive pathologic margins. In women 70 yo or older w/ clinically negative LN and ER (+) cancer, can pursue breast-conserving therapy plus tamoxifen or aromatase inhibitor w/out irradiation. (Intergroup CALCGB/RTOG/ECOG study)
        ii. *Initial w/u*: hx, physical, CBC, LFTs, CXR, B diagnostic mammography, bx results for estrogen/progesterone receptors, HER2/neu expression.
            • If bone or abdominal sx or elevated alkaline phosphatase, obtain bone scan a/o abdominal CT/MRI as appropriate (some will get CT of c/a/p if > 1 cm).
            • For clinical stage I/II cancer, assess axillary LN status; perform SLNBx and complete axillary dissection if SLNBx +. For level I and level II dissections, at least 10 LNs are required for accurate staging. Only dissect level III if gross dz in I or II.
                ◦ Still, consider as optional if esp. favorable tumors, if adjuvant therapy is unlikely to help pt, elderly pts, and those w/ serious comorbidities (BINV-B).
            • In literature regarding tx of neoplasms w/ "favorable histology," this refers to tubular (almost always HER2/neu non-overexpressed, ER (+)), colloid. Medullary risk of metastasis is equal to other high-grade carcinomas; do not treat as favorable histology.
            • *SLNBx*: must have clinically negative axilla, or negative core or FNA bx of suspicious nodes. If cannot indentify sentinel LN or if is (+) for metastasis, a full axillary LN dissection indicated or axillary RT is given. Internal mammary node excision is optional if sentinel nodes identified in internal mammary chain.
    b. *Stage III and inflammatory BrCA*
        i. "Inoperable" locally advanced.
            • *Tx*: anthracycline-based + taxane neoadjuvant chemotx indicated. Follow w/ total mastectomy and axillary LN dissection or lumpectomy and axillary dissection and adjuvant XRT *and* postop hormonal therapy. Some have advocated option of chemo/XRT alone. If inoperable, palliative XRT may be considered along w/ hormonal tx if hormone receptor (+) or unknown.
    c. *Stage IV* (metastatic or recurrent)
        i. Eval w/ H&P, CBC, LFT, CXR, bone scan, x-rays of abn areas of bone scan, +/– CT/MRI of chest and abdomen, bx of any possible site of recurrence. PET is optional.
        ii. *Tx*:
            • *Local recurrence only* (*note*: consider all for chemo/endocrine tx):
                ◦ If previous mastectomy, then resect local recurrence if able to get clear margins and give XRT if prior irradiation doesn't preclude. If unresectable, consider XRT if no limiting prior irradiation.
                ◦ If previous breast-conserving therapy, perform total mastectomy.
            • *Systemic recurrence* (all get chemo/endocrine tx unless toxicity significantly impairs quality of life).
            • *Bone metastasis*: bisphosphonate, calcium citrate, vitamin D if expect survival > 3 mo, and Cr < 3.

6. *Radiation*
    a. *Indicated if*:
        i. Tumor size > 5 cm.
        ii. 4 or more (+) LNs.
        iii. Stage I or II dz managed w/ breast conservation surgery or advanced DCIS tx'd w/ WLE.

AJCC TNM Classification for Breast Carcinoma

Primary Tumor (T)	Regional Lymph Nodes (N)–Clinical & Pathological	Distant Metastasis (M)
Tx – Primary tumor can't be assessed	Nx – Regional LN's can't be assessed	Mx – Presence of distant mets can't be assessed
T0 – No evidence of primary tumor	N0 – No regional LN mets	M0 – No distant mets
Tis – Carcinoma in situ	N1 – Mets to 1–3 movable ipsilateral axillary LN's or internal mammary detected by SLNbx N1mi – micrometastases – > 0.2 mm and < 2.0 mm	M1 – Distant mets
T1 – ≤ 2 cm in greatest dimension	N2 – Mets to 4–9 ipsilateral axillary LN's clinically fixed or matted OR ipsilateral internal mammary in absence of axillary disease	
T2 – > 2 but ≤ 5 cm	N3 – Mets to > 10 axillary LN's OR ipsilateral internal mammary LN's in presence of axillary disease OR ipsilateral supraclavicular LN's	
T3 – > 5 cm		
T4 – Direct extension to chest wall or skin; includes inflammatory carcinoma		

AJCC Staging for Breast Carcinoma (2009 Version)

Stage	TNM	5-Year Survival
0	TisN0M0	92.7
I	T1N0M0 T0-1N1mi	87.8
IIa	T0N1M0 T1N1M0 T2N0M0	81.4
IIb	T2N1M0 T3N0M0	74.0
IIIa	T0N2M0 T1N2M0 T2N2M0 T3N12M0	66.7
IIIb	T4, Any N, M0	41.0
IIIc	Any T, N3, M0	49.3
IV	Any T, Any N, M1	14.8

  iv. Locally advanced/inflammatory breast CA refractory to neoadjuvant chemotherapy.
b. Usu. 50 Gy w/ local 10- to 15-Gy boost, starting 2–4 wk postop, and lasting ~ 6 wk, 5 d/wk.
7. *Sentinel lymph node*
  a. *Indications*
    i. Early, nonmulticentric invasive breast CA (< 4.5 cm), clinically node (–), *w/out* neoadjuvant chemo/XRT.
    ii. *Certain cases of DCIS*: > 2.5 cm, comedo, multifocal/multicentric, high grade.
  b. *Contraindications*
    i. Palpable axillary LAD.
    ii. Tumors > 5 cm (multiple drainage routes probable).
    iii. Previous axillary surgery or neoadjuvant chemotx or XRT.
    iv. Large bx cavity (> 6 cm); cavity drainage may be different than tumor drainage.
  c. *Technique*
    i. Inject subareolar (generally the highest sensitivity) or peritumoral.
    ii. Blue dye (isosulfan blue, methylene blue, vital blue dye). Methylene blue assoc. w/ rare cases of anaphylaxis; also skin necrosis if inject too superficially. Inject 5 min preop if lateral to nipple, or 10–15 min preop if medial to nipple.
    iii. Technetium-99m. Inject 30 min to 24 h preop.
8. *Axillary dissection*
  a. Assists w/ staging and local control, but not survival.
  b. Perform level I, II axillary dissection for stage I, II cancer if SLN not performed. The Auchincloss modification of Patey's MRM has been the standard for several decades, and does not resect pectoralis minor or level III nodes unless those nodes are clinically involved.
9. *F/u*
  a. Regular physical exam and MGM. If breast-conserving tx used, then first MGM is 6 mo after surgery. LFTs, tumor markers, and routine bone scans not utilized.
  b. If on tamoxifen, get annual pelvic exams and expedited exams for vaginal spotting.
  c. If on aromatase inhibitors, monitor bone health w/ DEXA scan or other modalities.
C. Carcinoid
1. *General*: arise from enterochromaffin cells (neural crest origin), and variably secrete vasoactive substances (5-HT/serotonin, histamine, dopamine, substance P, prostaglandins, etc.).
2. *Appendiceal* (40%)
  a. Appendectomy sufficient for tumors < 1.5 cm in diameter w/out evidence of spread.
  b. Right hemicolectomy indicated if tumor > 1.5 cm in diameter or gross evidence of spread to lymph nodes, mesoappendix, etc.
3. *Rectal* (15%)
  a. Diameter < 1 cm → local excision.
  b. Diameter 1–2 cm → wide local excision; if invade muscularis propria → LAR or APR.
  c. Diameter > 2 cm → regional excision; majority succumb to systemic dz and thus sphincter-sparing is generally advocated.
4. *Pulmonary* (11%): as blood flow bypasses liver, more likely to manifest w/ carcinoid syndrome.
5. *Small intestine* (27%)
  a. Wide resection indicated; 70% metastatic to lymph nodes.
  b. 40% assoc. w/ second GI malignancy.
6. *Metastatic*
  a. *Medical tx*:
    i. Octreotide (note, operations on pts w/ metastatic carcinoid can induce *carcinoid crisis*, which is managed w/ IV octreotide drip)
    ii. Loperamide, diphenoxylate

      iii. Albuterol

      iv. H$_2$ blockers

      v. Cyproheptadine (serotonin receptor antagonist)

D. Colorectal

1. Decreased w/ fiber, calcium, omega-fatty acids possibly. Increased risk w/ fatty diets, possibly due to effects of additional bile salts in gut. 94% spontaneous, 5% HNPCC, 1% FAP.

  a. *Genetics*: loss of APC, DCC, p53, K-ras most common

  b. *Syndromes*

    i. *Familial adenomatous polyposis* (FAP)

- Loss of APC gene on chromosome 5q. Autosomal dominant, 20% spontaneous. 100% CRCa by age 40 yo. Dx requires > 100 polyps, and vast majority of pts will have many more.

- Begin surveillance in puberty w/ flex-sig. Recommend total colectomy by 20 yo.

- Assoc. w/ small intestinal (duodenal/ampullary) tumors as well; need routine EGD.

- *Gardner's syndrome*: FAP + desmoid tumors (treat w/ sulindac, taxmoxifen, or resection) +/− osteomas (classically in mandible).

- *Turcot's syndrome*: FAP + brain tumors

    ii. *Lynch syndrome* (hereditary nonpolyposis colon CA [HNPCC])

- 5% of population, autosomal dominant, assoc. w/ DNA mismatch repair genes, right colon cancers, and metachronous cancers.

- Amsterdam criteria: at least 3 1st-degree relatives over 2 generations, w/ at least 1 before 50 yo.

- *Bethesda criteria*: similar in principle to Amsterdam criteria but less stringent.

- Lynch I—no assoc. extra-colonic malignancies.

- Lynch II—assoc. w/ ovarian, endometrial, cholangiocarcinoma, a/o gastric CA.

- Surveillance colonoscopy at 25 yo or 10 yr before age of earliest CRCA in family.

- Operation should be subtotal colectomy (and TAH/BSO if no longer able or desires fertility).

    iii. *Polyps*

- *Hyperplastic*: most common colonic polyp, but no concerns for malignant transformation as w/ adenomatous polyps.

- *Hamartomas*: ectopic nonneoplastic tissue, assoc. w/ below:

    ◦ *Peutz-Jeghers*—in addition to GI hamartomas, have perioral hyperpigmented lesions, overall increased risk in GI cancer (not from hamartomas, though—usu. duodenal or colonic) as well as breast, biliary, possibly reproductive.

    ◦ *Cronkhite-Canada*—hamartomas + nail/hair atrophy/alopecia + hypopigmentation.

    ◦ *Juvenile polyposis*—polyps w/ no increased malignant potential, but pts do have increased overall risk of other neoplasia(s). Recommend routine colonic surveillance and total colectomy if cancer arises.

    ◦ *Adenomatous*—malignant potential, more so if villous than tubular; remove endoscopically.

      ■ If carcinoma in situ present, no further intervention other than surveillance colonoscopy.

      ■ If carcinoma invades muscularis mucosa, 8.5–20% (+) LN. *Options*:

        ▫ Do standard cancer procedure.

        ▫ If pedunculated (nonsessile), well-differentiated, no vascular/lymphatic invasion, and has clear margin on stalk for > 5 mm, can offer close surveillance colonoscopy.

- If tubular adenoma, < 1 cm, usu. f/u colonoscopy in 5–10 yr. If villous, > 1 cm, or 3–10 adenomas removed, then repeat colonoscopy in 3 yr.
  - If sessile, villous, and can't be entirely removed via endoscopy, perform segmental resection. If > ~ 7 cm, generally need celiotomy. If lower, can attempt transrectal resection.
  - If have invasive carcinoma w/ < 2-mm margin, or lymphovascular invasion, or poorly differentitated, then colectomy indicated.

2. Rectal 43%, sigmoid 25%, ascending 18%, transverse 9%, descending 5%. (c/c → 83% polyps in left colon, but only 61% of cancer w/ 55% total in rectum).

3. *Right-sided tumors*—less common, tend to grow larger before producing sx, generally present w/ bleeding/anemia, but SBO, biliopancreatic-like sx (RUQ pain, nausea) can occur.

4. *Left-sided tumors*—more common, can present like diverticulitis, fistula.

5. Rectal CA most commonly presents w/ hematochezia, but tenesmus, rectal pain, urgency, or mucous discharge can occur as well as fistula-in-ano.
   a. Assess if sphincters can be spared w/ U/S (TRUS or EUS) or MRI.
   b. May be able to spare (i.e., LAR) if proximal to last 3–5 cm of rectum (10 from anal verge). Neoadjuvant radiation +/– chemo may downsize tumor to allow easier resection; ~ 5000 cGy over 6 wk w/ 5-FU during first and last wks reduces depth of wall invasion and lessens LN involvement in ~ 70%.

6. Regardless of location, all CRCA can present w/ change in bowel movements. Colonoscopic eval is gold standard. Obstructive CA generally merits segmental colectomy w/ end colostomy. Bleeding or obstructive CA get metastatic w/u; includes LFTs (if LFT abnormal, get liver CT or MRI) and CEA. Preop, get baseline CEA; will need to follow every 4 mo postop to survey for recurrence or metastasis. Also get preop CT if tumor is in rectum or if > 4 cm (higher risk for invasion into adjacent structures).

7. Chemotherapy consider for stage II or III tumors—FOLFOX; add Avastin if stage IV.

8. *Radiation therapy*: effective in rectal tumors (w/in 12 cm from anal verge) in decreasing local recurrence and prolonging dz-free survival. Pts w/ locally advanced rectal CA (≥ T3) should get neoadjuvant chemoradiation prior to surigical resection.
   a. *Advantage to postop XRT*: good perfusion provides high oxygen tension, which facilitates radiation injury by free radical damage.
   b. *Disadvantages to postop XRT instead of preop*: increased small bowel in XRT field and creation of a relatively hypoxic field. Further, postop XRT in pts post-LAR is sphincter dysfunction and fecal incontinence.

AJCC TNM Classification for Colorectal Carcinoma

Primary Tumor (T)	Regional Lymph Nodes (N)	Distant Metastasis (M)
T1 – Invades submucosa	N0 – No LN mets	M0 – No distant mets
T2 – Invades muscularis propria	N1a – Mets in 1 LN's N1b – Mets in 2–3 LN's N1c – Tumor in subserosa, mesentery or nonperitonealized pericolic tissues without LN mets	M1a – Distant mets present
T3 – Invades subserosa, but no further than nonperitonealized paracolic fat	N2a – Mets in 4–6 LN's N2b – Mets in = & LN's	
T4 – Invades peritoneal cavity or contiguous organs		

AJCC Staging for Colorectal Carcinoma (2009 Version)

Stage	TNM	5-Year Survival	5-Year Survival
0	TisN0M0	Colon	Rectal
I	T1N0M0 T2N0M0	74.0	74.1
IIa	T3N0M0	66.5	64.5
IIb	T4aN0M0	58.6	51.6
IIc	T4bN0M0	37.3	32.3
IIIa	T1-T2N1/N1cM0 T1N2aM0	73.1	74.0
IIIb	T3-T4aN1/N1cM0 T2-3N2aM0 T1-T2N2bM0	46.3	45.0
IIIc	T4aN2aM0 T3-4aN2bM0 T4bN1-N2M0	28.0	33.4
IV	Any T, Any N, M1a-b	5.7	6.0

Colorectal Tx Based on Stage

Stage	Definition	Tx Based on Stage
I	T1 or T2	Surgery (see chart below for appropriate procedure)
II	Invasive to local area or contiguous structures, but no (+) LN. T3 or T4	Surgery + FOLFOX
III	LN (+)	Surgery +FOLFOX
IV	Metastatic	FOLFOX +/− Avastin; surgery for obstruction/symptomatic lesions

Colorectal Surgical Tx Based on Location

Location	Procedure
Ascending	Right hemicolectomy (distal 4–6 cm of TI to transverse colon supplied by right branch of middle colic a.)
Transverse	Extended right hemicolectomy. Divide right and middle colic aa's at their origin, then remove colon supplied by them
Splenic flexure	Segmental colectomy
Descending	Left hemicolectomy (from splenic flexure to rectosigmoid junction)
Sigmoid	Segmental colectomy

Location	Procedure
Prox 1–⅔ of rectum (5–6 cm above dentate line, or ~10 cm above anal verge)	LAR: removal of sigmoid colon *and* proximal rectum w/ anastamosis in pelvis below the peritoneal reflection
Mid-rectum	LAR or APR: excision of rectum and anus w/ permanent closure of perineum and creation of end colostomy. Must do APR if involves anal sphincters, rectovaginal septum
Lower rectum	APR or transanal excision. Latter feasible if tumor is mobile, < 4cm in diam, are T1-2, N0 on US/MRI, well or mod differentiated, involve <40% of rectal wall, and are located w/in 6 cm of anal verge

Note: some advocate the "no-touch technique" for intraoperative handling of specimen: first close off venous outflow and obliterate the lumen of cancerous segment before resecting/touching specimen. This has not proven to improve outcome in any measure.

E. **Esophagus**
   1. *Epidemiology/etiology*: fastest-growing cancer in United States (4% of CA), but 9th most common CA worldwide.
      a. SCC traditionally more common than adenocarcinoma, but the latter has been increasing much faster in incidence in the United States (70% new dx's in United States).
      b. *Risk factors for SCC*: highest endemicity in N. China, Iran, Russia, India, and S. Africa. In the United States, blacks more affected than whites, Hispanics. Excessive intake of nitrates/ nitrosamines, alcohol, tobacco (smoking), and deficiencies in vitamins A, C, B$_2$, as well as acha- lasia, esophageal strictures/webs, prior radiation, tylosis assoc. w/ esophageal SCC.
      c. Primary risk factor for esophageal adenocarcinoma is Barrett's esophagus (malignant transfor- mation rate 1–2% per yr).
   2. *Staging and w/u*:
      a. CT chest and abdomen (some advocate PET scan; good to eval for metastatic dz).
      b. Endoscopic U/S (best means to determine depth of invasion and local LN; provide tissue dx).
      c. Bronchoscopy for upper ⅔ lesions (r/o fistula).
      d. CT head a/o bone scan if sx are suggestive; cervical LAD should be biopsied.
      e. Consider bronchoscopy, thoracoscopy, a/o laparoscopy to determine if metastatic dz present.
   3. *Tx*:
      a. *Contraindications*: distant mets, enlarged mediastinal or celiac (not paraesophageal) LN, esophagobronchial fistula. Most upper ⅓ cancers are nonresectable.
      b. *Neoadjuvant therapy*: cisplatinum + 5-FU concomitant w/ XRT of 4500 rad may be of benefit for ≥ T2 tumors.
      c. *Surgery*: Optimize nutrition (i.e., TPN).
         i. Celiotomy, should first check for metastatic dz—most commonly will be to liver or celiac nodes. If (+), then only resect if other palliative interventions are not feasible.
         ii. *Subtotal esophagectomy*: distal tumors (i.e., at GE junction) appropriately managed w/ Ivor-Lewis (or Tanner-Lewis modification). Need right thoracotomy (mobilize esophagus, anastamose stomach to esophagus in chest). If proximal esophageal margin (+) for can- cer, perform total esophagectomy w/ cervical anastamosis. 10-cm margins are desirable in esophageal tumors as they tend to spread horizontally.

  iii. *Total esophagectomy*: proximal (cervical, upper esophageal) neoplasms are more appropriately managed this way. Esophageal mobilization may be approached in 2 ways:
- Mobilize esophagus via right thoracotomy and bring conduit substernally or through posterior mediastinum to neck.
- Transhiatal esophagectomy, avoiding thoracotomy. Disadvantage of this is less thorough periesophageal lymphadenectomy, risk of injuring blood vessels or tracheobronchial tree.
- *Note*: Cervical anastamosis leaks more frequently than intrathoracic anastamosis (12% vs 5%), but mortality w/ cervical leak is far less than than w/ intrathoracic leak (2% vs 50%).

  iv. *Conduit*: stomach preferred (easy to mobilize, good blood supply; preserve right gastroepiploic; important to do pyloromyotomy/plasty to avoid stasis), followed by colon. Free jejunal grafts rarely utilized.

 d. *Adjuvant therapy*: XRT only recommended if (+) margins or residual dz. No proven advantage w/ adjuvant chemotx.

 e. *Palliative tx*:
  i. *Dilation* (caveat = perforation risk).
  ii. *Laser*: reported use in Japan for cure in superficial, in situ lesions as well as for palliation.
  iii. *Self-expanding stents* (oral or operative insertion)—facilitate pureed diet.
  iv. *Chemoradiation palliation*: SCCA more responsive than adenoca, and upper ½ lesions have less morbidity (esp. N/V).

 4. *Prognosis*: if able to perform R0 resection, anticipate 15–20% 5-yr survival. However, less than 60% of pts w/ locoregional dz can be fully resected.

F. Gastric (adenocarcinoma: GIST and lymphoma are discussed in separate sections)

 1. *Epidemiology/etiology*: overall decreasing in United States although cardia/GE junction CA increasing. *Wide geographic variation*: Japan, Costa Rica, Korea >> United States, W Europe. In United States, non-Caucasian (African Americans, Native Americans, Hispanic) males at increased risk gastritis, EBV, h/o operation for benign peptic ulcers. *H. pylori* risk factor for distal cancers and MALT, but could be protective against proximal CA. HNPCC is genetic risk factor.

 2. *Pathology*: 95% in United States = adenocarcinoma. GIST, lymphoma, carcinoid, SCCA in remainder. Most often found on lesser curve. 10% *linitis plastica* (malignancy spreads beyond gross mass) w/ esp. poor prognosis.

 a. *Lauren classification*:
  i. *Intestinal*: from mucosal glands, usu. more distal, and in older pts, often assoc. w/ *H. pylori*, atrophic gastritis.
  ii. *Diffuse*: from lamina propria, more invasive (transmural, across submosa, and in lymphatics—more frequent peritoneal mets), usu. more proximal and in younger pts.

 3. *Dx*:
 a. *Clinical*: generally presents w/ abdominal pain, wt loss. Anemia common. Advanced dz may manifest w/ dysphagia (prox. tumor) or gastric outlet obstruction (distal tumor).
  i. *Eponymic signs of metastasis include*: supraclavicular (usu. left) lymphadenopathy—*Virchow's node*; periumbilical met/mass—*Sister Mary Joseph's nodule*; ovarian drop met—*Krukenberg tumor*; prerectal drop met—*Blumer's shelf*.
  ii. *Acanthosis nigricans*: velvety, hyperpigmented, hyperkeratotic skin changes, usu. of axilla and groin classically assoc. w/ internal malignancy. Gastric CA is the most common malignancy found w/ this, although in some series lung CA is seen as frequently; many other cancers (i.e., pancreatic, endometrial, etc.) have reportedly been assoc. w/ acanthosis nigricans, as have nonmalignant conditions (i.e., metabolic syndrome). "Tripe palms" refers to similar changes in the palms.
 b. *Advanced*: EGD w/ bx is cornerstone. EUS useful to eval. depth and LN status (~ 75% accurate). CT scan to determine if unresectable (visceral metastases, malignant ascites). Diagnostic laparoscopy more sensitive regarding resectability,,esp. when combined w/ peritoneal washings.

 4. *Staging*: AJCC/UICC more widely used than Japanese system (see p. 78).

5. *Tx*:
   a. *Surgery*
      i. *Partial/total gastrectomy w/ gross margin of 6 cm is mainstay*; decide surgery by region involved.
         - *GE junction*: most common. Often very advanced. Siewert classification, 3 types:
           - *Type I*: originate in distal esophagus; assoc. w/ Barrett's esophagus. Need gastric pull-up to neck or Ivor-Lewis esophagogastrectomy.
           - *Type II*: adenocarcinoma of gastric cardia; w/in 2 cm of squamocolumnar junction. Total or proximal subtotal gastrectomy. Former has advantage of less esophagitis w/ plus Roux-en-Y reconstruction, and LNs along lesser curve are more easily removed.
           - *Type III*: subcardial infiltrating GE junction; tx same as type II.
         - *Midbody*: 15–30% of cases. To achieve adequate margin, total gastrectomy usu. indicated.
         - *Distal*: ~ 35%. Total vs distal subtotal gastrectomy have similar survival, w/ latter having better quality of life and should be performed if able to achieve adequate margins.
      ii. *Endoscopic mucosal resection* (EMR)
         - More frequently performed in Japan than in United States. Appropriate candidates have T1 tumors (confined to mucosa), which are well differentiated and polypoid or fungating or w/ elevated borders (Borrmann type I, IIa/b). Serial pathology sections should be performed after excision. If invades into submucosa but not beyond, pylorus-preserving gastrectomy may be appropriate.
      iii. *Lymphadenectomy classification* (not part of AJCC, but commonly described)
         - Japanese reports of improved survival in extended lympadenectomy, esp. in stage II/III dz, and authors recommend level of LN resection 1 level higher than involved nodes. Translates into a D2 resection for most cases, and certain centers in the United States have approached levels of success near those in Japan w/ no increased morbidity over D1 resections; most centers in United States and Europe though have experienced increased M&M w/ D2 vs D1 resections, so not uniformly recommended except for select specialist centers.
         - *D1*: removal of all LN w/in 3 cm of primary tumor (perigastric).
         - *D2*: D1 + removal of all hepatic, splenic, celiac, and left gastric LNs.
         - *D3*: total gastrectomy + omentectomy + splenectomy + distal pancreatectomy + porta hepatic + periaortic lymphadenectomy.
      iv. *Reconstruction options*:
         - *Subtotal gastrectomy*: BI, BII (ante- or retrocolic), or Roux-en-Y gastrojejunostomy (ante- or retrocolic). Roux-en-Y easier than BI w/ less risk of anastomotic tension, and less risk of bile reflux than w/ BII (w/ Roux limb > 40 cm).
         - *Total gastrectomy*: of Roux-en-Y esophagojejunostomy, pouch, or jejunal interposition, the first is usu. the easiest to perform w/ the least morbidity.
         - Lawrence-Hunt (jejunal) pouch.
   b. *Neoadjuvant therapy*: MAGIC trial: periop use of ECF (epirubicin/cisplatin/5-FU) [Chua YJ, et al., *Ann Surg Onc* 2007;14(10):2687–90.] Improved 5-yr overall survival compared to surgery alone for = T2 tumors. Similarly, combination chemoradiotherapy w/ XRT show some benefit in ongoing studies.
   c. *Palliative options*: Chemotx, XRT, resection, or endoscopic laser ablation/dilation/stenting may be appropriate alone or in various combinations.

AJCC/UICC TMN Classification for Gastric Carcinoma

Primary Tumor (T)	Regional Lymph Nodes (N)	Distant Metastasis (M)
Tx – Unknown	Nx – Unknown	Mx – Unknown
T0 – No tumor	N0 – No LN mets	M0 – No mets
Tis – In situ, no invasion of lamina propria	N1 – 1–2 (+) LNs	M1 – Distant mets
T1a – Invades lamina propria T1b – Invades submucosa	N2 – 3–6 (+) LNs	
T2 – Invades muscularis propria	N3a – 7–15 (+) LNs N3b – 16 (+) LN's	
T3 – Penetrates subserosa		
T4a – Invades serosa, but not adjacent structures T4b – Invades adjacent structures		

*Additional descriptors for gastric cancer:
  Histologic Grade (G): Gx= can't assess; G1= well-differentiated; G2= mod differentiated; G3= poorly diff.; G4= undifferentiated.
  Residual Tumor (R): Rx=can't assess; R0= no residual tumor; R1= microscopic residual tumor; R2= macroscopic residual tumor.

AJCC Staging for Gastric Carcinoma

Stage	TNM	5-Year Survival
0	TisN0M0	
Ia	T1N0M0	70.8
Ib	T2N0M0 T1N1M0	57.4
IIa	T1N2M0 T2N1M0 T3N0M0	45.5
IIb	T1N3M0 T2N2M0 T3N1M0 T4aN0M0	32.8
IIIa	T2N3M0 T3N2M0 T4aN1M0	19.8
IIIb	T3N3M0 T4aN2M0 T4bN0-1M0	14.0
IIIc	T4aN3M0 T4bN2-3M0	9.2
IV	Any T, Any N, M1	4.0

G. **Gastrointestinal stromal tumors** (GIST)
   1. A form of soft-tissue sarcoma, assoc. w/ mutation of c-KIT/CD117 (tyrosine kinase receptor protein).
      a. Not all are CD117 (+), however.
      b. Rarely spread by lymphatics, much more commonly to liver or elsewhere in abdomen.
      c. *Location*: stomach > small intestine > colon.

2. *Dx*: w/u should include CT or MRI of abdomen, CXR or CT chest, possibly EUS. Bx depends on index of suspicion or plans for neoadjuvant tx to facilitate surgery. As tumor is friable, care should be taken to not violate tissues unnecessarily.

3. *Staging*: TNM + mitotic rate; size and mitotic rate most important for determining likelihood or recurrence.

4. *Tx*:

   a. *Neoadjuvant therapy*: reserved for tumors which appear only marginally resectable (read about c-KIT tyrosine kinase inhibitors, below); optimal response require up to 6 mo.

   b. *Surgery*: mainstay of tx.

   c. *Adjuvant therapy*: Gleevec (imatinib mesylate) is an inhibitor of c-KIT (as well as platelet-derived growth factor and Bcr-Abl receptor) tyrosine kinases; 50% response rate. FDA-approved for pts at high risk of recurrence ($\geq$ 5 cm, high mitotic rate, small bowel origin), unresectable a/o metastatic tumors. Sunitinib malate (Sutent) is FDA approved for GIST tumors resistant to imatinib.

5. *Prognosis*: historically, overall 50% 5-yr survival; however, limited data on survival after initiation of imatinib therapy.

H. Hepatobiliary

1. *Hepatocellular carcinoma*

   a. *Etiology*: worldwide, most common lethal malignancy in men. Incidence rising rapidly in United States due to epidemic hepatitis C (up to ⅓ develop chronic dz, of which up to ⅓ develop cirrhosis, of which experience up to 2% chance/yr of developing HCC). Other risk factors include toxins (aflatoxin, polyvinyl chloride, etc.).

   b. *Dx*: frequently presents w/ jaundice and nonspecific constitutional sx. Alpha-fetoprotein (AFP) elevated in ~ 75%. Bx appropriate for any solid hepatic lesion w/ elevated AFP (> normal but < 400 ng/mL if hepatitis B surface antigen [−], or > 4000 if hepatitis B surface antigen [+]).

   c. *Staging*:

      i. T1 = solitary tumor, no vascular invasion. T2 = single or multiple tumors, none > 5 cm, none w/ vascular invasion. T3 = multiple tumors > 5 cm, or any involving branch of portal/hepatic vein. T4 = direct invasion of any organ other than gallbladder. N, M status based simply on presence/absence of LN/distant spread.

      ii. Multiple histologic types, of which fibrolamellar has the best prognosis, and is less frequently assoc. w/ cirrhosis.

   d. *Tx*:

      i. *Surgical*:

         • *Resection*: method of choice for peripheral lesions in Child's A cirrhotics.
           ○ Hepatic reserve physiology largely determines resectability. See Chapter 14 for details of evaluation of liver function such as indocyanine green and MEGX. Preop portal vein embolization of planned resection area may be of benefit to induce hypertrophy of remaining hepatic parenchyma, and thus postop hepatic function.

         • *Transplant*: method of choice if Child's B or C, and if single tumor < 5 cm or up to 3 tumors, none of which are > 3 cm in diameter, and no evidence of extrahepatic spread.

      ii. *Other*

         • Ablation
           ○ *Radiofrequency* (RFA): of limited success if near large vessel due to "heat sink" phenomenon.

         • Embolization

         • Arterial infusion

   e. *Postop*

      i. *Prognosis*: overall 5-yr survival is ~ 35% after resection, and up to 75% after transplantation.

      ii. *Surveillance*: liver CT/MRI along w/ AFP levels (if initially elevated) should be followed frequently for 2 yr, then annually if normal.

2. *Cholangiocarcinoma* ("Klatskin tumor" refers to neoplasm at bifurcation of extrahepatic bile duct)
   a. *Risk factors* include choledocholithiais, hepatolithiasis, choledochal cysts, nitrosamines, hepatic flukes (i.e., *Fasciola* spp.), ulcerative colitis, HNPCC, and sclerosing cholangitis.
   b. *W/u:*
      i. CT and ERCP generally obtained. Like pancreatic adenocarcinoma, CEA and CA 19-9 may be elevated.
      ii. *Usu. unresectable. Criteria for unresectability include:* (+) LN outside hepatic pedicle; distant metastasis; bilateral extension into secondary hepatic ducts; bilateral extension into hepatic parenchyma; combination of vascular involvement w/ contralateral ductal spread.
   c. *Surgery:*
      i. *Lower third* (distal): pancreaticoduodenectomy (Whipple).
      ii. *Middle third:* local excision (remove GB and CBD from hepatic duct to pancreas) and LN dissection. Reconstruct w/ hepaticojejunostomy.
      iii. *Upper third* (proximal): bile duct resection beginning distally, including GB and LN in porta hepatis, possibly along w/ caudate lobe (controversial). Reconstruct w/ hepaticojejunostomy.
   d. *Adjuvant tx:* XRT +/− 5-FU may be of some benefit; limited data.
3. *Gallbladder carcinoma:*
   a. *Risk factors* include cholelithiasis, gallbladder polyps (solitary polyp > 1 cm greater risk than multiple or smaller polyps), porcelain gallbladder (mucosal calcification higher risk than uniform, transmural calcification), and typhoid carrier state.
   b. *Management:*
      i. *Surgery:*
         • Regardless of operation performed, bile spillage significantly worsens outcome. As bile spillage is also increased in gallbladder cancer operations, *strong consideration should be given to open cholecystectomy in all suspected cases of gallbladder cancer.*
         • Known gallbladder carcinoma should undergo staging laparoscopy, as ~ ½ have metastatic dz.
         • If does not penetrate muscularis (T1), cholecystectomy is adequate.
         • If invades muscularis or deeper (stage ≥ T2), lymphadenectomy (portal, periductal, right celiac, posterior pancreaticoduodenal) should be added to liver parenchyma excision (IVb/V), typically w/ 2+ cm margins beyond palpated or imaged tumor. Some recommend consideration of port site excision as well.
      ii. *Adjuvant tx:* chemotx (5-FU) + XRT recommended for all, except T1, N0 pts.

I. **Lung**
1. *Lung cancer* = number 1 cause of cancer death in United States; tobacco smoking = number 1 risk factor.
   a. *Histological types:* adenocarcinoma (50%), squamous cell (30%), small cell (20%), large cell (10%).

AJCC TNM Classification for Lung Carcinoma

Primary Tumor (T)	Regional Lymph Nodes (N)	Distant Metastasis (M)
Tx – Primary tumor cannot be assessed *OR*, tumor proven by malignant cells in sputum or bronchial washings, but not seen by imaging or bronchoscopy.	Nx – Regional LN's cannot be assessed	Mx – Presence of distant met(s) cannot be established
T0 – No evidence of primary tumor	N0 – No regional LN mets	M0 – No distant met(s)
Tis – Carcinoma in situ	N1 – Mets to ipsilateral peribronchial *a/o* ipsilateral hilar LN's, and intrapulmonary nodes involved by direct extension of the primary tumor (ipsilateral parynchymal spread only)	M1a – Tumor nodule in contralateral lobe with pleural nodules or malignant pleural or pericardial effusion M1b – Distant mets

Primary Tumor (T)	Regional Lymph Nodes (N)	Distant Metastasis (M)
T1 – ≤ 3 cm in greatest dimension, surrounded by lung/pleura, w/out bronchoscopic evidence of invasion more proximal than lobar bronchus	N2 – Mets to ipsilateral mediastinal a/o subcarinal LN's	
T2 – 3–7 cm in greatest dimension OR invading visceral pleura OR involving main bronchus ≥ 2 cm distal to carina OR associated with atelectasis or obstructive pneumonitis that extends to the hilar region but doesn't involve whole lung T2a – 3–5 cm T2b – 5–7 cm	N3 – Mets to contralateral mediastinal, or contralateral hilar, or any scalene or supraclavicular LN's	
T3 – > 7 cm OR any size that directly invades chest wall (including superior sulcus), diaphragm, mediastinal pleura, parietal pericardium; OR in main bronchus < 2 cm distal from carina; OR associated atelectasis or obstructive pneumonitis of entire lung		
T4 – Invades vital structures of heart, great vessels, trachea, recurrent laryngeal n. esophagus, vertebral body, carina, satellite tumor nodules in different ipsilateral lobe		

AJCC Staging for Lung Carcinoma

Stage	TNM	Median Survival (Months)
0	TisN0M0	
Ia	T1N0M0	115
Ib	T2aN0M0	76
IIa	T2bN0M0 T1N1M0 T2aN1M0	47
IIb	T2bN1M0 T3N0M0	24
IIIa	T1N2M0 T2a-bN2M0 T3N1-2M0 T4N0-1M0	17
IIIb	T1N3M0 T2N3M0 T3N3M0 T4N2-3M0	10
IV	Any T, Any N, M1	7

2. *Lung cancer management*:

   a. *Non-small cell* (NSCLC—adenocarcinoma, squamous cell, large cell, bronchoalveolar, etc.):

      i. *Presentation/dx*: freq. presents w/ cough and constitutional sx such as wt loss or fatigue; SCCA may also cause hypercalcemia. Imaging should include CT of chest/liver/adrenals. *Tissue dx*: percutaneous, broncoscopic, or thoracoscopic means (FNA, brushings, etc.). Mediastinoscopy standard for mediastinal LN; should be considered for central T1 tumors and all T2 or T3 tumors. 40% of pts present w/ metastatic dz.

      ii. *Tx*: surgical resection (lobectomy +/− mediastinal lymphadectomy) gold standard for curative tx of stage I and II cancers. Prohibitive operative risk pts may be offered XRT for stage I and II dz; RFA is other option for small (i.e., < 3 cm) peripheral lesions. Adjuvant chemotx (i.e., cisplatin) standard for T2+ or N1+ dz. T3 and stage III tumor management is individualized, but usu. involves neoadjuvant chemotherapy. *Surgery is not recommended as primary tx for N2–3 or M1 dz*, although resection of a solitary brain metastasis may favorably impact survival.

   b. *Small cell lung cancer* (SCLC):

      i. *Presentation/dx*: similar for NSCLC (above), except that frequently manifest paraneoplastic syndrome(s) such as Eaton-Lambert (proximal LE asthenia), Cushing's syndrome, and SIADH. In addition to w/u listed for NSCLC, obtain MRI of head and bone scan, +/− bone marrow bx. ⅔ of pts present w/ metastases, and the majority of the remainder have locally unresectable dz.

      ii. *Tx*:
      - SCLC is exceptionally chemo-sensitive; all pts are given chemotx +/− XRT may be added for relatively local/limited dz.
      - Surgical resection is indicated for less than 5% of pts w/ SCLC (rarely limited to T1/T2 and N0).

3. *Prognosis*: overall, 15% 5-yr survival. However, stage I non-small cell w/ appropriate tx has > 70–90% 10-yr survival; only 10% of pts are dx'd this early, however. Some have advocated screening high-risk pts w/ chest CT to identify these cancers early, thus improving survival.

J. **Lymphoma**

1. *Hodgkin lymphoma*

   a. *Presentation*:

      i. A = *asymptomatic*, B = *symptomatic* (fever, night sweats, pain, pruritis).

      ii. *Staging*: I = 1 area or 2 contiguous areas on same side of diaphragm. II = 2 noncontiguous areas on same side of diaphragm. III = both sides of diaphragm involved. IV = liver, marrow, lung, or other nonlymphoid tissue except spleen.
      - Staging celiotomy rarely indicated w/ high-resolution CT scanners, but still may be indicated for stage Ia or IIa (may avoid chemotx if can prove not more advanced). Contraindicated if have B sx, if XRT not an option, or if have (+) marrow, mediastinal LAD, or other extranodal dz.
        - 2 liver bx's. Splenectomy. Lymphadenectomy of suspicious LNs, as well as LN bx of splenic hilum, porta hepatic, celiac trunk, para-aortic/caval/iliac. Clip areas of suspicious LNs. In females, ovaripexy to assist w/ XRT management.

   b. *Dx*: dependent on tissue (intact LN); Reed-Sternberg cells diagnostic.

   c. *Tx*: CHOP chemotx (**c**yclophosphamide, **h**ydroxydaunomycin [doxorubicin], **O**ncovin [vincristine], and **p**rednisone) + rituximab standard. Assoc. w/ infertility, esp. young males. XRT may given instead if stage Ia, IIa.

2. *Non-Hodgkin lymphoma*

   a. Presentation same as above, need tissue dx.

   b. Worse prognosis than Hodgkin. Usu. systemic at dx.

   c. *Tx*: XRT and MOAP chemotx (vincristine, cyclophosphamide, prednisone, adriamycin).

3. *Gastric lymphoma*

   a. Most common site of primary lymphoma in GI tract.

   b. *Dx*:

    i. Endoscopy w/ bx's and EUS appropriate for initial dx. Subsequent evaluation should include: *H. pylori* histologic and serologic testing; CT of chest and abdomen; bx of bone marrow and any identified LAD appropriate to assess extent of dz.

    ii. Dx appropriate if lymphoma appears to be sole or primary locus of dz. ~ 2% of all lymphomas, ~ 15% of all gastric malignancies. Most commonly B-cell lymphoma > MALT > other.

  c. *Tx*:

    i. Early MALT (**m**ucosa-**a**ssociated **l**ymphoid **t**umors—now termed extranodal marginal zone lymphomas of MALT type) and potentially early diffuse large B-cell lymphoma should be treated for *H. pylori*, which may induce remission (effective in ⅔ of localized MALT lymphomas). F/u serial endoscopy mandatory.

      • Positive nodal status, transmural extension, and certain genetic markers (as well as *H. pylori*-negative MALT cases) likely to fail this management; XRT usu. tx'd w/ chemotx used for antibiotic-resistant MALT tumors (surgery reserved for failure of XRT and chemo).

    ii. B-cell gastric lymphoma appropriately tx w/ chemotherapy (CHOP + rituximab) +/– XRT w/ > 80% dz-free 5-yr survival rate for early stage dz. Main risk of chemotx is perforation (~ 5%). XRT useful for tumors less than 3 cm in size, markedly less so if > 6 cm.

    iii. Uncommonly, surgery may be pursued for localized dz in some institutions, or recommended for cases resistant to chemotherapy; surgical resection, even w/ positive margins, can be of benefit in such select cases.

4. *Intestinal lymphoma*

  a. Second most common site of GI lymphoma. In adults, represents up to 25% of all small bowel malignancies and is the most common small bowel malignancy in children under 10 yo. Frequently mimics celiac or tropical sprue as malabsorptive dz (also increased incidence in pt w/ celiac dz as well as AIDS), but also causes bleeding, obstruction, or perforation. Generally located in lymphoid-rich ileum.

  b. *Dx*: histological—Kiel classification subtypes into low-, intermediate-, and high-grade lesions.

  c. *Tx*:

    i. As w/ small bowel adenocarcinoma (most common small bowel malignancy; tx w/ resection, which if is in duodenum right of SMA means Whipple), resection of bowel and lymph-containing mesentery is indicated. Duodenal lymphoma may require pancreaticoduodenectomy. Obtain frozen section to confirm clear margins; tumor widely infiltrates submucosa.

    ii. Unlike small bowel adenocarcinoma, adjunctive chemotx such as CHOP (particularly for intermediate- and high-grade dz) and XRT is often indicated.

5. *Thyroid lymphoma*

  a. Rare. Typically presents as rapidly growing goitrous mass +/– fever, dysphagia, a/o dysphonia. Increased risk after Hashimoto's thyroiditis. Non-Hodgkin B-cell most common subtype, followed by MALT tumors.

  b. *Dx*: U/S, FNA, CT of head/neck, chest, abdomen.

  c. *Tx*:

    i. Chemotx w/ CHOP alone yields good survival rates for B-cell tumors.

    ii. Surgery (near-total or total thyroidectomy) may provide some additional survival benefit to CHOP, but assoc. w/ significantly higher complications due to edema, anatomic distortion. Not consistently recommended.

    iii. MALT tumors of thyroid often may be treated w/ XRT alone.

K. Occult primary

1. Represents up to 10% of all malignant dx's. Most commonly involves liver, lungs, lymph nodes, a/o bone. Primary site ultimately found in < ⅓ of cases.

2. *3 broad categories*: (1) adenocarcinoma and other nonsquamous carcinoma (majority of cases); (2) squamous cell carcinoma; (3) neuroendocrine tumors.

  a. *W/u may be aided by*:

    i. PET/CT

ii. *Immunohistochemical stains*: cytokeratins (CK7, CK20)—patterns of (+) and (−) status helpful for evaluating carcinomas such as lung/breast/endometrium/ovary/urothelium/thyroid/pancreas/colon.

iii. *Other*:

- *Axillary lymphatic adenocarcinoma in female*: often from breast CA. Consider breast imaging, including MRI.

- *Supraclavicular SCCA*: likely from head/neck source; obtain head/neck CT, panendoscopy (nasopharyngoscopy, bronchoscopy, direct laryngoscopy, esophagoscopy).

- *Mediastinal lymphatic adenocarcinoma*: possible germ cell tumor; get β-hCG, AFP, LDH levels.

- *Bone scan as indicated by sx*.

- *Adenocarcinoma or poorly differentiated carcinoma in men*, particularly in retroperitoneum: also consider testicular U/S, PSA, CA-125, β-hCG, AFP, LDH.

- *Neuroendocrine tumors*: octreotide scan may be of benefit.

3. *Tx*: based on presumptive primary. Regional lymphadenectomy and XRT generally appropriate for adenocarcinoma or squamous cell carcinomas. Chemotherapy appropriate for histologic type may result in significant response in 10–50% of pts. Overall median survival little more than 6 mo.

L. Pancreas

1. *Pancreatic adenocarcinoma*

a. *Epidemiology/etiology*:

i. Main risk factors are male gender, age over 60 yo, and cigarette smoking.

ii. Almost always has mutation of codon 12 of K-ras oncogene, but p53 tumor suppressor gene also mutated in up to 75% of cases. p16 and BRCA mutation linked to some cases as well.

iii. Familial cases assoc. w/ HNPCC (see section D. above on colorectal cancer), familial (*BRCA2* mutation) breast CA, ataxia-telangectasia, familial atypical multiple mole melanoma syndrome, and Peutz-Jeghers syndrome.

b. *Dx*: classically presents w/ wt loss and painless jaundice. Helical CT scan is generally modality of choice for making dx. If CT doesn't demonstrate mass, ERCP/EUS can be useful (even if classic "double duct" sign of CBD and pancreatic duct stricture is absent), particularly if brushings are obtained. However, tissue dx is not required before pursuing surgery for pancreatic head mass.

c. *Staging*

i. Considered unresectable if involves SMA, celiac axis, or invades posteriorly on preop CT. Distant metastasis (including para-aortic or celiac LNs) is a contraindication for surgery. Involvement of portal vein or SMV means borderline resectability to most surgeons, but this is controversial, as is direct invasion of adrenal, kidney, or colon. Many surgeons will proceed w/ laparoscopy (to look for peritoneal implants, etc.) if CT doesn't demonstrate evidence of unresectability or metastasis, and then open for pancreatic resection if still no evidence of spread.

d. *Tx*:

i. *Neoadjuvant*: consider in tumors that appear to be nonmetastatic, but locally advanced to make them potentially resectable. Pursuing neoadjuvant tx is one of the few indications for obtaining tissue bx before intervening.

ii. *Surgical*

- *Curative* (pancreaticoduodenectomy ["Whipple" operation]); appropriate for < 20% of pts. "Pylorus-preserving" Whipple has not been proven to improve postop gastric emptying. Nor has extensive lymphadenectomy beyond peripancreatic LNs been proven to improve survival in the United States.

- *Palliative*

  ◦ *Biliary bypass*: hepaticojejunostomy. Preop stenting only recommended if evidence of cholangitis or severely symptomatic (i.e., pruritic) and surgery is not imminent.

  ◦ *Duodenal bypass*: only about ¼ of pts will develop duodenal obstruction, thus gastrojejunostomy is usu. reserved for pts w/ no evidence of distant metastasis who are therefore more likely to survive long enough to become symptomatic from obstruction.

    iii. *Adjuvant*:

- *Chemotx*: gemcitabine agent of choice for metastatic dz. May have some role as adjuvant tx.
- *Radiation*: when given w/ 5-FU, *may* be of benefit in some cases (not proven).

  e. *Prognosis*: after resection, median survival just over 15 mo (5-yr survival 20%). If metastasis, 3–6 mo.

2. *Intraductal papillary mucinous neoplasms*

  a. First described in 1980s.

  b. Usu. present in 7th–9th decade of life, slightly more often in men, and are usu. in the pancreatic head.

  c. Subtypes include main-duct, branch-duct, or combined IPMNs. Increased risk of malignancy w/ main-duct IPMN. Commonly mucin will be found at the ampulla of Vater.

  d. Small, branch-duct IPMNS w/out solid component can be managed conservatively; otherwise, tx is pancreas resection.

3. *Mucinous cystic neoplasm*

  a. Lesions w/ increasing malignant potential w/ age, formerly referred to as cystadenoma or cystadenocarcinoma.

  b. Typically occur in 5th–6th decade of life, more commonly in women, and tend to be located in body or tail of pancreas.

  c. Unlike IPMNs (above), these do *not* communicate w/ duct. Characteristically have thick wall w/ ovarian stroma.

  d. Tx is most often w/ distal pancreatectomy.

4. *Serous cystic neoplasm*

  a. Account for ¼ of cystic neoplasms of the pancreas, and are seen more commonly in pts w/ von Hippel-Lindau dz.

  b. Differentiate from mucinous variety by aspiration of contents for mucin (if find mucin, consider malignant or premalignant).

    i. Also, on CT, serous cystic neoplasms characteristically have a much thinner wall than mucinous cystic neoplasms; they also often demonstrate a "sunburst" pattern of calcification w/ in a central scar on CT.

    ii. These tumors may have honeycomb appearance w/ thin septa dividing tumor into microcysts.

    iii. These tumors have clear demarcation between cyst and pancreatic parenchyma (unlike MCN).

    iv. These tumors do not communicate w/ pancreatic duct).

  c. Almost always benign ($< 1/_{10,000}$ contain a malignancy). WHO refers to more common benign variant as *serous cystadenoma* and the rare malignant type *serous cystadenocarcinoma*.

  d. More common in females (2:1) and assoc. w/ von Hippel-Lindau dz; usu. present in 7th decade.

  e. *Tx*: resection is curative, and is primarily performed to avoid sx assoc. w/ mass effect of large tumors, as malignancy is exceedingly rare.

5. *Insulinoma*

  a. *Pathology*: most common pancreatic endocrine tumor, followed by gastrinoma.

    i. Majority sporadic, solitary, benign (85%), less than 2 cm, and equally distributed throughout pancreas.

    ii. > 3 cm or angioinvasive more likely malignant. Mets most often in surrounding lymphatics and liver. Multiple tumors suspect for MEN I.

  b. *Dx*:

    i. *Whipple's triad suggestive*: sx of hypoglycemia w/ rest or exercise, glucose < 45 during sx, and relief of sx w/ glucose administration.

    ii. *Hypoglycemia w/ insulin*: glucose ratio > 0.4 indicative.

    iii. *To r/o factitious dz*: check for elevated C-peptide, proinsulin (not seen if factitious). Can also screen for anti-insulin antibodies and sulfonylureas to r/o factitious hypoglycemia.

    iv. Nesidioblastosis may have identical presentation, but usu. presents early in life (often in infancy), and is not assoc. w/ any mass.

    c. *Localization*:

       i. Gold standard = intraop 10 MHz U/S and palpation; 96–100% successful.

       ii. Spiral CT and gadolinium MRI are primarily to r/o hepatic mets; only 45% successful in locating primary, and neither good if < 1 cm. U/S and somatostatin receptor scintigraphy also have been used, but results are no better. Rarely, calcium gluconate injection and selective venous sampling used 88–100% (sensitive).

    d. *Tx*:

       i. *Medical*: diet change and diazoxide generally not effective.

       ii. *Surgical* tx = enucleation. Some give IV secretin afterwards to identify ductal leak.

         • Subtotal pancreatectomy (enucleation of tumor if in head and distal pancreatectomy) indicated for MEN I pts and familial pts who often have multifocal dz. Subtotal resection also indicated for nesidioblastosis.

6. *Gastrinoma* (Zollinger-Ellison syndrome)

    a. 2nd most common islet cell tumor (after insulinoma), most common pancreatic tumor in MEN syndrome, and most common symptomatic malignant endocrine pancreatic neoplasm. 75% sporadic, 25% MEN I syndrome. Malignancy not based on pathology, but behavior. Initially reported rates of 60–90% malignancy have decreased in recent years to ~ ⅓ of cases (except in MEN I cases—85% LN mets, prognostic significance of LN mets uncertain, however). Large (> 3 cm), sporadic tumors most prone to hepatic mets.

    b. Usu. presents as abdominal pain, w/ ⅔ having diarrhea, and 15% w/ diarrhea alone. N/V not uncommon. GI bleeding in 10%.

       i. Diarrhea stops or significantly decreases w/ NGT aspiration, an important distinguishing feature (i.e., from carcinoid or VIPomas).

       ii. May present as persistent, virulent peptic ulcer (esp. if persist after tx for *H. pylori* or H_2 blockade) or GERD w/ severe esophagitis.

       iii. Also consider dx if pt has other indicators of MEN I (hypercalcemia, elevated PTH, pituitary tumor).

    c. *Dx must include hypergastrinemia in presence of increased gastric acid secretion.*

       i. Fasting gastrin level usu. not above 100 pg/cc in normal pts, but occasionally non-ZES pts will have levels up to 1000 pg/cc; > 1000 pg/cc is essentially diagnostic in pts w/ acid secretion. Significant hypergastrinemia (enough to cause ZES) rarely may also be caused by certain ovarian tumors.

       ii. Basal acid output (BAO) normally < 5 mEq/h. ZES produces a BAO of > 15 mEq/h, or a ratio of BAO to maximum AO > 0.6. Usu., gastric pH < 2.5 for in ZES.

       iii. *If unsure of dx, may administer secretin provocation test*: check fasting gastrin level, then give 2 CU/kg IV of secretin, then recheck gastrin at 2, 5, 10, and 20 min; paradoxical increase in gastrin > 200 pg/mL is 87% sensitive (most false negative results from *H. pylori*) and 100% specific.

       iv. *Differential dx for hypergastrinemia*:

         • *Excess stimulation*

           ○ ZES, antral G-cell hyperplasia (+/– pheochromocytoma), pyloric obstruction

         • *Insufficient gastrin inhibition*

           ○ Atrophic gastritis

           ○ Pernicious anemia

           ○ Gastric carcinoma

           ○ Vitiligo

           ○ H_2 blockers, PPI

           ○ Antral-exclusion operations (also, retained antrum in duodenal stump after Billroth II)

           ○ Vagotomy

         • *Decreased metabolic processing of gastrin*

           ○ Chronic renal failure

           ○ Small bowel resection (usu. transient)

- *Miscellaneous*
    - Rheumatoid arthritis
  d. *Localization*:
    i. > 50% in duodenum (45–60% of all, 60–80% in MEN I), 60–90% in gastrinoma triangle (junction of D2 and D3, junction of cystic duct and CBD, junction of head and neck of pancreas). Rarely in renal capsule, ovarian malignancies.
    ii. ^{111}In-octeotide scintigraphy most useful test. CT scan and arteriogram each miss 50%; venous sampling not helpful.
  e. Preop prep should include NGT, PPI (titrate to gastric acid output to < 5 mEq/h).
  f. Palliative care includes tumor debulking, PPI, somatostatin; consider total gastrectomy.

7. *Glucagonoma*
  a. Assoc. w/ "migratory necrolytic erythema" (related to amino acid deficiency), wt loss, diabetes, VTE. Almost always malignant w/ 70% having metastatic dz, and only 30% cure rate; octreotide can be used for palliation of sx.
  b. *Dx*: confirmed w/ elevated glucagon level, which can be provoked w/ secretin. Normal upper limit is 150–190 pg/cc.
  c. Localization typically achieved via enhanced CT, MRI, or angiography. Most often in body or tail.
  d. Preop prep should included TPN w/ amino acid supplementation, octreotide prn sx.
  e. *Tx*: surgical excision of primary (and mets, if any).
  f. ~ 30% of cases assoc. w/ postop thrombotic complications; consider use of periop anticoagulants.

8. *VIPoma*
  a. *"Werner-Morrison syndrome," or WDHA syndrome*: watery (secretory) diarrhea, hypokalemia, achlorhydria.
    i. Diarrhea is secretory (not related to intake), high volume (dx unlikely if < 700 cc/d) and persists w/ NGT aspiration and H$_2$ blockers (unlike most cases of gastrinoma), but is consistent feature along w/ hypokalemia. Other features more variable, and may also include cutaneous flushing, hypercalcemia, a/o hyperglycemia.
    ii. ~ ½ metastatic at dx.
  b. Dx confirmed w/ elevated VIP and diarrhea (consider gastrinoma, carcinoid, or infectious source if VIP normal). Upper limit of normal is 200 pg/cc.
  c. Localization via enhanced CT, MRI, or angiography. Up to 10% intrathoracic; consider chest CT if initial studies (–).
  d. Preop prep should include octreotide to assist w/ fluid management.
  e. *Tx*: distal pancreatectomy is sufficient for most; if no tumor found, also examine other retroperitoneal tissues such as adrenals. Debulking of tissue is indicated even if metastatic, and octreotide can be used for palliation as well.

9. *PPoma*
  a. Equal distribution in pancreas.
  b. No assoc. clinical syndromes.
  c. Tx = surgical resection.

10. *Somatostatinoma*
  a. Gallstones, steatorrhea, pancreatitis, diabetes mellitus are present w/ variable consistency (i.e., 10% have hypo-, not hyperglycemia). Rarely assoc. w/ neurofibromatosis. 70–90% malignant.
  b. Localization may be procured via CT, MRI, angiography, a/o somatostatin-receptor scintigraphy. Most situated in pancreatic tail and generally large enough to localize w/out difficulty.
  c. *Tx*: surgical resection (distal pancreatectomy, not enucleation). Debulking of mets (usu. hepatic) indicated. Simultaneous cholecystectomy is indicated even if gallbladder w/out stones as cholelithiasis eventually develops in the majority of cases.

M. Sarcoma—soft tissue (for osteosarcoma, see Chapter 19; for GIST tumor, see section G. above)
1. *Rare cancers* (0.6% of malignancies in United States) arising from mesenchyma.

2. *Distribution*: Location (~ ½ in extremities) 33% lower extremity; 16% viscera; 15% retroperitoneal/intraabdominal; 14% upper extremity; 10% trunk; 12% other. Histopathology 20–25% liposarcoma; 19% leiomyosarcoma; 18% malignant fibrous histocytoma (MFH) (*Note: many sources rank MFH as most common type*); 10% fibrosarcoma; 7% synovial; 4% malignant peripheral nerve tumor (MPNT); 22% other.

3. *Behavior*:

   a. *Locally*: locally compress structures, expanding from w/in pseudocapsule.

   b. *Metastatic*:

      i. Almost always spread hematogenously; *exceptions*: clear cell (only 30% hematogenous), fibrohistiocytoma, synovial, epithelioid (15% LN; consider SLNBx).

      ii. Lung usu. involved in metastasis (exception = GI sarcomas → liver).

4. *Risk factors*:

   a. *Environmental* (possible): radiation, trauma, pesticides/herbicides, infectious agents.

   b. *Genetic*: Li-Fraumeni syndrome, neurofibromatosis, familial adenomatous polyposis.

5. *Dx and grading*:

   a. *Bx*: bear in mind future potential definitive procedures when orienting bx. Core-needle bx more likely than FNA to give definitive pathology. Open bx in the extremity can be performed w/ pneumatic tourniquet after exsanguination of the limb. Small incision directly over lesion, oriented along Langer's lines or axis of limb. < 5 cm: *excisional bx*. > 5 cm: *incisional bx*. Frozen and permanent pathology are indicated. Meticulous hemostasis is important to diminish risk of seeding from postop hematoma.

   b. *Radiographic*: MRI is the standard for dx, staging, and surveillance. CXR/CT are important adjuncts for detecting pulmonary metastases. Low grade → CXR and MRI of tumor. High grade → chest CT and MRI of tumor.

      i. T1 ≤ 5 cm in greatest dimension.

      ii. T1a tumor above superficial fascia.

      iii. T1b tumor invading or deep to superficial fascia.

      iv. T2 > 5 cm in greatest dimension.

      v. T2a tumor above superficial fascia.

      vi. T3b tumor invading or deep to superficial fascia.

      vii. N1 regional lymph node metastasis. (*Note:* sarcoma is unique in that N1 dz as well as M1 dz constitutes stage IV.)

      viii. M1 distant metastasis.

   c. FNCLCC Histologic Grading System

      i. Based on 3 parameters and scored as follows:

         • Differentiation (1–3)

         • Mitotic activity (1–3)

         • Extent of necrosis (0–2)

      ii. Scores are summed to designate a grade:

         • Grade 1: 2 or 3

         • Grade 2: 4 or 5

         • Grade 3: 6–8

6. *Tx*:

   a. *Extremity/trunk*: < 5 cm → excision w/ negative margins (attempt 1- to 2-cm gross margin). > 5 cm, *low grade* → excision and postop external beam radiation (EBRT), 50 Gy. > 5 cm, *high grade* → excision w/ periop brachytherapy (BRT) or postop EBRT. > 10 cm, *high grade* → consider preop EBRT tx; complete excision and BRT or EBRT—appropriate chemo: antracyclin a/o ifosfamide.

      i. Currently, ~ 90% of pts are able to undergo limb-sparing surgery, not amputations.

      ii. Compartment resection does not improve survival.

      iii. Reconstruct vessels in thigh. Sacrifice sensory nerves, but not motor if possible.

      iv. In shoulder, popliteal region do amputation or limb salvage + XRT.

v. In hand/feet, do local amputation.

vi. *Viscera*: bowel resection. If incomplete, give postop EBRT-morbid.

vii. *Retroperitoneal/intraabdominal*: bx not indicated for suspicious retroperitoneal mass unless suspect lymphoma or germ-cell tumor, contemplate neoadjuvant tx, dx if suspect unresectable dz, or suspect metastases from another primary. Instead, go directly to excision of mass.

b. *Metastatic dz*: consider metastatectomy on case-by-case basis.

c. *Adjuvant tx*:

i. *Radiotherapy*: preop generally advantageous over postop (smaller field, may reduce intraop seeding, may facilitate dissection). Chief disadvantage is impairment of wound healing (wait 3–6 wk post-XRT to operate); if give XRT postop, also wait 3–6 wk. Usual XRT dose = 50 Gy. If anticipate close margins, consider brachy tx. Consider postop XRT if margins < 1 cm, but should be standard for resectable high-grade sarcoma.

ii. *Chemotherapy*: doxorubicin, anthracycline, ifosfamide, etc., appears to benefit pts w/ large, high-grade tumors.

7. *Surveillance*:

a. F/u w/ physical exams, regional imaging, and CXRs or chest CTs.

b. Resect or amputate local recurrence (56% 5-yr survival).

c. Chemo may be of some benefit for disseminated dz (ifosfamide, adriamycin).

8. *Prognosis*:

a. 56% 5-yr survival overall.

b. Grade most important (> 5–6 mitoses in 30 HPF is *high grade*); extremities better than retroperitoneum. Margins only important for local recurrence. In primary extremity dz overall *low grade* dz → 90% 10-yr survival, *high grade* dz → 55% 10-yr survival.

N. Skin cancers

1. *Melanoma*

a. 3% of skin cancers, 67% skin cancer mortality. Assoc. w/ mutations in p16 (INK4a), CDK4, and B-RAF.

b. *Management*:

AJCC TNM Classification for Melanoma

Primary Tumor (T)	Regional Lymph Nodes (N)	Distant Metastasis (M)
Tx – No evidence of primary or unknown primary	Nx – Minimal requirements to assess regional nodes cannot be met	Mx – Minimal requirements to assess the presence of distant mets cannot be met
T0 – Atypical melanocytic hyperplasia (Clark I), not a malignant lesion	N0 – No regional LN involvement	M0 – No known distal mets
Tis – Melanoma in situ	N1 – Metastasis limited to 1 LN N1a – Clinically occult/microscopic N1b – Clinically evident/macroscopic	M1 – Distant metastasis M1a – to skin, subcutaneous tissue, or distant LN M1b – To lung M1c – To other viscera or any distant metastasis w/ elevated LDH
T1 – < 1 mm thick T1a – No ulceration and mitosis < 1/mm² T1b – W/ ulceration or mitoses ≥ 1/ mm²	N2 – Metastasis in 2–3 regional LN *or* intralymphatic regional metastasis w/out LN metastasis N2a – Microscopic only N2b – Macroscopic (clinically evident) N2c – Satellite or in-transit metastasis, but no LN metastasis	

(Continued)

AJCC TNM Classification for Melanoma (*Continued*)

Primary Tumor (T)	Regional Lymph Nodes (N)	Distant Metastasis (M)
T2 – 1.01–2 mm thick T2a – No ulceration T2b – W/ ulceration	N3 – Metastasis in 4+ regional LN, *or* matted LN, *or* in-transit metastasis/satellite metastasis plus regional LN metastasis	
T3 – 2.01–4 mm thick T3a – No ulceration T3b – W/ ulceration		
T4 – > 4 mm thick T4a – No ulceration T4b – W/ ulceration		

i. *W/u*:
- If palpable LN in region, consider FNA; if inguinal LAD, consider pelvic CT.
- If evidence of regional spread, consider CXR and LDH, PET scan.
- If CNS sx, consider head CT/MRI.

ii. *Wide local excision*:
- *In situ*: 0.5-cm margins (*note*: in situ dz is the only level of melanoma appropriate for Mohs)
- Depth < 1 mm: 1-cm margins
- Depth 1.01–2 mm: 1- to 2-cm margins
- Depth 2.01–4 mm: 2-cm margins
- Depth > 4 mm: 2-cm margins (some advocate 3-cm if able)

iii. *Lymph nodes*:
- *Indications for SLNBx*: stage Ib, II. (Primary cutaneous melanoma w/ Breslow thickness > 1 mm; lesions < 1 mm w/ invasion of reticular dermis to Clark's level IV; poor prognostic indicators [ulceration, regression, lymphovascular space invasion]).
- *Indication for regional lymph node dissection*: regional LN metastasis (established by FNA or SLNBx).
  - Unlike many other cancers (e.g., breast), regional lymphadenectomy may prolong survival in addition to decreasing rate of local recurrence. Adequate numbers of LN for dissection: groin = 10; axilla (level I–III), neck = 15.
  - *Iliac/obturator LN dissection:* indicated if Cloquet's node (+), if pelvic CT or PET (+), or (more controversial) if 3+ superficial groin LN (+).

iv. *Adjuvant tx*:
- *Immunotherapy*:
  - *IL-2*: FDA approved for metastatic dz since 1998; long-term response in only 6%, though.
  - *IFN-α2b*: FDA approved for stage IIb–III dz. May increase dz-free survival in limited subsets of pts; probably appropriate for pts w/ local dz > 4 mm thick or w/ (+) regional LN metastasis.
- *Chemotx*: dacarbazine, temozolomide most frequently used in clinical trials for metastatic dz.
- *Radiation*: consider for stage III pts w/ 4+ LN, particularly in head/neck or if recurrent dz.

v. *Special circumstances*:
- *Ear*: generally requires resection of underlying cartilage and reconstruction.
- *Face*: lymphatic drainage frequently involves parotid; operative surgeon should be prepared for parotidectomy.
- *Trunk*: Sappey's line imperfectly predicts the lymph node drainage. Lymphoscintigraphy should be used to demonstrate drainage pattern.

- *Subungual*: requires amputation of distal phalanx along w/ sufficient dorsal skin to achieve recommended margins; volar skin used to fashion flap. 40% 5-yr survival.
- *Anus*: very poor prognosis. Excision to clear margins is recommended if able to preserve sphincters; otherwise, APR is performed, but the extra morbidity w/ this operation does not improve overall survival.
- *Distant metastasis*: resection of isolated distant metastasis is often appropriate; consider HILP/infusion w/ melphalin for in-transit mets.

    vi. *F/u*:
- Complete hx and physical q 6 mo for several years, then annually.
- CXR, LDH, LFT q 6 mo, depending on circumstances, may be appropriate.

2. *Squamous cell carcinoma* (SCCA)
   a. *Risk factors* include immunosuppression and UVA exposure. Somewhat unique to SCCA (not seen in BCCA, below), is risk of tumor in areas of chronic inflammation (i.e., Marjolin's ulcer).
   b. *Prognosis*:
      i. If < 2 cm in diameter, 5% local recurrence, 7% distant spread
      ii. If > 2 cm in diameter, recurrence doubles, distant spread triples
   c. *Tx*:
      i. *Precursor lesions* (actinic keratosis, etc.): cryotherapy, topical 5-FU, curettage, dermabrasion, CO_2 laser, etc., may be utilized.
      ii. For SCCA, surgical resection preferred, generally w/ 4-mm margins appropriate for tumors < 2 cm in diameter. For tumors > 2 cm in diameter, 10-mm margins may be more appropriate.
      iii. Mohs surgery or XRT may be appropriate around critical structures such as eye, nose, ear, and mouth.
      iv. Regional lymph node involvement merits lymphadenectomy.
      v. Adjuvant XRT if > 1 LN (+), (+) margins, which cannot be resected further, or perineural tumor involvement.

3. *Basal cell carcinoma* (BCCA)
   a. *Risk factors* similar to those for SCCA. Pts w/ Gorlin syndrome (autosomal dominant: multiple BCCAs, odontogenic keratocysts, and palmar/plantar pitting) and nevus sebaceous of Jadassohn also at increased risk.
   b. *Most common skin cancer w/ several variants*:
      i. Nodular—most common form.
      ii. Aggressive variants include morpheaform, infiltrative, and sclerosing—more likely to recur.
   c. *Tx*: same as for squamous cell carcinoma. 10-mm margins should be considered for aggressive variants, regardless of size.

4. *Merkel cell carcinoma*
   a. Aggressive neuroendocrine tumor from pressure receptors; ¼ to ⅓ locally recur, and the same proportion have either regional lymph node spread a/o distant metastasis. Classically encountered on the face of older white males.
   b. Histopathologically difficult to distinguish from small cell lung cancer. Get screening CXR to evaluate for the latter; staining for cytokeratin-20 also helps differentiate from small cell lung cancer.
   c. *Tx*:
      i. WLE w/ 2- to 3-cm margins (or Mohs surgery) recommended.
      ii. SLNBx should be performed unless clinically positive dz prompts lymphadenectomy instead.
      iii. XRT recommended by many if either (+) LN (in addition to lymphadectomy) or if no SLNBx done.

5. *Kaposi's sarcoma*
   a. Spindle-cell malignancy assoc. w/ human herpes virus 8, primarily in immunosuppressed persons, although a variety of clinical and epidemiological forms exist. Most commonly encountered in the skin (almost invariably) or GI tract.
   b. *Tx*: excision (rarely performed), XRT, cryotherapy, or local injection of chemotherapeutic agent. Therapy is generally considered palliative (i.e., for GI hemorrhage).

O. Thymoma (see Chapter 6)

CHAPTER 11

ENDOCRINE

I. THYROID (BENIGN AND NEOPLASIA)

A. Embryology and anatomy

1. *Embryology*: descends from foramen cecum at base of tongue (branchial pouches I and II). Joins ultimobranchial bodies IV and V.

2. *Vascular*:

   a. Inferior thyroid artery arises from thyrocervical trunk, runs close to recurrent laryngeal, and also feeds parathyroids.

   b. Superior thyroid is first branch of external carotid. In minority of persons, an ima thyroidea arises from aortic arch.

   c. Superior, middle, and inferior thyroid veins drain into internal jugular.

3. *Nerves*:

   a. Internal branch of sup. laryngeal nerve provides sensation to larynx.

   b. External branch of sup. laryngeal nerve gives motor supply to tense larynx.

   c. Recurrent laryngeal inn. all other muscles of larynx.

B. Physiology

1. *Thyroid-stimulating hormone* (TSH) secreted by anterior pituitary, stimulates thyroid growth, uptake and organification of iodine, and releases of T_3 and T_4 from thyroglobulin.

   a. TSH release prompted by $\uparrow$ hypothalamic thyrotropin-releasing hormone (TRH) a/o $\downarrow T_3$.

   b. Catecholamines and ß-hCG also stimulate thyroid function.

   c. TSH $\downarrow$ by (−) from $\uparrow T_3$ and T_4. Glucocorticoids, prolonged starvation also $\downarrow$ thyroid function.

   d. *Wolff–Chaikoff effect*: transient $\uparrow$ in iodine organification followed by $\downarrow$ thyroid activity in response to large doses of iodine.

2. *Follicular cells*:

   a. Predominant thyroid cell type. Traps iodine by complexing w/ tyrosine to form monoiodotyrosine (MIT) or diiodotyrosine (DIT), stored intracellularly to thyroglobulin.

   b. *In periphery*:

      i. $T_3 \uparrow\uparrow$ biologically active than T_4, binding directly to nuclear receptors.

      ii. Majority of peripheral T_3 derived from T_4 peripherally.

      • Conversion $\downarrow$ by certain drugs (corticosteroids, propranolol, PTU) and clinical states (sepsis, brain death?) → clinical hypothyroidism.

      iii. Half-life of $T_3 \sim 10$ h. Half-life of $T_4 \sim 7$ d. Body usu. has > 1 wk worth of biologically active hormone in periphery.

      iv. Thyroxine-binding globulin (TBG) transports ~ 80% of thyroid hormones. Hormones unable to act on cells while bound.

      • During pregnancy (hyperestrogenemia), TBG levels $\uparrow$, leading to $\uparrow$ plasma *bound* T_4. As *free* T_4 is unchanged, pt remains clinically euthyroid.

3. *Pharmacology*:

   a. *Thioamides*: inhibit organification of iodine and oxidation to MIT/DIT. *Risks*: agranulocytosis (< 1%), hepatic dysfunction, rash, and arthralgias.

      i. *Methimazole* (Tapazole)

      • *Advantage*: once daily dosing.

      • *Disadvantage*: crosses placenta, contraindicated in pregnancy.

      ii. *Propylthiouracil* (PTU):

      • *Advantage*: additional action of inhibiting peripheral conversion of T_4 to T_3; useful for more rapid control of hyperthyroid sx vs methimazole.

    b. *Lugol's solution*: high concentration of inorganic iodine. Helps control vascularity of thyroid, preparing Graves' pts for surgery.

    c. *Corticosteroids*: ↓ peripheral conversion of T_4 to T_3 (like PTU and beta antagonists).

    d. *Beta antagonists*: ↓ end-organ manifestations of thyrotoxicosis (HTN, tachycardia, tremor). Additionally, propanolol ↓ peripheral conversion of T_4 to T_3 (like PTU and corticosteroids).

4. *Laboratory assessment of follicular physiology*:

    a. *TSH*: most sensitive assay of thyroid function, gen. reflecting pathology before sx.

    b. *Total T_4*: affected by levels of serum protein, which bind much of the T_4

    c. *Free T_4 index*: serum free T_4 difficult to measure directly, so the index is calculated using the levels of total T_4 (above) and the T_3 resin uptake test (below).

    d. *T_3 resin uptake test* (indirectly measures free T_4): low levels of available (measured) T_3 indicate low levels of free T_4 (means lots of binding sites were unoccupied by T_4, thus available to bind T_3). Conversely, high levels of measured (free, available) T_3 indicate large levels of T_4 (occupying binding sites, making the T_3 free to be measured).

    e. *Radioactive iodine uptake* (RAIU): used to distinguish hyperthyroidism (low TSH and increased RAIU) from subacute thyroiditis (low TSH and low RAIU).

    f. *Thyroid autoantibodies*

        i. *Thyroid antimicrosomal antibodies*: Hashimoto's dz, Graves' dz

        ii. *Antibodies to TSH receptor*: Graves' dz

        iii. *Thyroglobulin antibodies*: assoc. w/ Hashimoto's dz

    g. *Thyroglobulin*: synthesized by follicular cells. Useful for surveillance in pts after thyroid ablation for cancer.

5. *C cells*:

    a. Neural crest cells that migrate into superolateral areas of thyroid during development.

    b. Produce calcitonin, which inhibits osteoclast liberation of calcium from bone (effect = decrease calcium level, though effects often not clinically significant). Calcitonin release stimulated by hypercalcemia, alcohol, a/o pentagastrin.

    c. May transform into medullary thyroid carcinoma. Elevated risk MEN IIa, IIb. Serum marker = calcitonin, not thyroglobulin

C. Benign disease

1. *Graves' dz*: indications for surgery → contraindication to RAI (pregnant, child) or question of CA.

    a. *Presentation*: hyperthyroid sx such as tachycardia, weakness, and tremors may be present along with, classically, proptosis.

    b. *Dx*: Circulating TSH low, serum T_4 a/o T_3 elevated, along w/ FTI, thyroid radioactive iodine uptake. Often diffuse goiter, exophthalmos, and high titers of thyroid antibodies.

    c. *Tx*:

        i. *Antithyroid meds*: best for pts who are young, pregnant, or lactating.

        ii. *Radioactive iodine*: for older pts w/out above concerns, pts w/ toxic multinodular goiter.

        iii. *Surgery* (subtotal thyroidectomy): for children/young adults w/ severe dz or those who want rapid response; also if unable to exclude cancer, or for tx of endemic goiter or hyperfunctioning adenoma.

2. *Goiter*: "Endemic form" from iodine deficiency, in 12% of world's population, rare in United States. 3–4% of United States population has goiter, usu. from multinodular goiter.

    a. Physical exam, TSH, T_4 levels.

    b. FNA bx should be procured on single, dominant, or particularly large nodules.

        i. 20% of "indeterminate" are actually malignant, whereas "benign" readings have only 1–2% false negative rate.

        ii. If h/o neck irradiation, forego FNA; 40% will have malignancy, w/ less than half in the most suspicious nodule. For the same reason, forego FNA if family hx of thyroid cancer. Substernal goiters should not be assayed w/ FNA.

    c. *Tx*:

        i. *Medical*:

- TSH suppression w/ thyroxine does not predictably decrease goiter size, may actually induce hyperthyroidism. Only considered for young pts (less risk of arrythmias and osteoporosis) w/ small goiters who desire nonoperative management.
- Radioactive iodine more effective than TSH suppression, may induce hyperthyroidism in ~ 5%. Hypothyroidism in ~ 1/4 after tx. Respiratory embarrassment may worsen w/ RAI. Best for pts too ill to have surgery. Exception: substernal goiter—always operate due to airway concerns. addressed surgically because of airway concerns.

   ii. *Surgical*:

- For enlarging/large, symptomatic (respiratory compromise, dysphagia, SVC obstruction), or substernal goiters. Also if FNA → malignancy concerns, or pt has cosmetic concerns.
- Total or subtotal thyroidectomy considered, may be pursued, depending on size, symmetry, pt desire regarding supplemental exogenous thyroxine vs risk of recurrence.

3. *Thyroiditis*

   a. *Hashimoto's* (chronic lymphocytic; autoimmune): most common cause of hypothyroidism, although euthyroid state or even thyrotoxicosis may be transiently present. 15× common in women. Thyroid usu. enlarged, may be tender. Histopath: Askanazy cells, lymphocytic infiltrate. *Dx:* ↑ serum thyroid Ab titers. ↑ risk lymphoma. No tx necessary if euthyroid and no goiter. If enlarged (non-nodular) and no compressive sx, suppressive medications OK. Surgery (subtotal thyroidectomy) indicated for compressive sx; to r/o malignancy; cosmesis.

   b. *Suppurative*: rare, may follow URI in children. Often fever, dysphagia, neck pain. *Tx:* I&D. Recurrent cases should be evaluated w/ barium swallow to r/o piriform sinus fistula.

   c. *Riedel's* (struma): hard, w/ fibrosis. Assoc. w/ sclerosing cholangitis, retroperitoneal fibrosis. Bx to r/o anaplastic carcinoma. Usu. hypothyroid. Surgery poss. needed to decompress trachea.

   d. *Subacute* (deQuervain's; granulomatous): usu. young women, +/− assoc. w/ recent viral illness. Often fever, palpitation, asthenia, malaise, wt loss, thyroid swelling. May mimic Graves' dz. *Labs:* ↑ ESR and serum gamma-globulin w/ ↓ RAIU, but normal; elevated thyroid hormone levels. Often resolves spontaneously; relief poss. accelerated w/ ASA a/o corticosteroids.

D. Neoplastic disease

1. *General*:

   a. Best prognostic indicator for mortality age > 40–50 yo. *Other concerning factors*: very young age (< 15 yo), fam h/o thyroid CA or MEN II syndrome (other familial hx syndromes such as FAP, Gardner's, or Cowden's, increase risk as well), hx of head/neck irradiation, large (> 4 cm) nodule, or U/S findings of irregular border or microcalcifications.

   b. W/u should include neck U/S w/ FNA.

   c. Invasive thyroid carcinoma of any size usu. tx'd w/ total/near-total thyroidectomy.

   d. *Complications* (rates for experienced endocrine surgeons):

      i. *Recurrent laryngeal nerve damage* (persistent): ~ 3% after total, ~ 2% after subtotal thyroidectomy.

      ii. *Hypoparathyroidism*: ~ 2.5% after total, < 0.5% after subtotal thyroidectomy.

      iii. *Hypothyroidism*: note, performing "only" a lobectomy may still result in hypothyroidism; pts should be counseled on this preop.

2. *Papillary*:

   a. 80% of thyroid cancers, gen. best prognosis. Type most assoc. w/ h/o head/neck irradiation.

   b. *Pathology*: concentric calcifications in psammoma bodies. Often multicentric. Mets usu. via lymphatics.

   c. *Tx*:

      i. Total thyroidectomy usual. Mod rad neck dissection (and level VI/central neck dissection as thyroid cancer usu. spreads here first) if clinically (+) nodes.

      ii. Lobectomy + isthmusectomy may be done in *absence* of the following: size ≥ 1 cm; fam h/o of thyroid CA; personal h/o of head/neck irradiation; clinically or histologically (+) lymph nodes; (+) margins; grossly multifocal dz; aggressive variant of papillary cancer (i.e., columnar cell, tall cell, oxyphilic, insular, or poorly differentiated).

3. *Follicular*:
   a. Unlike other thyroid neoplasms, malignancy cannot be determined w/ FNA; 80% of "follicular neoplasms" from FNA turn out to be benign.
   b. Unlike other thyroid neoplasms, metastasizes primarily hematogenously, not via lymphatics. Usu. metastasizes to bone.
   c. *Tx*: If FNA dx of follicular neoplasm and no evidence of metastasis, thyroid lobectomy and waiting for final path is reasonable (if pt willing to undergo poss. 2nd operation). Completion thyroid done if path = malignancy.

4. *Hürthle cell* (oxyphilic cell carcinoma):
   a. Usu. considered a follicular variant, but more commonly spreads to LN, concentrates iodine less well, and slightly worse prognosis than standard follicular carcinoma.
   b. *Tx*: similar for follicular carcinoma.

5. *Medullary*:
   a. From Clara, or "C," cells, secrete calcitonin. 80% sporadic, but may be familial, or assoc. w/ MEN II (latter 2 both assoc. w/ RET proto-oncogene). May have flushing, diarrhea (similar to carcinoid syndrome) a/o Cushing's syndrome. Metastasizes to LNs (stage IV if outside level VI), bone, lung, and liver.
   b. *Preop*:
      i. Calcium or pentagastrin stimulation can sometimes detect occult tumor.
      ii. Baseline serum markers of calcitonin, CEA.
      iii. For RET proto-oncogene (+) pts, r/o hyperparathyroidism, pheochromocytoma.
   c. *Operative*:
      i. Total thyroidectomy and central neck dissection for all pts w/ MTC.
      ii. Consider additional dissection (levels II–V) if tumor > 1 cm (or 0.5 cm in MEN IIb pts) or (+) LN metastasis in level VI.
   d. *Postop*:
      i. Does not uptake iodine; follow w/ calcitonin levels.
      ii. Adjuvant XRT not useful, but chemotx may be considered in palliative setting.

6. *Anaplastic*:
   a. Least common, uniformly lethal. Mean age at dx older (65 yo) than other thyroid cancers. Assoc. w/ p53 mutation. Stage IV by definition. At dx, up to half have metastasized (usu. lung), most are locally unresectable. Death frequently (~ ½) from airway compromise. Median survival ~ 6 mo.
   b. *Tx*:
      i. If CXR and CT scans suggest resectable dz, total thyroidectomy and selective LN dissection are appropriate for local control.
      ii. For unresectable tumor (majority), consider prophylactic tracheostomy.
      iii. Postop, pt should be referred for adjunctive care (i.e., combination hyperfractionated XRT and doxorubicin).

7. *Lymphoma*:
   a. More common after Hashimoto's thyroiditis.
   b. *Tx*: CHOP +/– thyroidectomy.

8. *Metastatic*:
   a. Renal cell CA followed by breast CA most common source of metastasis.
   b. MACIS (**M**etastasis, **A**ge, **C**ompleteless of Resection, **I**nvasion, **S**ize) score < 6 = 20-yr survival of 99%; > 8 = 20-yr survival < 25%.

E. **Thyroid nodules** [from *Consensus Statement of Diagnosis, Treatment, and Surveillance of Patients with Differentiated Thyroid Cancer*, 16 Jul 04]
   1. *W/u*: U/S and FNA (need 2 slides w/ 6 clusters w/ 10+ cells each) should be employed. Scintigraphic scans unnecessary.

2. *Therapy*:
   a. *Operative*: differentiated thyroid carcinoma gen. an indication for complete thyroidectomy w/ compartmental nodal dissection.
   b. *Adjuvant*: check TSH and TG 3 wks postop. TSH > 30 required to benefit from I-131 ablation; all Hürthle cell carcinomas should be ablated. Pt should follow low-iodine diet for 2 wk prior to ablation. Synthroid is begun the day following ablation, then baseline total body scan 1 wk after ablation.

3. *Surveillance*: protocol depends if low or high risk.
   a. *Low risk*: near total thyroidectomy and I-131 ablation; no clinical evidence of tumor; TG < 1 ng/mL on Synthroid; tumor < 4 cm, not of virulent subtype, no evidence of distant metastases; stage I and < 45 yo or stage II and > 45 yo; MACIS score < 6.
   b. *6-mo f/u: low risk*—stimulated TG (rTSH or off Synthroid), no I-131.
      i. If TG > 2 ng/mL, U/S of neck w/ bx if abnormality seen.
      ii. If bulky dz present, repeat surgery, followed by I-131 ablation.
      iii. If U/S negative, repeat I-131 ablation.
   c. *6-mo f/u: high risk*—Synthroid withdrawal w/ TG measurement.
      i. If TG > 2 ng/mL or significant rise from suppressed level → U/S neck w/ bx if abnormality seen.
      ii. If bulky dz present, repeat surgery, followed by I-131 ablation.
      iii. If U/S negative, repeat I-131 ablation.
   d. *12-mo f/u*:
      i. *If negative 6-mo evaluation*:
         • No scans, keep TSH suppressed and reevaluate at 12 mo.
      ii. *If positive 6-mo evaluation*:
         • Stimulated TG (rTSH or off Synthroid), no I-131 scan.
         • If TG > 2 ng/mL, U/S neck w/ bx if abnormality seen.
         • If bulky dz present, repeat surgery, followed by I-131 ablation.
         • If U/S negative, repeat I-131 ablation.
   e. *Ongoing f/u*: Low risk w/ 2 negative f/u evals → annual suppressed TG; follow low but (+) TG. High risk w/ 2 negative f/u evals → annual suppressed TG; if TG > 2 ng/mL, obtain stimulated TG to see if there is further rise.
   f. *If suspect residual or recurrent dz*, pursue 1 tx w/ I-131, and if negative postablation, regard tumor now as "I-negative." Consider further eval w/ FDG PET under elevated TSH condition (rTSH or off Synthroid).

II. PARATHYROID

A. Embryology, anatomy, and physiology

1. *Embryology*: Superior thyroids from 4th branchial pouch, and counterintuitively, the inferior parathyroids arise from the 3rd branchial pouch, and migrate caudally w/ the thymus, less constant in ultimate location.

2. *Anatomy*:
   a. Superior parathyroids usu. posterior to recurrent laryngeal nerve; inferior parathyroids are anterior to nerve.
   b. Blood supply generally from inferior thyroid artery of thyrocervical trunk.
      i. Unilateral adenomas feeding artery may be larger than contralateral, and useful for locating the gland.
   c. *Supernumerary glands*:
      i. 85% of pts have 4 glands. 10–15% of pts have supernumary glands. Most often in thyroid or thymus.

3. *Physiology*:
   a. *Parathyroid hormone*:
      i. Secreted by parathyroid chief cells in response to hypocalcemia levels.
      ii. In *bone*, stimulate osteoclasts and inhibit osteoblasts.

iii. In the *kidney*:
- Increases distal nephron reabsorption of calcium.
- Decreases proximal renal tubule resorption of bicarbonate, increasing chloride resorption.
  - *Chloride* : phosphorus ratio > 33 suggestive of hyperparathryoidism.

iv. In the *gut*, PTH works indirectly through 1,25 dihydroxy vitamin D (PTH stimulates its hydroxylation from 25-hydroxy vitamin D in the kidney), promoting gut absorption of Ca, phosphorus.

b. *Vitamin D*
i. D_3 (cholecalciferol): from UV-mediated activation of 7-dehydrocholesterol in skin and subsequently undergoes up to 2 hydroxylations:
- *Liver* (first): to 25-hydroxycholecalciferol.
- *Kidney* (second): to 1,25-dihydroxycholecalciferol.

ii. D_2 (ergocalciferol): most common form in foods.

c. *Calcitonin*: secreted by parafollicular cells; elevated in pts w/ medullary thyroid cancer. Stimulates calcium deposition in bone (net effect to decrease serum calcium levels), but is less clinically significant than PTH.

B. **Hyperparathyroidism**
1. *Primary*: elevated parathyroid hormone not caused by stimuli such as low serum calcium (i.e., parathyroid adenoma, hyperplasia, carcinoma).
2. *Secondary*: elevated parathyroid hormone in response to appropriate stimuli (i.e., low serum calcium).
3. *Tertiary*: persistence of elevated parathyroid hormone after initial stimuli have been removed. Often assoc. w/ renal transplantation.

C. **Localization:** Sestamibi and U/S useful for localization, pre- and intraop, respectively. Look for hidden *superior* parathyroid glands in tracheoesophageal groove along carotid sheath. Look for hidden *inferior* parathyroid glands in thymus.

D. **Surgery** (indicated if dx made as estimated long-term complications of asymptomatic dz ~ 20%)
1. *Adenoma* (80%): excise, bx at least 1–2 other glands.
2. *Hyperplasia* (15%—seen w/ MEN I, MEN IIa): remove 3.5 glands (or all, w/ reimplantation of 0.5 in forearm).
3. *Carcinoma* (5%): en bloc resection w/ thyroid lobe, regional lymphadenectomy
4. *Intraop key that offending gland has been removed*: decrease in rapid PTH assay.
5. *Calciphylaxis may also be indication*:
   a. Results from dermal arteriolar calcification and patchy skin necrosis.
   b. Dx based on hx, exam, and calcium × phosphorus product ≥ 70.
   c. Skin lesions fail to heal skin grafts—most often amputation and 3.5 gland parathyroidectomy w/ 0.5 gland reimplant indicated.
6. When removing parathyroid for primarily parathyroid problem, if need to reimplant, do so in arm. If removing for other reason (i.e., vascular compromise from thyroidectomy), implant in SCM.

E. **Hypoparathyroidism**
1. Almost always from surgical removal of glands (i.e., thyroidectomy complication); sx from hypocalcemia, though hyperphosphatemia common as well.
2. *Tx*:
   a. Usu. hypoparathyroidism after thyroidectomy is transient (1–3 wk).
   b. *If pt has tetany*:
      i. Ensure adequate airway protection.
      ii. Calcium gluconate IV bolus (10–20 mL of 10% solution), then gtt 1 mL/kg/h (using 50 mL of 10% calcium gluconate in 500 mL of D_5W).
      iii. If refractory, check Mg. If low, give $MgSO_4$, 2–4 g/d IV.
   c. *Asymptomatic low-ionized calcium level*:

      i. Oral calcium, such as CitraCal (400 mg PO two to four times per day).

      ii. Add vitamin D (1,25 dihydroxycholecalciferol), 25,000–200,000 IU/d, if need to give above more frequently than two times per day.

      iii. Low-phosphorus diet (eliminate dairy, consider adding aluminum hydroxide gel).

III. PITUITARY

A. Embryology and vasculature

1. *Regions*:

    a. *Hypothalamus*: releases TRH, GHRH, GnRH, CRH into median eminence, through neurohypophysis to adenohypophysis.

    b. *Posterior pituitary* (neurohypophysis): releases:

      i. ADH in supraoptic nucei, regulated by osmolar receptors in hypothalamus (effects, mechanism).

      ii. Oxytocin in paraventricular nuclei in hypothalamus (effects, mechanism?).

    c. *Anterior pituituary*: ACTH, GH, LH, FSH, TSH, prolactin.

B. Specific tumors

1. *Prolactinomas*

    a. *Dopamine*: inhibits prolactin secretion (bromocriptine effect).

      i. *Bromocriptine*: for prolactinomas, possibly for TSH-, FSH/LH-secreting tumors

2. *Acromegaly* (growth hormone tumor)

3. *Nonfunctional tumors*: can cause *decrease* in adenohypophyseal hormones and mass effect such as bitemporal hemianopsia

C. Syndromes:

1. *Sheehan's syndrome*: postpartum infarction and necrosis of pituitary (etiology thought in part to be due from pituitary ischemia from obstetric hemorrhage a/o DIC). Sx (lactational failure, amenorrhea, adrenal insufficiency, hypothyroidism, etc.) may present soon after delivery or up to 20 yr postpartum. Certain aspects (i.e., gonadotropic) of pituitary function may be relatively spared. DI occurs in ~ 1% of cases.

IV. ADRENAL (BENIGN AND NEOPLASIA)

A. Embryology and vasculature: adrenal cortex develops from mesoderm whereas medulla is of neuroendocrine origin. Arterial supply from inferior phrenic, aorta, and renal arteries. Venous drainage on right directly into IVC via multiple short veins, venous drainage on left into renal vein.

B. Adrenal insufficiency and perioperative management

1. To prevent, hydrocortisone 100 mg IV on induction, and q 8 h to total of 3 doses.

C. Syndromes:

1. *Cushing's syndrome* (hypercortisolism):

    a. Most often from exogenous cortisol intake, followed by pituitary ACTH adenoma (Cushing's dz). Ectopic causes include medullary thyroid CA, thymomas, lung CA.

    b. *W/u*:

      i. *1st*:

- Draw 24-h urine free cortisol.
- Abstain from alcohol for 2 mo prior if possible.
- Good to exclude hypercortisolism from depression, obesity.

      ii. *2nd*:

- Get *low*-dose overnight dexamethasone suppression test; negative-feedback on pituitary.
- 1 mg dexamethasone at 2300, check plasma cortisol at 0800.
- Normal pts will suppress cortisol to < 3–5 mcg/100 cc; Cushing's pts will usu. not suppress.
- False (+) possible w/ obesity, alcoholic, phenytoin, rifampin, estrogens, tamoxifen.
- If still unsure, can confirm w/ CRH/dexamethasone suppression test.

- Good for partially suppressible pituitary adenomas and nonsuppressible ectopic/adrenal lesions.
- 0.5 mg dexamethasone q 6 h × 48 h, then 0800 bolus of CRH. Check cortisol at 15 min; 1.4 mcg/100 cc diagnostic for Cushing's syndrome.
- If does suppress, then problem is from excess ACTH (pituitary) = Cushing's dz = most common noniatrogenic cause.
- If does not suppress, then either have nonsuppressed pituitary or nonpituitary cause; go to next step.

iii. *3rd*:
- Get serum ACTH.
- Normal = 10–100 pg/cc. If < 5, nearly pathognomonic for primary adrenal d/o.
- If low, then primary adrenal problem (adenoma, hyperplasia, carcinoma).
- If high, from pituitary (Cushing's dz—usu. 15–500) or ectopic source—often > 1000—go to next step (high-dose dexamethasone test).

iv. *4th*:
- If serum ACTH high, get *high*-dose overnight dexamethasone suppression test.
- 2 mg dexamethasone PO q 6 h × 48 h, w/ 24-h urine for free cortisol and and 17-OH steroids on second day. Also, can simply give 8 mg at 2400.
- Cortisol will suppress if due to pituitary adenoma but not if from primary adrenal problem or ectopic ACTH source.
- If suppresses, means pituitary source.
- If doesn't suppress, means ectopic ACTH is problem. If still equivocal, go to CRH test.

v. *5th*:
- Get CRH test.
- 1 mcg/kg ovine CRH given over 30 sec, then check plasma ACTH and cortisol q 15 min for 1 h.
- If ACTH-independent, peak ACTH response will be < 10 pg/cc.
- If ACTH-dependent, peak ACTH response > 30 pg/cc.
- More useful perhaps is that w/ Cushing's dz, ACTH should increase > 35% whereas ectopic ACTH-producers rarely demonstrate any rise.
- If ACTH increases, then pituitary adenoma.
- If ACTH doesn't change, then ectopic ACTH producer.

vi. *Note*: MIR and NP-59 scintigraphy can localize adrenal tumors, differentiating from hyperplasia.

c. *Etiology* (after exogenous administration)
   i. Cushing's dz (pituitary adenoma) 68%, ectopic ACTH 12%, adrenal adenoma 10%, adrenal carcinoma 8%, adrenal cortical hyperplasia 1%, ectopic CRH < 1%, alcoholism < 1%. [Orth, DN. *N Engl J Med* 1995;332:791–803.]
   ii. *Cushing's dz*: tx w/ transsphenoidal resection +/− XRT.
   iii. *Adrenal adenoma*: adrenalectomy (if < 6 cm, can do posterior approach or laparoscopically) open anterior approach if > 6 cm or suspect carcinoma.
   iv. *Adrenal carcinoma*: suggested by rapid progression of sx, wt gain, *virilization*, and elevated urinary 17-ketosteroids and plasma DHEA sulfate. Differentiation from CAH by presence of hypercortisolism.
   - Only 50% produce hypercortisolism/Cushing's.
   - MRI T-2 adrenal-to-liver ratio helpful:
     - *Adenomas* 0.7–1.4
     - *Carcinoma* (including metastatic dz) 1.4–3.0
     - *Pheochromocytoma* > 3.0
   v. *Hyperplasia*: bilateral adrenalectomy (medical tx not first choice).
   vi. *Pediatric*: most often adrenocortical neoplasia (adenoma vs carcinoma).

- Both carcinoma and congenital adrenal hyperplasia may cause virilization; latter typically assoc. w/ hypotension and hyperkalemia, however. See Chapter 18.
- If < 15 yo, usu. malignant.
- *Tx*: adrenalectomy.

2. *Addison's disease* (hypocortisolism)
   a. *Sx*:
      i. *Chronic*: hyperpigmentation (most noticeable in non-sun-exposed areas), orthostatic hypotension.
      ii. *Acute* (Addisonian crisis): hypotension, abdominal pain, N/V, fever, lethargy, hyperkalemia, hypoglycemia, altered MS, possible seizures, metabolic acidosis.
   b. Critically ill pts may be relatively cortisol-insufficient. Consider stress-dose hydrocortisone.
      i. *UCSF protocol*: check baseline cortisol, then give 0.25 mg cosyntropin, then wait 45 min and draw another cortisol. Normal if either test > 20 or if increase > 7.
   c. *Etiology*:
      i. *Most often autoimmune* (may be assoc. w/ vitiligo, type I DM, Hashimoto's thyroiditis, etc., in autoimmune polyendocrine syndrome; Addison's + Hashimoto's referred to as Schmidt syndrome).
      ii. *Hemorrhage* (e.g., Waterhouse-Friedrichsen syndrome), infection (adrenal TB).

3. *Conn's syndrome* (primary hyperaldosteronism)
   a. Classically high Na, low K, but 20% w/ normal K.
   b. *Check renin level*: "Primary" = decreased renin. "Secondary" = elevated renin.
   c. *Etiology*: aldosterone-producing adenoma >> bilateral adrenal hyperplasia >> adrenal carcinoma (secondary causes include renal artery stenosis, CHF, cirrhosis, pregnancy).
   d. Suspect if diastolic HTN + K < 3.5 (< 3.0 if on diuretic).
   e. Check 24-h urine K and upright PRA and PAC.
   f. *Screening (+) if 2 of 3*:
      i. Spontaneous hypokalemia w/ inappropriate kaliuresis (> 30 mEq/d).
      ii. Plasma renin activity (PRA) < 3.0 ng/cc/h.
      iii. Plasma aldosterone concentration : plasma renin concentration ratio > 20.
   g. *Confirmation*
      i. Supplement w/ KCl.
      ii. High Na diet for 5 d, then . . .
      iii. Check 24-h urine aldosterone, Na, cortisol and upright PRA, serum K.
      iv. If elevated aldosterone, dx of primary hyperaldosteronism confirmed.
      v. Venous sampling, look for aldosterone : cortisol > 4:1.
   h. *Source of primary aldosteronism*:
      i. First get adrenal CT or MRI.
         - Unilateral mass > 1 cm → dx = adenoma → unilateral adrenalectomy (give spironolactone, K preop).
         - Otherwise, can get posture studies.
            - If fall in aldosterone and 18-OH > 100 ng/gl → APA, consider to localize:
               - Iodocholesterol (NP-59)
               - Adrenal venous sampling
               - Dexamethasone suppression
            - In general, bilateral adrenalectomy for adenomas is not performed, as resulting adrenal insufficiency is difficult to tx.
      ii. Idiopathic dz tx'd w/ spironolactone, triamterene, amiloride, or nifedipine.

4. *Incidentalomas*
   a. *Indications for resection*:

   i. Diameter > 4 cm.

   ii. Elevated 24-h urine free cortisol +/– (+) low-dose dexamethasone suppression test.

   iii. *Elevated aldosterone* : renin ratio.

   iv. Elevated urine *or* plasma metanephrines.

   v. Noncontrast CT w/ > 10 Hounsfield units *and* . . .

   - Delayed enhanced CT w/ < 50% contrast washout at 15 min *or* . . .
   - Chemical shift MRI w/ no signal drop on out-of-phase MRI.

   vi. Significant interval growth.

5. *Pheochromocytoma*

   a. *Pathology*:

      i. Derived from neural crest cells. Produce epinephrine *and* norepinephrine. Epinephrine-producing cells are located near adrenal cortex, dependent on cortisol for norepi → epi conversion. Extraadrenal pheochromocytomas usu. do not secrete epinephrine.

      ii. May be assoc. w/ MEN IIa, IIb (check calcium, calcitonin in addition to metanephrines); von Recklinghausen's dz (neurofibromatosis); Bourneville's dz (tuberous sclerosis); Sturge-Weber (meningofacial angiomatosis); von Hippel-Lindau (hemangioblastomas in retina, CNS, +/– renal cell CA).

      iii. Extraadrenal pheochromocytomas are referred to as paragangliomas. Typically along aorta and iliac bifurcation along sympathetic chain; rarely in bladder, causing hypertensive crises w/ micturation. Often multicentric, malignant in ~ 50%, more common in children, may be assoc. w/ the dz's above as well as Carney's triad (gastric epithelioid, pulmonary chondroma, paraganglioma). Cervical chemodectomas rarely functional, usu. (–) for chromaffin staining.

      iv. Malignancy is based on behavior, not histology.

      v. *Related tumors*:

         - *Neuroblastoma*: immature derivative of sympathoadrenal tissue, see Chapter 18.
         - *Ganglioneuroblastoma*: from immature ganglia cells.

   b. *Dx*:

      i. *T2-weighted MRI*: suspicious mass > liver ratio > 3 (< 1.4 = adenoma; 1.4–3 = carcinoma).

      ii. Clonidine will not suppress catecholamines < 500 pg/mL after 3 h w/ pheo.

   c. *Localization*:

      i. T2-weighted MRI have unique high-intensity signal.

      ii. [131]Iodine or ^{123}I-tagged metaiodobenzylguanidine (MIBG) may be used, but requires preparation w/ Lugol's solution.

   d. *Tx*:

      i. Surgery indicated for all; laparoscopic approach increasingly accepted.

      ii. Control venous drainage first, minimize handling of gland.

      iii. Preop prep w/ alpha blocker (phenoxybenzamine) indicated for all, followed by addition of beta blocker if tachycardic. Ensure pt appropriately fluid-loaded before OR. Phentolamine useful intraop IV alpha blocker.

6. *Congenital adrenal hyperplasia (CAH):* see Chapter 18.

7. *Nelson's syndrome*

   a. Rapid enlargement of pituitary adenoma.

   b. 10% of postbilateral adrenalectomy.

   c. Visual disturbances, elevated ACTH, hyperpigmentation.

   d. Tx w/ surgery or irradiation although results frequently disappointing.

CHAPTER 12

PROXIMAL GI AND ACUTE ABDOMEN

I. STOMACH

A. Anatomy and physiology

1. *Vasculature*:

   a. *Arterial*: celiac axis perfuses left and right gastric a.'s (latter comes from hepatic a.), as well as left (from splenic a.) and right (from gastroduodenal a.) gastroepiploic a.'s, which also contributes to short gastric a.'s. Most common anomaly is aberrant left hepatic a. originating from the left gastric a. (instead of the proper hepatic a.); thus proximal division of left gastric a. could potentially lead to left hepatic ischemia.

   b. *Venous*: right gastric and left gastric (coronary) veins drain into portal vein, and left gastroepiploic vein drains into splenic vein (which empties into portal vein). All other venous drainage nonportal.

2. *Vagus nerve anatomy and physiology*:

   a. *Anatomy*:

      i. *Anterior* (left) vagus gives early hepatic branch to supply liver, gallbladder, and duodenum. Main trunk of anterior vagus runs parallel to lesser curve of stomach approximately 1 cm into lesser omentum w/ branches going directly into stomach wall. At incisura, main trunk divides into smaller branches, which supply antrum and pylorus.

      ii. *Posterior* (right) vagus is larger and lies posterior and to right of esophagus in fatty tissue. Branches run to celiac axis and often to stomach fundus (this latter branch may arise in the thorax and is liable to be missed during vagotomy). Has variable position; may lie adjacent to esophagus or the anterior surface of aorta, or in between. Can palpate the lesser curve at the left gastric artery and apply caudal pressure to produce a "bowstring" effect of the nerve. Complete vagotomy hinges on division proximal to hepatic and celiac branches.

   b. *Physiology*: see section F. below on postvagotomy syndromes.

3. *Regions*:

   a. *Cardia*: Glandular elements predominantly secrete mucus.

   b. *Fundus and body*: contain *parietal cells (chief cells)*, which produce intrinsic factor (necessary for B_{12} absorption in small intestine), hydrochloric acid, and pepsinogen. Angle of His relates the fundus to the left esophagus. *Angularis incisura* relates the body to the antrum.

   c. *Antrum*: Contains *G cells* which make gastrin as well as *D cells*, which produce somatostatin.

B. Peptic ulcer disease (gastric)

1. 10% in United States harbor cancer. 85% colonized w/ *H. pylori*. Surgery reserved for cases refractory to medical therapy (3–6 mo), obstruction, hemorrhage, or perforation. Divided into 5 types: overall 10% represent malignancy. Risk ~ 5% if under 1 cm.

2. *Helicobacter pylori*:

   a. *Medication options*:

      i. H_2 blocker or PPI × 2 wk PLUS

      ii. Bismuth subsalicylate 525 mg PO four times per day × 2 wk PLUS

      iii. Metronidazole 250 mg PO four times per day × 2 wk PLUS

      iv. Tetracycline 500 mg PO four times per day × 2 wk

      v. *Note*: alternate abx include combination of clarithromycin 500 mg PO two times per day and 1 of the following: tetracycline *or* metronidazole *or* amoxicillin 1000 mg PO two times per day [Howden CS, Hunt RH. *AJG* 1998;93:2336.]

   b. *Type I*: lesser curvature, near incisura, *not* assoc. w/ high acid levels (many hypochlorhydric), assoc. w/ blood group A. Small, punched-out lesions, account for 60% of all gastric ulcers.

      i. *Tx*: distal gastrectomy (including ulcer) w/ Billroth I is primary. Billroth II is an acceptable alternative. Mortality ~ 3%, recurrence ~ 3%. Ulcer excision w/ highly selective or parietal cell vagotomy sometimes performed w/ mortality ~ 1%, but recurrence 5–25%.

   c. *Type II*: combination of duodenal and gastric (usu. near incisura) *are* assoc. w/ high acid levels, assoc. w/ blood group O. Account for ~ 25% of gastric ulcers.

      i. *Tx*: truncal vagotomy and antrectomy (including the ulcer), B-I preferred, but B-II acceptable reconstruction. Mortality 2%, recurrence 2%. Highly selective vagotomy w/ ulcer excision meets w/ recurrence 25%.

   d. *Type III*: prepyloric (may be multiple and usu. w/in 2–3 cm of pylorus) *are* assoc. w/ high acid levels. 15% of gastric ulcers.

      i. *Tx*: truncal vagotomy and antrectomy (including the ulcer), B-I preferred, but B-II acceptable reconstruction. Mortality 2%, recurrence 2%. Highly selective vagotomy w/ ulcer excision meets w/ recurrence 44%.

   e. *Type IV*: "Csendes ulcer," high on lesser curvature, w/in 1–2 cm of GE junction, *not* assoc. w/ high acid levels. Small, punched-out lesions, often assoc. w/ dysphagia and GERD.

      i. *Tx*: variable. If < 2 cm from GE junction, can perform distal gastrectomy along lesser curve w/ ulcer and Roux-en-Y esophagogastrojejunostomy (Csendes procedure) may be an appropriate. Ulcers > 2 cm from GE junction may be amenable to distal gastrectomy w/ vertical extension along lesser curvature to incorporate the ulcer (Pauchet, Shoemaker procedure) followed by B-I reconstruction. If large ulcer or much inflammation, a total or near-total (90%) gastrectomy w/ Roux-en-Y jejunal anastamosis is option. Less aggressive option: truncal vagotomy and antrectomy leaving ulcer in place (Kelling-Madlener procedure); multiple bx's should be taken if ulcer is not excised.

   f. *Type V*: may occur anywhere in stomach, assoc. w/ NSAID usage.

   g. *Emergent surgery*:

      i. Hemorrhage, perforation, or obstruction, or an otherwise unstable pt may dictate a lesser procedure than described above.

      • Intermittent bleeding from type I, II, or III ulcers → TV w/ distal gastric resection.

      • Life-threatening hemorrhage from type I, II, or III ulcers → bx and oversew/excise ulcer + TV drainage procedure.

      • Perforations (type I, II, III) in unstable pts, ulcer bx/excision w/ omentoplasty closure is indicated +/– vagotomy and drainage if pt tolerates the extra time.

         ○ *Note*: In the era of proton-pump inhibitors, pts w/ nonmalignant ulcers who have not been on PPI should be strongly considered to *not* have acid-reducing procedure; just repair the perforation, etc., then tx medically postop. Recurrence postop, after appropriate medical tx should receive an appropriate acid-decreasing procedure.

      • Hemorrhage in type IV ulcers can be emergently addressed w/ ligation of left gastric artery, bx/oversewing ulcer through high anterior gastrostomy. Vagotomy and drainage may be added if tolerated.

      • *Obstruction*: antrectomy and Billroth I (second choice, B-II). If severe scarring precludes these options, consider gastrojejunostomy.

C. Obesity surgery

   1. *Definitions*:

      a. *Overweight*: BMI > 25.

      b. *Obese*: BMI > 30 (traditionally considered 20% over ideal body wt).

      c. *Morbidly (severely) obese*: > 100 lb over ideal body wt *or* 2× or more than ideal body wt *or* BMI 40+ kg/m^2.

         i. Possibly represents up to 5% of United States population.

      d. *Super obese*: BMI > 50 (usu. 200 lb or more over ideal body wt).

   2. *Indication for surgery*: BMI > 40 kg/m^2 or > 35% kg/m^2 obesity-associated comorbidities (HTN, DM, DJD, OSA, depression) in psychologically stable pt who has failed dietary therapy.

      a. Proceed w/ particular caution if > 600 lb, nonambulatory, age > 60. Prader-Willi syndrome contraindication for surgery.

   3. *Surgical therapy*: 2 procedures recommended by NIH: LAP-BAND and Roux-en-Y gastric bypass.

      a. Restrictive

         i. *Adjustable gastric banding* (LAP-BAND):

            • Adjustable band is placed laparoscopically ~ 1 cm below GE junction. Hospital stay ~ 1 d.

            • Add saline to band periodically w/ goal of 1–2 kg wt loss/wk.

- Most pts experience loss of ~ 50% of excess wt for at least 3 yr.
- > ½ of pts' HTN, DM resolve.
  ii. *Vertical banded gastroplasty*
  b. *Restrictive > malabsorptive*
  i. *Roux-en-Y gastric bypass*:
  - Most common bariatric procedure performed in United States. Can be laparoscopic or open.
  - Create 15- to 30-mL (average = 20-mL) pouch and jejunal limb 75–150 cm long (longer limb = more wt loss). Primary risk is gastrojejunostomy leak (< 2%). Can do laparoscopically or open.
  - Hospital stay ~ 3 d.
  4. *Complications*:
  a. Most significant complication w/ bypass procedures is anastomotic leak, which frequently first manifests as tachycardia (fever, peritonitis may be absent).
  b. Most common complication w/ banding procedures is migration of port, which can result in gastric obstruction, and even strangulation.
  c. Pts at high risk for pulmonary and thrombotic complications. Aggressive prophylactic measures appropriate.

D. Gastric cancer (see Chapter 10)

E. Postgastrectomy syndromes
  1. Up to ¼ of pts develop attributable sx, the majority of which resolve w/ time a/o have unclear pathophysiologic basis. Reoperation is reserved for significant, refractory sx secondary to a well-defined, surgically amenable dx.
  2. *Dumping syndrome*
  a. *Due to absence of pyloric "brake" from partial/total gastrectomy broadly classified into 2 forms*:
  i. *Early* (more common):
  - Fluid shifts from osmotic load (~ 30 min postprandial) cause N/V, possible diarrhea, diaphoresis, tachycardia, palpitations, etc. GI sx more common than cardiovascular.
  - Particularly common after gastrectomy + *Billroth II* reconstruction.
  - *Dx*:
    - Clinical picture frequently obvious.
    - Gastric-emptying studies (nuclear medicine) a/o provocation w/ 200 cc bolus of 50% glucose solution to reproduce sx may be considered.
  - *Tx*:
    - Frequent small meals high in protein, fat, fiber, and low in carbohydrate (esp. sugars) usu. sufficient. Separation of liquids and solids may be helpful as well.
    - Octreotide (somatostatin analogue) demonstrated to significantly decrease sx, esp. diarrhea.
    - Surgery required in < 1%.
      - Interposition of iso- or antiperistaltic 10- to 20-cm jejunal limb between stomach and small bowel most frequently used.
      - Alternately, Roux-en-Y reconstruction has been described.
  ii. *Late* (less common):
  - Rebound hypoglycemia and possible tachycardia, diaphoresis, confusion occur ~ 2 h postprandially due to excessive release of insulin in response to rapid carbohydrate load in small intestine.
  - Treat w/ diet modifications as for early dumping syndrome. Addition of pectin a/o acarbose to diet may yield additional benefit. Jejunal interposition surgery as for early dumping syndrome reserved for severe, refractory cases (rare).
  3. *Afferent loop syndrome*
  a. Results from obstruction of afferent limb of *Billroth II*, and may mimic bile reflux gastritis, SBO/efferent limb obstruction, biliary dz, or pancreatitis. Mechanisms include kinking, internal herniation, anastomotic stricture, adhesions, or volvulus of afferent limb; antecolic limbs > 40 cm are predisposed to this complication.

b. Incompletely obstructed pts present w/ postprandial crescendo pain relieved w/ bilious vomiting (w/out ingested food) ½ to 1 h after meals. Megaloblastic anemia from bacterial stasis (bacteria bind w/ cyanocobalamin) may be seen. Elevation in LFTs a/o amylase may result from increase duodenal pressure. Complete obstruction may result in necrosis and perforation.

c. *Dx*:

   i. Plain films +/– upper barium study may suggest the dx.

   ii. HIDA scan likewise can be of benefit.

d. *Tx*: no effective medical solutions; surgical options include:

   i. Simply shortening the afferent limb or lysing adhesions (rarely performed).

   ii. Conversion to Billroth I anastamosis.

   iii. Conversion to Roux-en-Y.

   - Vagotomy should accompany Roux-en-Y to prevent marginal ulceration secondary to diversion of duodenal efflux.

4. *Retained antrum syndrome*

   a. Like the afferent loop syndrome above, this occurs exclusively in pts who have had *Billroth II* reconstruction after gastrectomy.

   b. Antral mucosa may extend up to 5 mm beyond pyloric musculature, and thus may be left in duodenal stump if gastrectomy does not extend far enough distally. W/ Billroth II reconstruction, this antral tissue is left exposed to alkaline secretions in the duodenal stump, w/ no buffering from acidic gastric juices. Resultingly, antral cells are stimulated to release large quantities of gastrin, leading to increased acid secretion by the parietal cells.

   c. Pts present w/ recurrent ulceration after *partial* gastrectomy and *Billroth II* reconstruction.

   d. *Dx*: although duodenal bx is the gold standard, a technetium scan may demonstrate abnormal uptake in duodenal stump.

   e. *Tx*: H₂ blockers or PPIs should be tried before considering surgical correction by either conversion to a Billroth I reconstruction or resection of retained antrum in duodenal stump.

5. *Efferent loop syndrome*

   a. Rare, usu. occurs after Billroth II reconstruction secondary to herniation of small bowel through mesocolic defect, although adhesions or other causes are occasionally responsible.

   b. Most often presents w/ intermittent abdominal (often LUQ) pain and distension, followed by bilious emesis, often w/ partially digested enteric contents.

   c. *Dx*: barium upper GI study demonstrates contrast in stomach, failing to pass through efferent limb.

   d. *Tx*: surgery is required to address causative problem—reduction of retroanastomotic hernia, closure of retroanastamotic space, lyse adhesions, revise anastamosis, etc.

6. *Bile (alkaline) reflux gastritis*

   a. Again, this occurs more commonly after Billroth II resection.

   b. Presents w/ intense epigastric pain and bilious vomiting, frequently w/ wt loss and microcytic anemia as well.

   c. *Dx*:

      i. Clinical hx suggestive.

      ii. HIDA scan useful to reveal bile flux into stomach/esophagus.

      iii. Endoscopy provides bx's as well as gastric aspirate for analysis (i.e., bile). Mucosa classically appears red and friable.

      iv. *Caveat*: difficult to correlate presence or magnitude of reflux w/ sx; many asymptomatic pts have evidence of bile reflux.

   d. *Tx*:

      i. *Medical* tx not effective.

      ii. *Surgical* tx of choice is conversion to Roux-en-Y w/ limb at least 40 cm long.

      - If have Billroth II (usu. the case), can divide just proximial to gastrojejunostomy (leave that anastamosis intact), and bring down the proximal end to jejunum as Roux limb.

7. *Metabolic*

   a. *Anemia*

      i. *Microcytic* (more common—affects ~ ⅓ gastrectomy pts)

         • Multifactorial (decreased intake, impaired absorption, poss. blood loss from inflamed mucosa).

         • *Tx*: oral iron supplementation.

      ii. *Megaloblastic* (less common)

         • Risk particularly high after > 50% gastric resection due to loss of intrinsic factor-facilitated B_{12} absorption in ileum. Check serum B_{12} level.

         • *Tx*: intramuscular B_{12} injections q 3 mo. Consider folate supplementation.

   b. *Osteoporosis/osteomalacia*

      i. From impaired calcium malabsorption secondary to physiologic duodenal bypass a/o fat malabsorption leading to decreased absorption of vitamin D.

      ii. *Tx*: oral calcium (1000–2000 mg/d) and vitamin D (500–5000 U/d).

   c. *Diarrhea*

      i. Steatorrhea from poor mixing of dietary fat w/ bile/pancreatic enzymes after effective duodenal bypass should be treated w/ pancreatic enzyme (and possibly fat-soluble vitamin) supplementation.

F. **Postvagotomy syndromes**

   1. *Diarrhea*

      a. 20–40% pts postvagotomy, but usu. abates after several months.

      b. Mechanism poorly understood, possibly related alterations in bile acid excretion/cycling.

      c. *Tx*:

         i. *Medical*: cholestyramine (4 g PO three times per day w/ meals) binds bile salts and may help in persistent cases.

         ii. *Surgical*: interposition of 10-cm reversed jejunal segment ~ 80 cm from ligament of Treitz is most commonly performed procedure, but is required in < 1% of vagotomy pts.

   2. *Gastroparesis*

      a. Occurs to variable degree after total, but not highly selective/parietal cell, vagotomy.

      b. Loss of antral pump results in *prolonged emptying of solids*.

      c. Loss of receptive relaxation results in *more rapid emptying of liquids*.

      d. Clinical sx range from subjective fullness to functional gastric outlet obstruction and bezoar formation.

      e. *Dx*: w/u may begin w/ contrast upper GI study or scintigraphy to evaluate gastric emptying, but should include upper endoscopy at some point to evaluate anastamosis.

      f. *Tx*: prokinetic agents such as metoclopramide (dopamine antagonist and acetylcholine-release potentiator) a/o erythromycin (activates motilin receptors) are given for established dx.

II. SMALL BOWEL

A. **General**

   1. *Average length 280 cm*: duodenum 20 cm, jejunum 105 cm, ileum 155 cm. Need at least 90–100 cm of small bowel to avoid short gut syndrome (parenteral nutrition dependence).

B. **Duodenum**

   1. *Common benign pathology*

      a. *Duodenal peptic ulcers*:

         i. *Tx*:

            • *Acute bleeding*:

               ◦ Mobilize via Kocher maneuver, apply manual pressure to posterior duodenal ulcer through anterior wall, then incise anterior surface of postpyloric duodenum ~ 2 cm. *Oversew in 3 locations*: superiorly and inferiorly in ulcer bed (targets gastroduodenal artery), and medially w/ U-stitch (targets transverse pancreatic artery). Close duodenum via pyloroplasty (read below), and add truncal vagotomy (gold standard) or HSV.

- *Chronic bleeding refractory to medical tx*:
  - Truncal vagotomy and antrectomy (send specimen to ensure parietal cells seen in proximal margin and resect at least 1 cm distal to pylorus) is standard.
- *Perforation* → (1) closure and omental patch +/– HSV *or* (2) closure and omental patch +/– TV
- *Obstruction* → (1) antrectomy and TV w/ B-I *or* (2) antrectomy and TV w/ B-II *or* (3) TV and Finney vs Jaboulay pyloroplasty *or* (4) TV and gastrojejunostomy
- *Intractability* → HSV (open vs laparoscopic)

C. Jejunum and ileum

1. *Benign pathology*

   a. *Crohn's disease*: see Chapter 13, section IB1. on inflammatory bowel dz.

   b. *Sprue*: malabsorptive dz that may mimic intestinal lymphoma (conversely, consider intestinal lymphoma in "sprue" cases that do not completely respond to therapy). Frequently present w/ diarrhea/steatorrhea, wt loss, anorexia, abdominal distension, and anemia (iron- and B_{12}/folate-deficient). *Malapsorption of 2 of the 3 needed for dx*: fat, xylose, B_{12}. Bx usu. pursued.

      i. *Celiac sprue*: due to reaction to gluten (a protein found in wheat), w/ some genetic predisposition. 80% improve w/ gluten-free diet. The remainder may have another concomitant problem (i.e., lactase-deficiency) or lymphoma. Correctly dx'd cases refractory to diet therapy may (~ 50%) respond to glucocorticoids.

      ii. *Tropical sprue*: thought to be of yet-to-be-determined infectious etiology. Tx w/ 2–4 wk of abx (i.e., tetracycline) and B_{12}/folate +/– iron supplementation.

   c. *Diverticular disease*:

      i. *False diverticula*: much less common than duodenal diverticula, decreasing in incidence in more distal bowel. Most frequently found along mesenteric border. Complications, such as bleeding, perforation, diverticulitis, and obstruction, are best tx'd w/ intestinal resection and re-anastomosis.

      ii. *True diverticula* (contains all 3 components of bowel wall, including *muscularis*):

         - *Meckel's diverticula*:
           - Most common congenital anomaly of small bowel, resulting from failure of obliteration of vitelline (omphalomesenteric) duct.
           - *Classically follows the "rule of 2s:"* found in 2% of population; located on antimesenteric border of bowel usu. w/in 2 feet (45–60 cm) of ileocecal valve; may have 2 or more types of mucosa in the diverticulum (i.e., gastric > pancreatic >> colon, etc.).
           - Although usu. an incidental finding, the most common complication is hemorrhage (esp. in children) due to ulceration of normal ileum adjacent to gastric-mucosa (hence acid-producing) diverticulum. Much less commonly, pts present w/ obstruction or diverticulitis (more common in adults).
           - *Dx*: imaging test of choice is a Tc-99m-pertechnetate scan, which highlights ectopic gastric mucosa. Most useful in pediatric population (adults have less ectopic gastric mucosa). Sensitivity enhanced w/ pentagastrin a/o H_2 blocker. In adults (or children w/ negative scans), a small-bowel follow-through contrast study may be more helpful.
           - *Tx*: any symptomatic Meckel's diverticulum should be resected; incidentally found diverticula in children (and possibly adults [more controversial]) should probably be resected as well. If the adjacent ileum is bleeding, a segmental bowel resection and anastamosis is required; otherwise, depending on the width of the diverticulum, it may be feasible to resect just the diverticulum and primarily close the bowel (hand-sewn or stapled method).

   d. *Short-gut syndrome*: sx may begin when < 120 cm of small bowel remain, and < 60 cm (often < 90 cm) requires TPN; intact ileocecal valve can lower threshold to ~ 45 cm. Numerous complications:

      i. *Diarrhea*: may be from hypergastrinemia (SB metabolizes gastrin) or bile acid malabsorption. Tx w/ fiber, H_2 blockers, PO opioids, a/o bile-acid binding medications as appropriate.

      ii. Malnutrition, fluid, and electrolyte deficiency.

iii. *Urolithiasis* (calcium oxalate): excess binding of free oxalate in the colon results from presence of excess bile salts in colon (facilitate absorption); low dietary citrate augments propensity toward stone formation. Prevention of urolithiasis is undertaken w/ cholestyramine (binds bile salts), increased PO citrate, and avoidance of high-oxalate foods:

- *High-oxalate foods*: beets, rhubarb, tofu, spinach, tomatoes, peanuts, nuts, poppy seeds, wheat germ, tea, cocoa/chocolate

- *Moderate-oxalate foods*: green beans, blueberries, blackberries, raspberries, strawberries, sweet potatoes, coffee, cocoa/chocolate

2. *Malignant*: most common small bowel tumors—adenocarcinoma, carcinoid, GIST, lymphoma

   a. *Adenocarcinoma*: predominantly occur in proximal small bowel (duodenum, proximal jejunum); tx w/ wide resection (10-cm margins) of bowel and mesentery.

   b. *Carcinoid*: see Chapter 10.

   c. *GIST*: see Chapter 10.

   d. *Lymphoma*: see Chapter 10.

III. THE ACUTE ABDOMEN

   A. Typically sudden onset of abdominal pain that lasts > 6 h w/out improvement is surgical.

   B. Adjunctive abx for most types of perforated or inflamed viscus has broad gram-negative and anaerobe coverage. Piperacillin/tazobactam, ampicillin/sulbactam popular choices. For pancreatitis, imipenem or meropenem have better penetration.

   C. General surgical causes
      1. Appendicitis, Meckel's diverticulitis, volvulus, SBO (in adults w/out h/o abdominal surgery, think about cancer, malrotation, internal hernias, Gallstone ileus, etc.), cholecystitis, pancreatitis, perforated peptic ulcer

   D. Vascular causes
      1. *AAA, mesenteric infarction, aortic dissection*

   E. Urologic causes
      1. *Urolithiasis, pyelonephritis*

   F. Gynecologic causes
      1. *Ectopic pregnancy, PID, mittelschmerz*

   G. Medical mimics
      1. *DKA, Addisonian crisis, porphyria, sickle cell crisis, malaria, gastroenteritis*

CHAPTER 13

DISTAL GI, IBD, GI HEMORRHAGE, FISTULAS, AND OBSTRUCTION

I. COLON

A. Anatomy and physiology

1. Average 150 cm long, maximum diameter in cecum (average 7.5 cm; 10–12 cm portends perforation).

2. *Vascular*: right, transverse colon supplied by SMA: ileocolic, right colic, middle colic arteries. Left colon and sigmoid supplied by IMA: left colic, sigmoid, and superior rectal/hemorrhoidal arteries. Marginal artery of Drummond is a collateral vessel forming an arc between the SMA and IMA circulation along the mesenteric border of the colon; most vulnerable watershed area is the splenic flexure. Arc of Riolan (meandering mesenteric artery) is collateral between proximal SMA and proximal IMA of significance in the event of obstruction of either.

3. Primary function is to resorb water from stool.

B. Benign pathology

1. *Inflammatory bowel dz*: poorly understood, probably from genetic (i.e., genes NOD2/CARD15) as well as environmental influences (i.e., luminal bacterial exposure—*smoking* is strongest known factor) and mucosal immune system defect. In approximately 10–15% of cases, clinical and histologic features insufficient to distinguish Crohn's dz from ulcerative colitis. In such cases ordering serum p-ANCA (more often positive w/ UC) and ASCA (more often positive w/ Crohn's) assays may be warranted. [Information on medical management of both Crohn's dz and ulcerative colitis below in part from: Isaacs KL, et al. State of the art: IBD therapy and clinical trials in IBD. *Inflamm Bowel Dis* 2005;11:S3–12.]

   a. *Crohn's dz*

      i. 50% involves small and large bowel, 30% exclusively small bowel, 20% exclusively large bowel.

      ii. Characterized by rectal sparing often, "skip lesions," transmural inflammation, linear ulcerations, "creeping" mesenteric fat, and granulomas. Smoking is risk factor. Incidence increasing.

      iii. *Medical management*:

      - *Aminosalicylates*: usu., active portion is bound to sulfa moiety until cleaved in the gut, activating it. Newer generations lack the sulfa component, making them better tolerated, able to be given in higher doses.

         ○ *Mesalamine/5-aminosalicylate/5-ASA (Pentasa*, slow-release) and *Asacol* (pH-dependent release) allow drug release in proximal gut, useful for small and large bowel dz. *Rowasa* is given as enema.

      - *Corticosteroids*: used to induce remission (not for maintenance), successful 70% of time after 1 mo. Tapered after improvement.

         ○ *Budesonide*: high topical potency, low systemic absorption w/ high first-pass effect. Its delivery is pH-dependent (due to coating), delivered to terminal ileum/cecum. Efficacy almost as good as prednisone.

      - *Immunosuppressant medications*

         ○ *6-mercaptopurine (6-MP)*: used as steroid-sparing drug to maintain remission, generally begun after corticosteroid-induced remission, w/ response lagging up to 4 mo. Potential myelosuppression warrants following CBC. Pancreatitis is another risk.

         ○ *Azathioprine (AZA, Imuran)*: precursor to 6-MP, can be used as alternate to 6-MP.

      - *Anti-TNF-α antibody*

         ○ *Infliximab*: chimeric mouse antibody to TNF-α, give for cases refractory to steroids or immunosuppressants ($^2/_3$ respond, $^1/_3$ remit). Side effects to infusion in ~ 20%, and repeated doses may result in antichemeric antibodies; often given w/ immuno-suppressants to prevent this.

   iv. *Surgical management*:

- Most pts will ultimately require some surgical intervention.
- *Indications for surgery* (in decreasing order of frequency): obstruction, internal fistula, perianal dz, abscess, perforation, toxic megacolon.
- Resection and anastamosis has lower complication rate than strictureplasty, but risk of short gut syndrome should be borne in mind if large segments involved. Risk of Crohn's recurrence is not affected by choice of resection vs strictureplasty. Only resect grossly involved bowel.

  b. *Ulcerative colitis*

   i. Idiopathic inflammatory condition of colon clinically characterized by episodic diarrhea and rectal bleeding.

   ii. Exclusively large bowel dz, although "backwash ileitis" may occur. Involves contiguous bowel, from anus retrograde. May lead to "lead pipe" colon. Microcrypts, pseudopolyps, mucosal ulceration.

   iii. *Medical management* (approach as a pyramid):

- ASA best agent for induction as well as maintenance of mild dz. Total dose more important than route (PO vs rectal). Higher doses of mesalamine (> 1.2 g/d) may additionally afford some protection against colorectal cancer for UC pts.
- Steroids are indicated for moderate dz.
- AZA (precursor to 6-MP) is an immunomodulator, indicated to induce remission for moderate to severe dz, provide maintenance, and help avoid steroids.
- Cyclosporine may be added for severe cases, usu. as last line before surgery.
- Non-FDA-approved adjuncts include fish oil, nicotine, probiotics, and biologics.

   iv. *Surgical management*:

- Less than 20% of pts after 20 yr of dz will have had surgery for UC.
- *Indications*: toxic megacolon, hemorrhage, perforation, failure of medical management, or malignancy. Dysplasia may be indication for surgery (esp. if assoc. w/ a lesion), but histologically can be difficult to differentiate from reactive atypia. Therefore, finding of dysplasia in acutely inflamed colon warrants repeat bx after inflammation subsides, according to some authors.
- *Procedure choice*:
  - *Three issues*: emergency or elective; should rectum be resected; should intestinal continuity be restored.
  - Total/subtotal colectomy and ileostomy usu. indicated for emergent indications (hemorrhage, perforation, etc.). < 15% will have continued sx after this, and a minority of these cases will need proctectomy.
  - Proctocolectomy w/ pouch-anal reconstruction is the usual procedure for elective cases.
    - Kock continent ileostomy rarely used for reconstruction anymore.
    - Ileostomy construction is safest procedure after proctocolectomy but requires appliance. *Indications* (contraindications for IPAA): Crohn's, prior extensive small bowel resection, perineal dz, anorectal dysfunction, malignancy in lower rectum, and poor systemic physiology.

2. *Diverticulitis*

  a. *Colonic diverticuli*: M = F; 10% at 40 yo, 75% by 80 yo; 10% right colon; 80% asx, 95% involve sigmoid, 65% in sigmoid only; 10–20% will develop hemorrhage or diverticulitis.

  b. *Diverticulitis*

   i. Will occur in 20% of pts > 40 yo, caused by inspissated stool obstructing neck, increasing intraluminal pressure.

   ii. 10–15% of cases will have free perforation, and generalized peritonitis; more common in immunosuppressed.

   iii. *Sx*: pain, esp. LLQ; F, malaise; change in bowel habits; urinary sx (frequency, nocturia) from pericystic inflammation. 3–5% will have colovesical fistula, may have pneumaturia or recurrent polymicrobial UTIs. TTP, guarding; ileus or bowel obstruction; palpable mass, esp. on pelvic or rectal exam; guaiac-positive stool. Check CBC, UA.

   iv. *Dx*: CT scan test of choice. Contrast enema less common. Flex sigmoidoscopy w/ minimal insufflation may be used to r/o perforated CRCA.

   v. If surgery not chosen/indicated, colonoscopy mandatory after acute phase if bleeding or possible CRCA radiographically.

   vi. *Tx*: cases can be broadly classified into uncomplicated and complicated.

- *Uncomplicated* (~ 75%): clinically, LLQ pain, fever, leukocytosis. Radiographically, CT w/ local inflammation w/out evidence of pericolonic abscess, bleeding, or free perforation.

  - Tx w/ bowel rest, IV vs oral abx (fluoroquinolone + metronidazole most commonly), and IV fluid resuscitation.

  - *Outpt*: if mild TTP, low-grade fever, can tx w/ oral abx 7–10 d; high-fiber diet w/ psyllium.

  - *Inpt*: NPO, IVF, +/– NGT.
    - Parenteral abx (for GNR and anaerobes) for 7–10 d, or until AF w/ normal WBC and NT exam.
    - Clear liquids, then low-residue diet 2–4 wk after acute attack; then high-fiber diet w/ psyllium. More effective for pain control than for decreasing complications.

  - Of those admitted, 50% will not be resolved w/ conservative therapy. 30% of inpts will develop free perforation. 9% will have urinary fistulas. 1% will have right-sided dz only.

  - If sx do not improve w/in 48 h, consider repeat CT scan w/ contrast. Abscess or extracolonic air/contrast suggest failure and need for operation.

- *Complicated* (~ 25%): clinically, peritonitis or obstruction. Radiographically, CT w/ perforation (or pneumoperitoneum on KUB), abscess, or fistula.

  - If no peritonitis, isolated abscess may be drained percutaneously, followed by semi-elective surgery.
    - Otherwise, surgical intervention indicated.

- *Other*:

  - *Before any surgery done after resolution of acute inflammation*, a preop colonoscopy is performed if possible to exclude the possibility of carcinoma, as 10–20% of cases initially diagnosed as diverticulitis ultimately are found to harbor neoplasm.

  - Most surgeons recommend surgery for any repeat episodes of diverticulitis, or any episode in pts under 50 yo, but this remains controversial.

  - *Surgical strategies*:
    - *Single stage*: usu. elective cases w/ prepped bowel; resect, primary anastamosis.
    - *Two stage*: if anastamosis not safe due to bowel edema or gross contamination. First resect colon, perform end colostomy and either mucous fistula or Hartmann pouch. (Alternatively: resection and anastamosis w/ prox diverting colostomy.) Reanastamosis after 2–6 mo.

II. ANORECTAL

A. Anatomy and physiology

1. *Rectum*: ~ 13 cm long, no taeniae (they merge together). Anterior $^1/_3$ of proximal rectum covered by peritoneum. Peritoneal fold/reflection ~ 7 cm from anal verge.

2. *Anal canal*: 4 cm from anal verge to anorectal ring proximally. Lined w/ columns of Morgagni, contains cryptoglandular structures significant in anal fistula dz.

3. Proximal to dentate line, pink, lined by columnar epithelium. Distal to dentate line, lined by paler squamous epithelium.

4. *Internal sphincter palpable* ~ 1.5 cm distal to dentate line, essentially a thickening of smooth (involuntary) circular rectal muscle.

5. *External sphincter palpable* just distal to internal sphincter (intersphincteric groove between the 2), consists of voluntary, striated muscle from pelvic floor (contiguous w/ levator ani and puborectalis). Innervated by internal pudendal nerve and S4.

6. *Vascular supply to anorectal region*:

   a. *Proximal rectum: superior rectal (superior hemorrhoidal) artery*—last branch of IMA.

   b. *Distal rectum/anus*:

      i. *Middle rectal (hemorrhoidal) artery*—branch of internal iliac (hypogastric) artery.

      ii. *Inferior rectal (hemorrhoidal) artery*—branch of pudendal artery (which comes off of hypogastric artery).

B. Benign pathology

1. *Hemorrhoids*

   a. Cushions of soft tissue and blood vessels at right anterior, left lateral, and right posterior locations, which aid in fecal continence.

   b. *Internal* (proximal to dentate line, relatively insensate):

      i. *Sx*: bleeding a/o prolapse. Anal fecal/mucus leakage, pruritus also possible.

      ii. *Grades*:
      * *First degree*: no prolapse
      * *Second degree*: spontaneously reduces
      * *Third degree*: requires manual reduction
      * *Fourth degree*: cannot be reduced (strangulated)

      iii. *Dx*: DRE, anoscopy, and, particularly if pt > 40 yo, anemic, unimpressive hemorrhoids, or significant family h/o colorectal cancer, proximal endoscopy is indicated.

      iv. *Tx*:
      * Dietary fiber supplementation.
      * Most second, third degree → banding, although other options (sclerotherapy, heater probe, etc.) exist. Avoid banding if immunocompromised, due to risk of sepsis.
      * Surgical hemorrhoidectomy if refractory or fourth degree internal hemorrhoids, and internal hemorrhoids w/ any of the following: symptomatic external hemorrhoids, fissure, fistula-in-ano, or large anal tags.

   c. *External* (distal to dentate line, covered w/ anoderm, sensate):

      i. *Sx* relatively minimal (hygiene-related, usu.), unless thrombose (severe pain).

      ii. *Tx*:
      * Conservative management (i.e., dietary modification) usu. sufficient.
      * Consider excision if symptomatic and other indication for internal hemorrhoidectomy.
      * Excise/evacuate thrombosed external hemorrhoids w/in 72 h of thrombosis.

2. *Anal fissure*

   a. Painful linear ulceration of anal mucosa, usu. posterior midline, often assoc. w/ sentinel tag. Less often at anterior midline. *Sx*: pain w/ defecation +/– blood on stool/toilet paper.

   b. *Dx*:

      i. External anal exam.

      ii. Invasive probing (anoscopy, etc.) usu. prohibitively painful in the clinic setting.

      iii. Location other than described above should prompt w/u for other etiology (i.e., Crohn's dz, STD, etc.).

   c. *Tx*:

      i. *Medical*
      * Early dz (i.e., w/in 3 wk of onset) → dietary fiber and Sitz baths.
      * Chronic lesions → above +/– topical NTG paste three times per day (0.2% preparation; side effect = HA). Try (2%) diltiazem if unable to tolerate NTG. Botox less frequently used: invasive, more expensive, poss. have higher recurrence rates.

    ii. *Surgical*

- Failure of conservative tx → lateral internal sphincterotomy. Main complication risk = incontinence.
- Anorectal advancement flap if failure of LIS or significant stenosis of the anal canal.

3. *Perirectal abscess*

   a. Begins in the intersphincteric plane at the level of the dentate line, often spreading in one or more of several directions.

     i. *Intersphincteric abscess*: abscess remains localized to original site. Often → dyschezia w/out obvious source.

     ii. *Perianal abscess*: caudad tracking of intersphincteric abscess toward external margin of anus; tender perianal mass. DDx should include thrombosed external hemorrhoid.

     iii. *Intermuscular abscess*: cephalad tracking of intersphincteric abscess w/in confines of rectal wall. Sx often vague, may require CT, U/S, or EUA for dx.

     iv. *Supralevator abscess*: cephalad tracking of intersphincteric abscess above levator. Sx often vague, may require CT, U/S, or EUA for dx.

     v. *Ischiorectal abscess*: spread of abscess across external sphincter into ischiorectal fossa (alternately, pus may repread across internal sphincter into anal canal).

     vi. *"Horseshoe abscess"*: circumferential spread of abscess in intersphincteric, supralevator, or ischiorectal spaces.

   b. *Dx*: H&P key. CT or other imaging occas. useful.

   c. *Tx*: wide incision and drainage.

     i. *Intersphincteric*: drain via division of internal sphincter at level of abscess.

     ii. *Perianal*: drain through incision in overlying skin.

     iii. *Intermuscular*: drain through incision through rectal/anal mucosa.

     iv. *Supralevator*: drain through incision through rectal mucosa.

     v. *Ischiorectal*: drain widely through incision through overlying skin and soft tissue. Spreading w/ hemostat, finger, etc., appropriate to break up loculations.

     vi. *Horseshoe*: drain through posterior midline incision extending from the coccygeal tip anteriorly to (but not through) the external sphincter. Counterincisions in the perineum for drainage may be appropriate.

4. *Perianal fistulas* (fistula-in-ano)

   a. ~ ¼ of perirectal abscesses develop this, less often from other dz (i.e., Crohn's dz).

     i. *Intersphincteric* (most common): usu. follows path of perianal abscess (caudad to anal margin), although may track cephalad. Remains in intersphincteric space, medial to external sphincter.

     ii. *Transsphincteric*: passes through external sphincter into ischiorectal fossa, ultimately opening into perineum.

     iii. *Suprasphincteric*: uncommon and difficult to tx. Courses cephalad over puborectalis/levator before turning downward to perineum. To open tract, must divide all muscles necessary for continence.

     iv. *Extrasphincteric*: rare, frequently due to noncryptoglandular dz (Crohn's, radiation, trauma, malignancy, etc.). Tract is lateral to both sphincter mechanisms, running from rectum to perineal skin.

   b. *Dx*

     i. Exam under anesthesia w/ anoscopy, palpation (for induration), and probing along dentate line. If can't identify internal opening, inject external opening w/ H_2O_2 a/o methylene blue through angiocatheter or pediatric feeding tube.

- *Goodsall rule*: if perineal opening anterior to line passing through ischial tuberosities, tract should pass to anal canal in a straight radial path (i.e., if skin opening is at 3 o'clock in the perineum, the anal canal opening should be roughly at 3 o'clock). If perineal opening posterior to the imaginary line, tract usu. courses around to open in the posterior midline anal canal. *Exception*: anterior fistula on the perineum > 3 cm (suggests prior horseshoe abscess) from anus frequently course to posterior midline, not in a straight radial path. Rule is more accurate for posterior than anterior abscesses. [Cirocco WC, Reilly JC, *Dis Colon Rectum* 1992 Jun;35(6):537–42.]

c. *Management*

   i. Drain source and fistula tract.

   ii. Intersphincteric fistulas → unroofed via division of interposed internal sphincter muscula-ture (fistulotomy) over a probe. To preserve continence, setons should be used if > ½ of the internal sphincter is involved (or for anterior fistulas in females).

   iii. *Large, complicated fistulas (or recurrent) above sphincter mechanisms can be approached w/*:

- Seton (i.e., thin Penrose drain that is sequentially tied tighter in outpt visits).
- Fibrin glue.
- Mucosal advancement flap: lift up rhomboid flap (wider at proximal base) including mucosa, submucosa, and internal sphincter, and advance to suture w/out tension over debrided base w/ fistulous opening ligated closed w/ absorbable suture.

5. *Rectal prolapse*:

a. Important to differentiate full-thickness/complete prolapse (procidentia), which has *circumfer-ential* folds, from mucosal prolapse, which has *radial* folds.

b. W/u should address cardiopulmonary status, and also include barium enema or colonoscopy (look for lead points), anorectal manometry, cinedefecography, EMG, and colon transit studies.

c. *Surgery*:

   i. *Transabdominal approach*: 0–5% recurrence.

- *Rectopexy*
  - Use for complete prolapse; contraindicated in pts w/ constipation.
  - Mobilize and fix rectum to presacral fascia.
  - Ripstein procedure is rectopexy w/ Marlex mesh. Ivalon sponge may be used instead. Complication assoc. w/ these procedures is erosion of foreign body into bowel. Instead, using permanent suture is preferred.
- *Resection and rectopexy* (Frykman-Goldberg procedure)
  - Use for complete prolapse w/ constipation.
  - Mobilize, resect redundant sigmoid colon, then suture rectal lateral ligaments to presacral fascia w/ permanent suture.
- *Total abdominal colectomy* (w/ ileorectostomy or ileodescending colostomy)
  - Use for slow transit (colonic inertia) constipation w/ prolapse.

   ii. *Perineal approach*: 10–25% recurrence—reserved for pts too frail for transabdominal operations.

- *Thiersch wire*
  - Places a nonabsorbable band (suture, tubing, etc.) SC around the anus as a cer-clage. Procedure does not treat underlying disorder, and is assoc. w/ complications such as fecal impaction and pelvic sepsis from erosion of the prosthetic. Rarely performed.
- *Delorme procedure*
  - Use for mucosal prolapse *or* low complete prolapse *or* internal intussusception.
  - Resect 10–25 cm of circumferential sleeve of rectal mucosa. Plicate underlying muscular wall w/ absorbable sutures. Reanastamose mucosal edges. Can do under local/spinal/epidural + sedation.
- *Perineal rectosigmoidectomy* (Altemeier procedure)
  - Use for complete prolapse in the elderly or otherwise poor surgical risk.
  - Make full-thickness incision 1–3 cm above dentate line (w/ rectum prolapsed). Divide and ligate mesentery of involved bowel. Transect bowel and anastamose free edges. Plicate levator ani anteriorly.

6. *Pilonidal disease* (L. *pilus* = "hair" + L. *nīdus* = "nest")

   a. Pattern of acute or chronic inflammatory changes generally in the soft tissues of gluteal cleft in young adults, thought to be due in part to hair follicles.

   b. *Tx*:

      i. *Acute*: I&D, then pack abscess or sinus cavity.

      ii. *Chronic*: division of sinus tracts, curettage, a/o excision of affected tissues. Marsupialization or flap coverage may be required.

7. *Hidradenitis suppurativa*: inflammatory process localized to regions of apocrine glands (axilla, perineum). Mild cases warrant trial of abx (i.e., doxycycline), but established dz generally requires excision followed by marsupialization or coverage w/ skin grafts or local flaps.

8. *Condyloma acuminatum* (Gk. *kŏndylos* = "knuckle" + L. *acūminātum* = "pointed")

   a. "Genital warts" resulting from infection w/ HPV (6, 11, 16, 18, etc.), assoc. w/ anal intercourse and HIV. Rarely grows to giant "Buschke-Löwenstein" tumors, which may harbor SCCA; tx = WLE. Poor surgical candidates → interferon/CO_2 laser/imiquimod.

   b. *Dx*: ddx—molluscum contagiosum (classically w/ umbilicated center), anal papillae, and secondary syphilis. Include anoscopy and proctoscopy to eval if in anal canal.

   c. *Tx*: recurrence is common.

      i. Sharp excision.

      ii. Topical podophyllin for perianal warts.

      iii. Bichloracetic acid may be used for perianal or intraanal warts.

      iv. Electrocautery excision a/o fulguration or CO_2 laser usage requires aspiration of vapors a/o masks.

III. APPENDIX

A. Anatomy and physiology

1. Blood supply from appendiceal artery from ileocolic artery from SMA.

2. Most commonly retrocecal position; find by tracing back taenia coli to confluence. Gravid uterus displaces cephalad.

B. Appendicitis

1. *Epidemiology/etiology*:

   a. M > F w/ bimodal age distribution, median age early 20s.

   b. From luminal obstruction most commonly from lymphoid hypertrophy (younger pts) > fecolith or stricture (older pts) > tumor.

2. *Presentation and dx*:

   a. *Clinical dx*: hx typically vague epigastric pain, gradually localizes, becomes more intense in RLQ, accompanied by N/V.

      i. Peritonitis inferred from pain w/ movement (i.e., walking) or pain w/ tapping heel.

      ii. Risk of rupture higher in very young and in elderly.

      iii. *Psoas sign*: pain w/ extension/hyperextension of right thigh.

      iv. *Obturator sign*: pain w/ passive external rotation of right hip w/ hip and knee flexed 90°.

      v. *Blumberg's sign*: eponym for rebound tenderness. *Note*: percussion may be just as useful, probably more humane (and specific for peritonitis).

      vi. *Rovsing's sign*: pain in RLQ w/ LLQ palpation.

   b. *Ddx*: urolithiasis, UTI (get *urinalysis* on all pts), gyn pathology (get *β-hCG* on all reproductive-age females, ectopic pregnancy, ovarian cyst, PID, etc.), diverticulitis, perforated peptic ulcer, IBD, etc.

   c. Radiographically, noncontrast helical CT (97% accurate) recommended for reproductive-age females, pts who will be observed, or those who may be d/c'd w/out reliable means for f/u (criteria: diameter > 6 mm, stranding in periappendiceal fat). U/S typically not useful except in children (criteria: diameter > 6 mm, no gas in lumen).

3. *Tx*:

   a. *Abx*: adjunctive role to surgery.

   b. Appendectomy.

    i. ~ 20% negative celiotomy rate generally acceptable. Higher rates seen in females of reproductive age. Lower negative rates seen in males.

- Finding of normal appendix should prompt intraop exploration for other sources such as Meckel's diverticulitis, Crohn's dz, sigmoid diverticulitis, perforated peptic ulcer, gynecologic source (i.e., PID, ovarian torsion), etc. Appendectomy should still be performed to diminish future diagnostic difficulty.

    ii. *Laparoscopic appendectomy*:

- W/ experience, takes the same or less time than open w/ equal or lower complication rate and less hospital time.
- Added benefit: look for other pathology if appendix normal and search for mets if appy tumor found.
- Advocated by many for reproductive-age females, for obese pts, and by some for pts over 50 yo.

    iii. In pregnancy, premature labor generally responds to tocolytics.

    iv. *For complicated appendicitis*:

- *Pregnant pts*: appendix rises above iliac crest by 5 mo. Clinical suspicion of appendicitis warrants surgical exploration (laparoscopic or open) regardless of gestational age.
- *Perforated*: important to adequately resuscitate before performing appendectomy. Maintain postop abx for a wk, or at least until pt is afebrile w/ normal WBC.
- *Abscess* (L. *abscessus* = "a going away" or "separating off"): percutaneously drain, perform interval appendectomy if pt responds to drainage and abx (otherwise need to operate sooner, despite increased risk of complications such as fistula).
- *Phlegmon* (Gr. *phlegmonē* = "inflammation"): inflammatory mass not amenable to percutaneous drainage. Unless pt has frank peritonitis, nonoperative management (NPO, IV abx) is reasonable. If pt does not improve w/in 48–72 h, operation indicated. Otherwise, interval appendectomy in 6–8 wk appropriate.

  c. *Postop care*:

    i. If purulent peritoneal fluid, close fascia only, leave skin open, keep on IV abx until AF, normal WBC.

    ii. If not ruptured or otherwise complicated, 1–2 doses of postop abx.

C. Appendiceal tumors

1. Malignancy found in ~ 1% of appendectomies. Carcinoid > malignant (metastatic > primary) > benign other. [Collins DC, *Am J Proctol*, 1963;14:365, and Schmutzer KJ et al., *Dis Colon Rectum*, 1975;18:324.]

2. *Carcinoid*: majority in distal $^1/_3$ of appendix, forming a discrete rounded tumor, and usu. < 1 cm.

3. Malignant (usu. metastatic adenocarcinoma, most often w/ primary colorectal CA). High incidence of synchronous and metachronous colorectal CA.

4. Frozen section should be performed on tumor, suspicious lymph nodes.

5. Appendectomy often adequate. Right hemicolectomy indicated for carcinoids > 1.5–2 cm in diameter (or those involving the base at junction w/ cecum), adenocarcinoma, and adenomas w/ uncertain margins/invasion.

IV. GI HEMORRHAGE

A. General

1. > 80% self-limited. > 80% of GI bleed admissions are for upper GI sources, ~ 15% for colon, ~ 3% small bowel.

2. < 10% require surgery. For hemodynamically significant bleeds, mortality is 5–12%.

3. Hematemesis characteristic of upper GI bleed. Melena, hematochezia may represent upper or lower GI bleeding.

4. Good PMHx and medications essential. In pts w/ alcoholic liver dz, 1st episode equally likely to be variceal or nonvariceal, but after 1 episode of variceal hemorrhage, subsequent bleeds have at least 70% probability of being variceal.

5. *Initial management*:

a. 2 large-bore IVs, begin infusion of (usu.) lactated Ringer's. Foley, OGT/NGT. If significant hematemesis, intubate.

b. *Identify source*:

   i. Lavage stomach through OGT/NGT. If returns blood or "coffee grounds" (or if present w/ hematemesis), prepare pt for emergency endoscopy. If lavage (–) but index of suspicion is high, upper endoscopy reasonable given that a competent or spastic pylorus can prevent return of blood on lavage from duodenal bleed.

   ii. If lavage (–) or otherwise upper source ruled out, manage for lower GI bleed (see section C. below).

B. *Upper* (proximal to ligament of Treitz; also see Chapter 15):

   1. *Peptic ulcer*

      a. Hemorrhage from stomach and duodenum equally common (together about ~ 50% of upper GI sources).

      b. Approximately ½ of cases due to *H. pylori* (~ $1/3$ due to NSAIDs). Highest risk ulcers for bleeding are in posterior duodenum.

      c. *Likelihood of endoscopic failure* (rebleeding):

         i. Visible vessel, 40–80%; nonbleeding clot, 20%; pigmented spot ulcer, 10%; clean ulcer, rare.

         ii. Ulcer size > 2 cm independent risk factor for rebleed.

      d. *Medical management*

         i. Cease NSAIDs, *H. pylori*, PPI/H_2 blocker tx as indicated for outpt management; rescope in 6 wk.

         ii. *Endoscopy*: electrocoagulation, LASER, injection (epinephrine, sclerosant).

         iii. 20% of pts fail initial endoscopic management, w/ virtually all rebleeding beginning w/in 4 d.

             • Repeat endoscopy successful in ~ ½.

      e. *Surgical management*

         i. Required for ~ 10% of ulcer bleeding, specifically failures of endoscopic management or significant transfusion requirement (i.e., > 4–6 U PRBCs per 24 h). Endoscopic findings (i.e., visible vessel) on initial endoscopy not necessarily absolute indication for surgery, but depends on capability of available endoscopist. Aggressive surgical intervention for elderly pts w/ high-risk lesions should be considered.

         ii. *Duodenal ulcer*:

             • Enter duodenum through duodenotomy. Generally, suture ligation of posterior wall ulcer w/ permanent suture, but u-stitch or 4-quadrant ligation around ulcer perimeter may be necessary, or even cephalad and caudad stitching of gastroduodenal artery.

             • If the pt is stable enough, an antisecretory procedure should be added (*controversial*—if pt has not previously been on PPIs or tx'd for *H. pylori*, many assert that medical management should be entertained given the current efficacy of medical tx).

                 ○ *Truncal vagotomy + antrectomy or pyloroplasty*: quick, 90% effective, but side effects include dumping syndrome and diarrhea.

                 ○ *Parietal cell vagotomy*: more time-consuming, but fewer side effects.

         iii. *Gastric ulcer*:

             • Ulcer excision should be included in any procedure, partially because up to 10% of all gastric ulcers are malignant (not a significant concern w/ duodenal ulcers).

                 ○ *Distal stomach* (most common—body/antrum/incisura):

                     ■ Distal gastrectomy + B-I or B-II reconstruction (add TV pt relatively stable).

                 ○ *Proximal stomach* (relatively rare):

                     ■ Subtotal or near-total gastrectomy (high morbidity)

                     ■ Local ulcer excision + distal gastrectomy (TV not necessary)

         iv. *H. pylori* ulcer

             • Controversial. Many advocate simply oversewing the ulcer and medically treating the pt, although recurrence rates vary considerably.

2. *Portal hypertension/varices*
   a. *Pathology and presentation*:
      i. Up to ¼ of cirrhotic pts have variceal bleeding at some point.
      ii. If no prior h/o variceal bleeding, a cirrhotic UGI hemorrhage is equally likely to be from peptic ulcers, gastritis, portal hypertensive gastropathy, or varices. After an initial variceal bleed, subsequent UGI hemorrhage ~ 75% likely to be from varices.
      iii. Variceal bleeding in a Child's C cirrhotic portends a 50% 30-d mortality, and 85% 1-yr mortality.
   b. *Medical tx* (80–90% effective):
      i. Pt should be moved to ICU, resuscitated, and prepared for upper endoscopy.
      ii. IV octreotide (somatostatin analogue) decreases splanchnic blood flow and is the medical adjunct of choice; vasopressin (+/– NTG) is often effective as well.
      iii. Endoscopic banding or sclerotherapy usu. effective.
         • *Exception*: sclerotherapy not good for gastric varices; surgery should be entertained if reasonable risk.
         • Sclerotherapy can be repeated 1–2 times in initial 48 h; if fails, Sengstaken-Blakemore tube should be inserted, and consideration for transjugular intrahepatic shunt (TIPS) or surgery. Mortality at this point likely exceeds 50%.
   c. *Surgical tx*: see Chapter 14.
3. *Acute gastric mucosal lesion* ("stress gastritis" or "stress ulceration")
   a. *Pathology and presentation*:
      i. Generally seen in ICU setting, presenting w/ drop in hematocrit, hematemesis, a/o coffee-ground appearance to NGT aspirate.
      ii. *Endoscopy*: pale mucosa, erosions, and petechiae.
   b. *Medical tx*:
      i. Prophylax w/ H_2 inhibitors or PPIs.
      ii. Endoscopic injection or coagulation may be useful for localized lesions, but dz usu. too diffuse.
      iii. Angiography (embolization vs vasopressin infusion) reserved for diffuse, refractory bleeding, but can be up to 80% (temporarily) effective if bleeding vessel can be found. Rebleeding common.
   c. *Surgical tx*:
      i. Rarely appropriate.
      ii. If only a few bleeding sites are found via gastrotomy (unusual), may be oversewed, followed by truncal vagotomy and drainage procedure.
      iii. More commonly, only appropriate surgical option is subtotal or near-total gastrectomy w/ Roux-en-Y gastrojejunostomy reconstruction. Mortality 60–90%.
4. *Mallory-Weiss tear*
   a. Tear in gastric mucosa near EG junction (most often lesser curvature), typically caused by intense retching/vomiting. ~ 10% of significant UGI hemorrhage. 90% self-limited, less if cirrhosis/coagulopathy.
   b. *Medical tx*:
      i. Endoscopy usu. can stop the bleeding w/ injection or coagulation.
      ii. Up to $1/3$ of pts rebleed after endoscopy w/in 24 h, but provision of PPI and correction of coagulopathy generally results in eventual cessation of bleeding.
   c. *Surgical tx*:
      i. Rarely needed. Oversewing of mucosal lesion through a cephalad gastrotomy effective.
5. *Dieulafoy lesion*
   a. Also known as "constant-caliber vessel," an unusu. large submucosal or mucosal artery in the stomach, not generally due to an overlying ulcer. Bleeding is frequently intense, but often self-limited.

    b. *Medical management*:

      i. Endoscopy to dx and identify vessel. Endoscopic tx prone to fail; endoscopist should mark the lesion w/ India ink to assist the surgeon (read below).

    c. *Surgical management*:

      i. Wedge resection of the involved gastric wall is appropriate management.

6. *Aortoenteric fistula*

    a. Most common at proximal suture line after aortic aneurysm repair, but cases due to spontaneous inflammatory erosion reported. Typically involves duodenum or proximal jejunum. Classically herald bleeding followed hours to days later by catastrophic bleeding.

    b. *Medical management*:

      i. Clinical suspicion should prompt upper endoscopy, which, if negative, should be followed by abdominal CT scan to look for an inflammatory process. If CT scan is negative (some argue *in lieu* of CT scan), angiography w/ lateral views should be the next step.

    c. *Surgical management*:

      i. Emergency celiotomy to achieve proximal aortic control followed by (typical scenario) removal of aortic graft and extraanatomic vascular bypass (i.e., axillary-bifemoral).

      ii. See Chapter 9 for more details.

C. *Lower* (distal to ligament of Treitz):

1. Irrigate via NGT to r/o UGI source, followed by anoscopy/proctoscopy to r/o anorectal source (ulcer, hemorrhoid, neoplasm, etc.), which may be controlled. Upper GI hemorrhage may bleed briskly enough to present w/ hematochezia and signs of volume depletion. Hemodynamically unstable pts w/ hematochezia should undergo emergent upper endoscopy as well.

2. Significant bleed should be evaluated w/ colonoscopy or angiography (sensitive to 0.5 cc/min) as most precise and can be used therapeutically (coagulation or vasopressin/embolization, respectively) as well. Angiography should be reserved for massive bleeds; colonoscopy more appropriate for lesser, more intermittent bleeds. Angiography can also be used therapeutically (embolization or vasopressin infusion) as a bridge to surgery, or in lieu of surgery in high-risk pts. Technetium Tc-99m RBC scintigraphy can detect bleeding as slow as 0.1 cc/min, but rarely specific enough to determine which side of the colon is bleeding; its primary use is guiding subsequent angiography or colonoscopy.

3. If unstable after attempts at resuscitation (ongoing hemorrhage, transfusion of 6 or more units of PRBCs, etc.), go to OR. If unable to localize (do not rely on Tc-99m RBC scan alone), then perform subtotal colectomy; no role for "blind" hemicolectomy.

4. *Diverticuli* most common etiology (~ 50%), w/ often self-limited but intense arterial bleeding. Right colon diverticuli more prone to bleeding than left. 75–90% stop spontaneously, 10% recur w/in 1 yr, over 25% recur w/in 5 yr.

    a. *Tx*: endoscopic tx not advised. Persistent bleeding should be treated w/ segmental colectomy.

5. *Angiodysplasia* (arteriovenous malformations) next most common (5–20%) cause of lower GI bleeding in all pts and the most common cause in pts over 50 yo. They bleed less severely (venous) than diverticuli but are more likely to recur (75%). More common in right than left colon, and appear as small, flat, red submucosal lesions. Assoc. w/ aortic stenosis, ESRD, and von Willebrand's dz.

    a. *Tx*: endoscopic tx initially effective in > 75%, but rebleed rate 10–15%. Hemicolectomy (usu. right) reserved for refractory bleeding.

6. *Neoplasms* (polyps, malignancies) may be responsible for up to 20% of lower GI bleeds; under 20 yo, juvenile polyps are second most common cause.

    a. *Tx*: bleeding after endoscopic polyp bx can often be controlled by endoscopy. Polyps or malignancies → surgery as appropriate.

7. *Inflammatory/infectious* causes such as ulcerative colitis, postradiation enteritis, and bacterial colitis are common. Less common causes include AIDS, CMV, and Kaposi's sarcoma.

    a. *Tx*: depends on source. Rectal bleeding from radiation → tx w/ topical of formalin, steroids, or sucralfate.

8. *Vascular* etiologies usu. from bowel ischemia, but inflammatory vasculitides possible. R/o aortoenteric fistula if h/o AAA.

     a. *Tx*: restore perfusion if ischemic, followed by revascularization procedure if indicated. See section B6. above on management of aortoenteric fistula.

  9. *Hemorrhoids* frequently noted in pts w/ GI bleeds, but responsible for < 5% of significant bleeds.

     a. *Tx*: surgical excision or banding of internal hemorrhoids.

D. "Obscure etiology" GI hemorrhage

  1. Small bowel is usual source of "obscure etiology" GI bleeding, and of 3% GI bleeding overall. ~ ½ due to angiodysplasia, except in pediatric population (*Meckel's diverticulum most common source of lower GI bleeding overall in children*). Other causes include tumor, IBD, hemobilia.

  2. W/u should follow algorithm for upper vs lower GI hemorrhage. If (–), a variety of modalities (CT scan, Meckel's scan [Tc-99m], capsule endoscopy, small bowel endoscopy, etc.) may be pursued.

V. FISTULAS

A. Management by "SLATE" steps.

  1. *Stabilization* (immediately):

     a. Rehydrate, correct anemia, and occasionally may give albumin as well to increase to 3.0 mg/dL.

     b. Drain abscesses, other interventions to reduce septic sources.

     c. Control drainage (sump catheter), stomadhesive, etc., to protect skin.

     d. *Provide nutrition*: 1.3–1.5 × BEE and 1.2–2.0 g/kg nitrogen/d. May need to shift to lipid-based rather than carbohydrate-based enteral feed, or even parenteral nutrition. High-output fistulas should be met w/ 2× RDA of water-soluble vitamins, esp. vitamin C.

     e. *Decrease volume*: NGT not beneficial. H_2 blockers or PPI should be initiated. Sandostatin as 100–600 mcg/d divided two to four times per day will not result in a higher closure rate, but has been shown to decrease time to closure in those who do spontaneously close; also makes fluid/electrolyte replacement less arduous. Pt should be NPO, w/ TPN.

  2. *Localize* (generally 7–10 d after dx):

     a. Water-soluble fistulogram via 5–8 pediatric feeding tube is single highest yield study. CT may be indicated if deep abscess suspected.

  3. *Assess*:

     a. *Define characteristics of fistula of prognostic importance w/ FRIENDS*:

       i. *Foreign body*: presence requires removal.

       ii. *Radiation*: less likely to heal spontaneously.

       iii. *Inflammation or Infection: either reduces rate of closure.*

       iv. *Epithelialization*: reduces rate of closure.

       v. *Neoplasia and Nutritional status*: cancer reduces rate of closure, and transferrin level > 200 at dx or after 3 wk therapy suggests reasonable spontaneous closure rate.

       vi. *Distal obstruction*: reduces rate of spontaneous closure.

       vii. *Site and Size* (length, width, and volume): most likely to heal (oropharyngeal, esophageal, duodenal stump, pancreaticobiliary, jejunal); least likely to heal (gastric, lateral duodenal ligament of Treitz, ileal). Tract length > 2 cm or bowel defect > 1 cm wide unlikely to close.

  4. *Therapy* (definitive): typically resect and reanastomose affected segment.

  5. *Ensure Healing*: continue nutritional support and gradually resume enteric feeding.

VI. BOWEL OBSTRUCTION

A. General principles: treat w/ bowel rest (NGT), resuscitation (IVF, Foley catheter).

  1. *Partial*: failure to improve after 3 d → OR.

  2. *Complete* (obstipated): all → OR.

B. Etiology: in United States postop adhesions are most common. In developing world, hernias are most common cause.

  1. *Mechanical*

     a. *Adhesions*: most often from pelvic operations, although any intraabdominal surgery can contribute.

     b. *Hernia* (inguinal, ventral, *internal*—know the surgical hx!).

c. *Neoplasm.*

d. *Volvulus*: more common outside United States. Higher incidence w/ age, institutionalization, psychotropic meds.

   i. *Sigmoid*:

- ~ 70% of colonic volvulus.
- *Plain films*: may show "coffee bean sign," or "bent inner tube" on AXR. Barium enema may show "bird's beak." CT scan rarely needed, but may reveal twisted mesentery.
- *Tx*: decompression via rectal tube place w/ proctoscopy or colonoscopy usu. adequate for immediate tx, should be followed by sigmoid resection during the same hospital stay as frequently recurs (~ ½). Peritonitis or failure of rectal tube decompression mandates emergent operation.

   ii. *Cecal volvulus*

- Compared w/ sigmoid volvulus, pts usu. younger and higher percentage are females.
- AXR often similar to colonic volvulus, but often evidence of SBO as well. Contrast enema can be useful to differentiate the 2 and look for colonic tumors.
- As not amenable to endoscopic decompression, the dx mandates surgery (tx = right hemicolectomy, as cecopexy frequently fails).

   iii. *Cecal bascule* (French *basculer* v. = "to tip over," *bascule* n. = "rocker, see-saw")

- Extremely rare. Involves the distal cecum "flopping" over the more proximal segment, due to adhesive band or excessively large pouch of cecum. Surgical therapy may involve lysis of adhesion a/o cecopexy, depending on pathology.

2. *Ileus*: most often due to inflammation (postop, abscess, sepsis), electrolyte abnormality (hypomagnesemia, hypokalemia, etc.), or medication (narcotics). Reverse the primary process.

3. *Ogilvie's syndrome* (colonic pseudoobstruction):

a. Physiologic colonic dilatation w/ clinical obstruction. Usu. assoc. w/ rx (i.e., narcotics), orthopaedic trauma (esp. pelvic or hip), or retroperitoneal inflammation.

b. *Dx*: clinical obstruction (although diarrhea may be present) w/ radiographic evidence of colonic dilatation (may be pancolonic or predominantly right-sided) and no evidence of mechanical blockage. Small bowel not involved as w/ ileus unless pt has incompetent ileocecal valve.

c. *Tx*: cessation of implicated factors (i.e., narcotics, calcium channel blockers, anticholinergics) if able. Cecal diameter > 10 cm ↑↑ risk of perforation (law of LaPlace) and mandates urgent intervention. Consider naloxone (0.4 mg IV) if narcotic-related.

   i. *Medical*:

- Rectal tube a/o colonoscopy to decompress colon.
- Neostigmine, 1–2.5 mg IV over 3 min may be successful and can be repeated in 30 min. Caveat is possibility of bradycardia: should be given in monitored (i.e., ICU) setting w/ atropine available (1 mg IV prn).

   ii. *Surgical*:

- Exploration is indicated for failure of above measures or if evidence of bowel ischemia or perforation (i.e., peritonitis) or cecal diameter > 10 cm postcolonoscopy.
- *Cecostomy*: performed if no evidence of colon necrosis (has been described under local anesthesia).
- Loop colostomy.
- Segmental resection w/ end ileostomy, mucous fistula: performed if necrosis encountered.

CHAPTER 14

HEPATOBILIARY AND PANCREAS

I. LIVER (NONBILIARY)

A. **Embryology and vasculature**: begins as ventral foregut bud. Portal vs 70% blood flow, 50% O_2. Hepatic a. usu. comes off celiac axis. Left hepatic a. may come off left gastric a., and right hepatic a. may come off SMA.

B. **Anatomy**:

1. *Couinaud system* describes 8 segments w/ independent arterial, venous, and biliary flow.

   a. Cantlie's line (from IVC to gallbladder fossa) divides liver into right, left lobes—corresponds internally w/ course of middle hepatic vein.

      i. Falciform ligament divides left lateral segments (II, III) from left medial segment (IV).

   b. Segments named in relation to hepatic vein drainage.

      i. Caudate lobe immediately anterior to IVC, w/ caudal aspect posterior to portal vein and cephalad aspect posterior to middle and left hepatic veins.

   c. Portal vein structures encased in fibrous sheath continuous w/ Glisson's capsule.

2. *Lobes and sections* (segments that compose them):

   a. *Right lobe*: V, VI, VII, VIII

      i. Right anterior segment: V, VIII

      ii. Right posterior segment: VI, VII

   b. *Left lobe*: II, III, IV

      i. Left lateral segment: II, III

      ii. Left medial segment: IV

C. **Physiology**

1. *Bilirubin*: direct increased when liver unable to normally excrete conjugated bilirubin and it leaks into systemic blood supply. Indirect increased when unable to conjugate/clear the pigment it receives. Icterus apparent w/ Tbili > 2 mg/dL.

2. *Alk phos*: bone, placenta, liver produces. Elevation suggests biliary obstruction if no bone dz or pregnancy.

3. *INR*: best indicator of synthetic liver function.

4. *Determining resectability of liver*:

   a. Best indicator of synthetic function of liver is INR.

   b. Indicators which generally preclude resection:

      - Bilirubin twice normal generally precludes surgery.
      - Child's-Pugh B or C (total score > 7)—mortality w/ A = 3.7% vs B, C = 16.7%.
      - Indocyanine green clearance at 15 min.
        - < 10% retention, any resection should be feasible; 10–20%, bisegmentectomy possible; 20–29%, do not recommend > unisegmentectomy.
      - Wedged hepatic pressure (hepatic venous gradient) > 10 mm Hg suggests nonresectable physiology.
      - Lidocaine metabolite (monoethylglycinexylidide [MEGX]) test
        - Metabolite decreases as functional liver mass decreases.
        - C_{13}-aminopyrine test is a breath test based on same principle.
      - Signs of portal hypertension (i.e., bleeding esophageal varices) are a relative contraindication to resection. [Franco et al., Resection of hepatocellular carcinomas. Results in 72 European patients with cirrhosis, *Gastroenterology* 1990; 98:733–8; Bismuth et al., Liver resection versus transplantation for hepatocellular carcinoma in cirrhotic patients, *Ann Surg* 1993;218:145–51; Bruix J et al., Surgical resection of hepatocellular carcinoma: prognostic value of preoperative portal pressure, *Gastroenterology* 1996;111:1018–22.]

D. Benign disease

1. *Cirrhosis*

   a. Scar tissue in liver parenchyma, leads to resistance to blood flow, w/ formation of portosystemic shunts (esophageal varices, hemorrhoids, umbilicus).

   b. *PEx*: jaundice, dark urine, peripheral edema, caput medusa, spider angiomata, gynecomastia, testicular atrophy, palmar erythema.

   c. Albumin, coag factors (fibrinogen, prothrombin, V, VII, IX, X) decreased.

   d. PT elevated w/ fat absorption (hence, vitamin K absorption) decreased, impaired due to biliary obstruction as well as synthetic abnormalities of coag factors.

   e. Cardiac output increased, SVR decreased, may lead to cardiac failure.

   f. See Table 14.1.

TABLE 14.1. Child-Pugh Classification

	1 Point	2 Points	3 Points
Encephalopathy	None	Moderate (I, II)	Severe (III, IV)
Ascites	None	Slight	Moderate
Bilirubin (mg/dL)	< 2.0	2.0–3.0	> 3.0
Albumin (g/dL)	> 3.5	2.8–3.5	< 2.8
INR	< 1.7	1.7–2.3	> 2.3

To calculate Child-Pugh class, add points from each row: A = 5–6, B = 7–9, C = 10–15.

2. Liver failure and portal hypertension

   a. *Relevant anatomy and physiology*

      i. *Anatomy*:
         - Portal vein results from SMV and splenic veins (splenic v. receives blood from IMV) confluence behind pancreatic neck. Left gastric (coronary) vein empties gastric lesser curvature and distal esophagus into portal vein near origin.
         - *Collaterals can develop in*: coronary/short gastric v.'s → azygous v. (esophagogastric varices); recanalized umbilical v. (from left portal v.) → epigastric v.'s (caput medusae); retroperitoneal v.'s; hemorrhoids.

      ii. *Physiology*:
         - Cirrhosis (hepatocellular necrosis resulting in fibrosis and nodular regeneration) results in hepatocellular failure and portal hypertension.
         - Portal pressure > 5–8 mm Hg stimulates formation of portosystemic collaterals.
         - Hepatic artery can increase in blood flow to compensate for decreased portal blood flow (buffer response), but the reverse is not true.
         - Advanced liver dz results in increased levels of endogenous vasodilators (prostacyclin, NO, etc.) w/ peripheral dilation and hyperdynamic state, activating sympathetics and renin-aldosterone axis.

   b. *Classification and etiology*

      i. *Prehepatic*:
         - Portal vein thrombosis (most common; in absence of hepatic dz, collateral flow to liver may develop, called cavernomatous transformation of portal vein).
         - Splenic vein thrombosis (left-sided or sinistral portal hypertension; usu. secondary to pancreatitis or pancreatic neoplasm). Isolated gastric varices result. Splenectomy alone curative.

      ii. *Intrahepatic*:
         - *Presinusoidal*: schistosomiasis most common; many nonalcoholic cirrhosis cases begin here also; primary biliary cirrhosis.

- *Sinusoidal*: alcoholic (deposits collagen in space of Disse); postnecrotic viral.
- *Postsinusoidal*: alcoholic (regenerating nodules compress hepatic veins); Budd-Chiari syndrome (hepatic vs thrombosis); right heart failure; constrictive pericarditis; vena caval web.

c. *Medical management*

i. *Ascites*

- *W/u*:
  - Paracentesis for cell count, cx, total protein, and albumin.
    - Serum-ascites albumin gradient (SAAG): $Alb_{serum} - Alb_{ascites}$
      - *SAAG > 1.1*: ascites assoc. w/ sinusoidal hypertension (cirrhosis, CHF, Budd-Chiari, etc.)
      - *SAAG < 1.1*: ascites assoc. w/ altered peritoneal permeability (infection, extrahepatic malignancy, other inflammatory d/o)
- *Nonoperative management*
  - *Salt-restriction* (impaired ability to clear free water; sodium-avid physiology). < 2 g/d.
  - *Aldosterone-antagonist* (spironolactone) crucial. 100–400 mg/d. Titrate up q wk prn.
    - Furosemide may be added for extra diuresis.
  - *Large-volume paracentesis* (LVP)—ensure INR < 2 and plt > 40,000 before procedure; give albumin (6 g/L) if > 5 L removed.
  - *TIPS* (not usu. offered if T_{bili} > 5, INR > 2, significant CHF, encephalopathy, or portal vs thrombosis).
    - Decreased recurrence compared to LVP.
    - Increased rate of encephalopathy.
    - Does not improve overall survival.
    - Best viewed as a bridge to transplantation.
  - *Spontaneous bacterial peritonitis*: prophylaxis (after an episode of SBP or GI hemorrhage) and tx (dx = > 250 PMNs/mm³ and single, nonanaerobic, bacterial species) is w/ FQ (ofloxacin, ciprofloxacin, etc.).
- *Operative management* (*Note*: refractory ascites has 25% 1-yr survival.)
  - Liver transplant is tx of choice (see Chapter 24 for more details).
  - *Shunts* (particularly partial shunts, read below): selective shunts are contraindicated.

ii. *Varices*

- *Prevention of bleeding*
  - Beta blockers (nonselective, such as propanolol or nadolol).
    - Don't prevent varices, but are indicated to prevent bleeding in already extant varices.
  - Titrate to reduce resting pulse by 25% or to 55 bpm.
    - Addition of nitrates may confer additional protection.
  - Endoscopic ligation.
    - Reserved for pts w/ large varices who cannot tolerate beta blockers.
    - Combined w/ beta blockers, effective for prevention of *recurrent* bleeding.
- *Tx of acute bleeding*
  - *Medications*:
    - *Octreotide* (has replaced vasopressin as DOC): 100 mcg IV bolus, then 250 IV mcg/h.
    - Beta blockade.
  - *Endoscopy*: may tx w/ banding or sclerotherapy.

- *TIPS* (see entry 2ci. above).
- *Sengstaken-Blakemore tube*: may be used to tamponade bleeding varices up to 48 h (useful as temporizing measure until transfer or surgery).

3. *Hepatic cysts*
   a. *Noninfectious*
      i. Usu. solitary. 50% of cases assoc. w/ polycystic renal dz.
      ii. Solitary lesions w/ cuboidal epithelium = cystadenomas = premalignant → resect.
      iii. Multiloculated cysts, if not echinococcal, are generally neoplastic.
      iv. Virtually no role for aspiration as simple cysts reaccumulate rapidly, neoplastic cysts mandate removal, and parasitic cysts are at risk of rupture.
      v. Most simple cysts can be managed w/ laparoscopic unroofing (~ $1/3$) of cyst, w/ placement of omentum in the cavity. Multiple cysts can also be unroofed w/ fenestrations created to drain underlying cysts.
   b. *Infectious*—echinococcosis (hydatid dz)
      i. Most common cause of acquired hepatic cysts, endemic in Greece, portions of Europe, South America, Australia, and southern and western Africa.
      ii. Usu. caused by *E. granulosus* (cystic dz), more rarely by *E. multilocularis* (alveolar dz, generally limited to Alaska and Canada and less amenable to surgery). Eggs in dog feces ingested by cows, sheep, etc., or humans, then filtered in liver, or more rarely, lungs.
      iii. Most pts present w/ abdominal pain, although symptoms of complications such as infection, anaphylaxis, biliary obstruction, etc. ~ $3/4$ of cysts are solitary and in right lobe.
      iv. *Dx*:
         - Eosinophilia and mildly elevated LFTs may be present.
         - Indirect hemagglutination test and Casoni skin test w/ ~ 85% sensitivity.
            - Latter actually can sensitize the pt to become falsely positive or anaphylactic in future assays.
         - Complement fixation ~ 70% sensitive.
         - Plain radiographs may demonstrate calcification of cyst walls in ½ of pts. CT scan, U/S, liver scan all ~ 100% sensitive. ERCP rarely demonstrates daughter cysts or "sand."
      v. *Tx*:
         - *Surgical resection is tx of choice.*
            - Liver resection/radical surgery and pericystectomy w/ similar mortality rates, but the former has lower recurrence rates. Laparoscopic pericystectomy often feasible for peripheral, readily accessible lesions.
            - Adjunctive pre- and postop benzimidazole is recommended.
            - Ablation via aspiration and injection of scolecite (hypertonic saline, chlorhexidine, 80% alcohol, 0.5% cetrimide; formalin no longer widely used). If bile is aspirated, sclerosants not used. Process repeated, then cyst unroofed. Anaphylaxis possible if ruptures or spills. Procedure rapidly waning in popularity. 80–90% effective.
            - Drainage or obliteration alternative tx.
            - Mebendazole recommended in early cases or cases not amenable to surgery.

4. *Hepatic infections*
   a. *Abscesses*
      i. *Pyogenic*
         - More common in United States, often multiple sites w/in liver.
         - Often from cholecystitis, appendicitis, obstructing pancreaticobiliary neoplasm, PID, trauma, and rarely colon cancer. Immunodeficiency increases risk.
         - Causative organisms *E. coli*, *Streptococcus* > *Bacteroides* > *Klebsiella*, *Enterococcus*.
         - Treat by drainage and abx.
      ii. *Amebic*
         - More common in developing world, usu. isolated lesion in right lobe of liver.

- More common in men and in younger pts (< 40 yo).
- 7–14 d of metronidazole is usual tx.
  - If no marked improvement or resolution w/in 48 h, may have wrong dx or may be superinfected → aspirate or drain.
  - Other indications for percutaneous drainage: rupture into thorax/abdomen; tx failure after 3–5 d of abx; bacterial superinfection; abscess in left liver lobe (risk of rupture into pericardium).

b. *Cholangitis*
   i. *Charcot's triad*—RUQ pain, jaundice, fever.
   ii. *Raynauld's pentad*—above plus shock, obtundation.
   iii. Mandates resuscitation w/ IVF, IV abx, and emergent decompression via ERCP.

c. *Parasitic*
   i. *Clonorchis sinensis, Opisthorchis viverrini*: flukes, which spend part of life cycle in biliary tree, endemic in portions of Asia (esp. China, Thailand, Korea, Vietnam, depending on species), acquired from eating raw freshwater fish. Although usu. asymptomatic, heavy infections can result in biliary obstruction and cholangitis. Tx of acute dz is w/ praziquantel or albendazole. Chronic infection is risk factor for cholangiocarcinoma.
   ii. *Fasciola hepatica, F. gigantica*: liver flukes w/ worldwide distribution, acquired by eating contaminated freshwater plants such as watercress. Although their life cycle varies from the *C. sinensis* and *O. viverrini*, they also can cause biliary obstruction and cholangitis. Unlike most trematodes, *Fasciola* is resistant to praziquantel: triclabendazole is the drug of choice.
   iii. *Ascaris*: roundworm rarely lodges in ampulla of Vater, causing pancreatitis and biliary obstruction.

d. Viral (e.g., hepatitis A, B, C, etc.). Chronic viral hepatitis a risk factor for hepatocellular carcinoma.

5. *Solid lesions*
   a. Check AFP, CEA, CA-19-9 for possibility of malignancy. U/S should be first radiographic test.
   b. *Hemangioma*
      i. Most common solid hepatic tumor; F > M, 6:1.
      ii. Majority are subcapsular. If greater than 4 cm, may be palpable or cause pain. Rupture is rare. Large lesions may act as AV fistula causing CHF. Kasabach-Merritt syndrome (thrombocytopenia from platelet sequestration) has been reported.
      iii. *Dx*:
         - *U/S*: well-defined, hyperechoic, hypervascular.
         - *CT*: peripheral enhancement w/ IV contrast.
         - *MRI*: T1 = isodense; T2 = hyperdense w/ peripheral enhancement w/ gadolinium. Tc-99m *RBC scan*: good test—sensitive, specific. Core needle bx contraindicated, but some assert FNA is acceptable risk.
      iv. *Tx*: Symptomatic lesions may be surgically removed; radiotherapy or embolization is reserved for poor surgical candidates. Pts w/ large lesions and h/o usage of estrogens should be counseled against continuing estrogen.
   c. *Focal nodular hyperplasia*
      i. 2× more common in females (avg. age at dx 40 yo). Like adenomas (below), genesis or enlargement may be linked to oral contraceptives. Unlike adenomas, no malignant potential.
      ii. Most pts are asx, though some complain of RUQ mass a/o discomfort.
      iii. *Dx*:
         - *U/S*: not helpful.
         - *CT*: w/ contrast often reveals characteristic central stellate scar.
         - *Angiography*: hypervascular pattern.
         - *MRI*: T1/T2 = isodense; T1 central low-signal scar that enhances w/ gadolinium. Tc-99m sulfur colloid scan: variable.
      iv. *Tx*: OCPs should be discontinued, and symptomatic lesions should be excised.

d. *Hepatic adenoma*

   i. Virtually limited to women and linked to OCP usage. Majority are solitary lesions, and about ½ are asx.; may progress to hepatocellular carcinoma.

   ii. Pts generally present w/ RUQ pain or intraabdominal hemorrhage; bleeding occurs more frequently during menstruation.

   iii. *Dx*:

   - *U/S*: not helpful; usu. increased blood flow.
   - *CT*: hypodense; contrast may yield heterogeneous appearance.
   - *Angiography*: ranges from hypovascular to hypervascular.
   - *MRI*: frequently hypodense, Tc-99m sulfur colloid scan: generally non-enhancing CT and U/S are nonspecific, and angiographic appearance ranges from avascular to hypervascular. FNA may be warranted, but not core needle bx.

   iv. *Tx*: as lesions may regress off of oral contraceptives, asx or mildly symptomatic lesions smaller than 6 cm may be observed off of OCPs. Lesions larger than 6 cm are more likely to bleed or be malignant and should be removed.

II. BILIARY

A. Biliary stricture

1. *Benign causes*: chronic pancreatitis, primary sclerosing cholangitis, acute cholangitis, trauma; most common iatrogenic from laparoscopic colectomy.

   a. Unrecognized injury may lead to cholangitis, secondary biliary cirrhosis, portal hypertension.

      i. Iatrogenic cases often present w/in 1 wk postop w/ pain, fever, and jaundice (Tbili > 2.5 mg/dL) from biloma/peritonitis.

      - CT or U/S-demonstrated bilomas should be perc drained. ERCP or sinogram can demonstrate anatomy. PTC may be useful to place stent.
      - Cystic duct leaks can be treated w/ perc drainage, +/– ERCP ampulla stent to decrease resistance.
      - Lateral bile duct injury can be stented w/ T tube.

B. Primary sclerosing cholangitis (PSC)

1. Progressive cholestatic dz characterized by stenosis and beading of intra- and extrahepatic biliary tree. Unlike PBC (see section C. below), more commonly affects men. ~ ½–¾ pts also have inflammatory bowel dz, but only ~ 5% of pts w/ IBD have PSC (some speculate abd colonic mucosal barrier may be linked to etiology). Often presents w/ abdominal pain, fever, hepatomegaly, pruritus, etc. Assoc. w/ HLA-DR8 and HLA-DR3. May lead to cholangiocarcinoma, particularly in pts w/ high EtOH ingestion.

2. *Dx*:

   a. Hyperbilirubinemia, perinuclear antineutrophil cytoplasmic antibodies (p-ANCA, ~ 75% seropositive) suggestive.

   b. *Radiology*:

      i. *U/S*: intra- and extrahepatic ductal dilatation, possible increased echogenicity (but normal in ½ of cases).

      ii. *MRI*: T2 imaging w/ wedge-shaped high signal intensity areas characteristic.

      iii. *Cholangiography*: multiple strictures and dilatations ("beading").

3. *Tx*:

   a. *Medical*: prednisone, methotrexate, cyclosporine, pentoxifylline, abx all reported.

      i. Ursodeoxycholic acid useful for sx related to hyperbilirubinemia as well. Extrahepatic strictures may be tx'd w/ balloon dilatation. Supplement fat-soluble vitamins.

   b. *Surgery*: drainage procedures (porto- or choledochoenterostomy) doomed to failure. Particularly in children, liver transplantation may provide good long-term relief.

C. Primary biliary cirrhosis (PBC)

1. Probable autoimmune condition affecting small-to-medium bile ducts w/ progressive cholestasis and ultimately liver failure. More common in *women* (unlike PSC above) and assoc. w/ HLA-DR8,

elevated levels of IgM, hepatic granulomas, increased ESR, frequent concurrent autoimmune conditions (autoimmune thyroiditis, scleroderma, etc.). 90+% w/ antimitochondrial (98% specific). Antinuclear Ab in 20–50%. Often initially presents w/ fatigue. 10% w/ severe pruritus that does not correlate well w/ degree of hyperbilirubinemia, thought to be related to increased production of endogenous opioids.

2. *Dx:*

   a. Hyperbilirubinemia, *antimitochondrial Ab*, etc., suggestive.

   b. *Radiographic findings*: U/S of liver demonstrates increased echogenicity. PTC/ERCP.

   c. Bx w/ nonsuppurative cholangitis w/ basement membrane damage, lymphocytic infiltration.

3. *Tx:*

   a. Ursodeoxycholic acid initial tx. Methotrexate, cyclosporine, corticosteroids, colchicines sometimes used. Pruritus tx'd w/ cholestyramine/colestipol. Rifampin, dronabinol, and plasmapheresis reported to be helpful as well. Refractory cases w/ cirrhosis are definitively tx'd w/ liver transplantation.

D. Congenital conditions

1. *Choledochal cysts*

   a. More common in Asia (partic. Japan) and women. Vast majority have long (> 1 cm) common channel (CBD and pancreatic duct).

   b. "Classic" presentation of RUQ pain, jaundice, and abdominal mass only occurs in ~ 10%.

   c. *Dx:*

      i. U/S or CT can procure dx, but cholangiography needed to establish type of cyst and facilitate operative planning.

   d. *Classification and tx* (note: all cysts are resected—given 25–30% lifetime cancer risk otherwise; also, simply draining into enteric limb assoc. w/ cholangitis)

      i. *Type I* (50%)—fusiform dilatation of entire CBD
         - *Tx*: cholecystectomy, resect extrahepatic biliary tract, Roux-en-Y hepaticojejunostomy.

      ii. *Type II* (< 10%)—saccular diverticulum of CBD
         - *Tx*: same as for type I.

      iii. *Type III* (< 10%)—intraduodenal choledochocele involving sphincter
         - *Tx*: excise, sphincteroplasty vs sphincteroplasty/sphincterotomy alone.

      iv. *Type IV* (35%)—intra- and extrahepatic cysts
         - Resect extrahepatic biliary tract, Roux-en-Y hepaticojejunostomy.
         - If cysts in 1 lobe only, consider lobectomy. If both lobes, transplant.

      v. *Type V* (< 10%)—intrahepatic cysts (Caroli dz)
         - Cholecystectomy w/ common bile duct exploration.
         - If cysts in 1 lobe only, consider lobectomy. If both lobes, transplant.

2. *Biliary atresia* (see Chapter 18)

E. Cholelithiasis and complications (move this or primary biliary)—C 416, etc.

1. *Cholelithiasis*: present in ~ 15% of United States population, usu. asymptomatic. Sx develop at rate of 1–2% per yr, reaching a plateau of about ~ 20%. Asymptomatic cholecystitis is not generally an indication for cholecystectomy except in some pt populations (i.e., heart bypass pts; they develop stones more frequently and have significant cholecystitis complications due to immunosuppression).

   a. *Cholecystitis*: 95% of cases related to gallstone impaction. RUQ pain and U/S demonstrating gallbladder wall thickening (> 3.5 mm) a/o pericholecystic fluid are diagnostic. Tx w/ abx and laparoscopic cholecystectomy (or open if unable to safely proceed laparoscopically). Intraop cholangiogram generally recommended if abnormal LFTs (particularly bilirubin and alkaline phosphatase) a/o dilated CBD (> 6 mm, although the normal diameter increases w/ age).

   b. *Acalculous cholecystitis*: accounts for 5% of cases of cholecystitis, generally occurs in older males who are critically ill; etiology possibly related to reperfusion injury or other inflammatory d/o. Dx is suggested by GB wall edema and pericholecystic fluid, but HIDA is test of choice. Gold standard is also laparoscopic cholecystectomy, although percutaneous cholecystostomy tube should be strongly considered for the unstable pt.

2. *Choledocholithiasis*
   a. *Primary*:
      i. Form in the biliary tree, not from the gallbladder.
      ii. Usu. brown pigment stones, which appear soft, "earthy," and are assoc. w/ chronic biliary stasis and infection.
      iii. Stasis may be from sphincter of Oddi dysfunction, papillary stenosis, or biliary stricture.
      iv. *Definitive tx depends on cause*:
         - *Hepaticojejunostomy*: use Roux-en-Y, w/ non-refluxing end-to-side anastamosis and limb length of at least 45 cm.
         - Sphincteroplasty.
   b. *Secondary*:
      i. Form in gallbladder, then pass into biliary tree. Usu. either cholesterol stones or black pigment stones.
      ii. Treat w/ cholecystectomy (and clearance of CBD w/ IOC/exploration or ERCP).
3. *Mirizzi syndrome*: compression of common hepatic duct by stone lodged in Hartmann's pouch or cystic duct.
4. *Biliary pancreatitis*: see section III. below on pancreas.
5. *Cholangitis*: medical emergency from bacterial infection of obstructed (cancer, stone, parasite, etc.) biliary system. Charcot's triad = fever, RUQ pain, jaundice. Raynold's pentad = fever, RUQ pain, jaundice, hypotension, altered mental status.
6. *Gallstone ileus*: results when cholecystoenteric fistula develops (usu. duodenum, occ. colon), allowing gallstone(s) to enter intestinal lumen. Point of obstruction is usu. ileocecal valve. Treat by milking stone back to normal bowel, then creating an enterotomy through which to deliver the stone. Most fistulas will close spontaneously, and the dissection required to perform chlolecystectomy and fistula is excision, which is generally not recommended during the initial surgery, particularly in unhealthy pts.
7. *Bouveret's syndrome*: gastric outlet caused by proximal migration of gallstone from fistula.
8. *Bile leak*: often presents w/ abdominal pain, possibly fevers a/o jaundice. Check LFTs and RUQ U/S or CT. If biloma present, can percutaneously drain. ERCP should demonstrate leak, and if involves cystic duct, stenting should decompress sufficiently to allow healing. Injuries to CBD or right/left typically require exploration.
   a. *Evaluation of jaundice*
      i. *After H&P, check bilirubin*:
         - Indirect *(unconjugated)* hyperbilirubinemia—*nonsurgical.*
            ○ Increased production (hemolysis, burns, transfusion rxn's).
            ○ Impaired hepatocyte uptake or conjugation (Gilbert's, Crigler-Najjar, viral hepatitis, neonatal jaundice, drug inhibition).
         - Direct *(conjugated)* hyperbilirubinemia—*usu. surgical.*
            ○ Impaired transport and excretion (Dubin-Johnson, Rotor's, cirrhosis, amyloidosis, cancer, hepatitis, pregnancy, TPN cholestasis).
            ○ Biliary obstruction (choledocholithiasis, Mirizzi's, benign stricture, periampullary CA, cholangiocarcinoma, primary sclerosing cholangitis, parasitic, Caroli's dz).
            ○ *Note*: high levels of indirect bilirubin eventually result in elevated direct bilirubin levels as well as after the bilirubin is conjugated.
         - *Direct hyperbilirubinemia w/u*:
            ○ If suspect intrahepatic dz, check hepatitis panel, liver bx, other tests.
            ○ If suspect common duct stones, check U/S.
               ■ If see dilated ducts, pursue ERCP for stone extraction.
               ■ If see normal ducts, some recommend MRCP.
            ○ If suspect malignant obstruction, check CT scan.
               ■ If see mass or dilated ducts and suspect proximal obstruction → ERCP.
               ■ If see mass or dilated ducts and suspect distal obstruction → PTC.

b. *ERCP*
   i. *Indications*
      - *Preop*:
        - ◦ Worsening biliary pancreatitis
        - ◦ Cholangitis
        - ◦ Stent placement for stricture (benign or malignant)
        - ◦ Symptomatic cholelithiasis in pts unfit for surgery
      - *Postop*:
        - ◦ Bile leak
        - ◦ Retained CBD stone
   ii. *Note*: open surgical papillotomy can be performed as well through duodenotomy. Key point is to perform papillotomy at 10 o'clock position to avoid bleeding.

III. PANCREAS

A. **Benign disease**
   1. *Acute pancreatitis*
      a. *Etiology*: gallstones, alcohol, trauma (including ERCP), hypercalcemia, hypertriglyceridemia, paramyxovirus (mumps), medications (diuretics [thiazides, furosemide], steroids, azathioprine, sulfonamides, NSAIDs), autoimmune (polyarteritis nodosa, SLE), scorpion envenomation [*Tityus trinitatus* of Trinidad; Bartholomew C, *BMJ*, 1970;1:666–8.] Rare causes include pancreas divisum, cystic fibrosis, pancreatic malignancy, helminth (i.e., *Ascaris*) obstruction, etc.
      b. *Presentation and w/u*:
         - *Clinical*: epigastric pain radiating to the back is classic. Hemorrhagic pancreatitis may (rarely) demonstrate Cullen's sign (periumbilical ecchymosis) or Grey Turner's sign (flank ecchymoses) or Fox's sign (inguinal ecchymosis).
         - *Biochemical*:
            - ◦ *Amylase*: generally rises w/in 2–12 h of sx onset, normalizing w/in 1 wk.
               - ■ *Hyperamylasemia ddx*: pancreatic injury or inflammation, small bowel injury, appendicitis, parotiditis, orchitis, hereditary macroamylasemia (molecule too large to be renally excreted), renal failure.
            - ◦ *Lipase*: generally rises w/in 4–8 h of sx onset, normalizing in 1–2 wk.
               - ■ Slightly more sensitive and specific for pancreatitis; no need to order lipase *and* amylase.
         - *Radiographic*: imaging not usu. needed for the dx. More commonly ordered if pt deteriorates, is thought to be septic, or fails to improve after a wk.
      c. *Scoring systems*:
         - Most cases are mild and resolve w/in several days.
         - Ranson's criteria (3+ predictive of severe attack w/ > 10% mortality; pt should be in ICU). See Table 14.2.

TABLE 14.2.   Ranson's Score for Pancreatitis

Nonbiliary Pancreatitis		Biliary Pancreatitis	
Initial	48 h	Initial	48 h
> 55 yo	Hct decrease > 10%	> 70 yo	Hct decrease > 10%
WBC > 16k / mm³	BUN increase > 5 mg/dL	WBC > 18k / mm³	BUN increase > 2 mg/dL
Glucose > 200 mg/dL	Ca^{++} < 8 mg/dL	Glucose > 220 mg/dL	Ca^{++} < 8 mg/dL
LDH > 350 IU/L	Fluid sequestration > 6 L	LDH > 40 IU/L	Fluid sequestration > 4 L
AST > 250 U / 100 mL	Base deficit > 4 mmol/L	AST > 250 U / 100 mL	Base deficit > 5 mmol/L
	PaO_2 > 55 mm Hg		

d. *Tx*: all cases are managed w/ the first 2 steps mentioned below. Moderate to severe cases, however, are biphasic. The first (inflammatory) phase is managed conservatively w/ these same first 2 stages, and surgery, which may actually worsen the inflammatory response, is avoided if possible. The second stage involves managing the sequelae, which are generally determined in the first 4–5 d; surgery and other invasive interventions are more frequently used in this phase.

   i. *NPO w/ NGT decompression* (some authors argue the latter is not necessary).

   - Nutritional support for prolonged cases has traditionally been via TPN; however, several studies now support enteric (at least trophic) feeds via nasojejunal tube both for alimentation and to prevent bacterial translocation.

   ii. *IVF resuscitation + Foley catheter.*

   iii. *Abx*: infected pancreatic necrosis merits tx w/ carbapenems, while prophylactic use (i.e., for sterile pancreatic necrosis) is controversial, w/ literature supporting both sides. One reasonable compromise is carbapenem usage if > 30% necrosis.

   iv. *ERCP*: reserved for biliary pancreatitis that deteriorates or fails to improve after 48 h.

   v. *Surgery*:

   - Delay surgery for after first 2 wk if at all possible; increased mortality w/ early operative intervention.

   - *Infected* pancreatic necrosis is the main indication for surgery, although some pts who fail to respond to optimal medical therapy may benefit from debridement. Many surgeons rely upon CT-guided FNA to determine if necrotic material is infected, while others base the decision to operate on clinical and radiographic evidence.

   - Pancreatic necrosectomy followed by temporary closure and planned redebridement in 24–48 h vs necrosectomy and placement of irrigation (i.e., Davol) drains are the 2 usual approaches.

   vi. *For cases of biliary pancreatitis*, cholecystectomy should be performed before discharge ($^1/_3$ of pts will have recurrence w/in 8 wk otherwise). In mild cases, surgery is generally undertaken once the pt is pain-free, w/ no abdominal tenderness; most also wait for normalization of amylase a/o lipase. If ERCP is not performed preop, intraop cholangiogram should be performed.

e. *Sequelae/complications*:

   i. *Acute fluid collection*: fluid around pancreas typically < < 4 wk following onset of inflammation that lacks capsular wall. If not infected, manage w/ observation, as most spontaneously resolve.

   ii. *Pancreatic pseudocyst*: fluid (pancreatic "juice") collection(s) in/around pancreas > 4 wk following onset of inflammation. Most resolve w/ time, but collections persisting > 6 wk or > 6 cm in diameter are more likely to require intervention to avoid complications such as infection, gastric compression, or hemosuccus pancreaticus. Drainage (cystgastrostomy, cystjejunostomy, or, rarely, cystduodenostomy) is performed once pseudocyst has substantial capsule.

   iii. *Pancreatic abscess*: infected peripancreatic fluid (either acute fluid collection or pseudocyst). Most are successfully managed w/ abx and percutaneous drainage.

   iv. *Pancreatic necrosis*: see section d. above on general treatment.

   v. *Pancreatic ascites*: direct communication of pancreatic duct from trauma or rupture of pancreatic pseudocyst. Management is usu. conservative, w/ percutaneous drainage, converting the condition to a *pancreatic fistula*.

   vi. *Pancreatic fistula* (see entry ii. on pancreatic pseudocyst and entry v. on pancreatic ascites above): initial tx is w/ TPN a/o nasojejunal feeds +/– IV octreotide, replacement of electrolytes (i.e., sodium, bicarbonate). Fistulas that persist beyond 6 wk despite appropriate medical tx are definitively managed w/ distal pancreatectomy (leak in tail), or Roux-en-Y limb (leak in head, body), although endoscopic stenting may be a viable option for some. If pancreatic duct is dilated (i.e., 8 mm), lateral pancreaticojejunostomy is often appropriate.

   vii. *Pancreatic pleural effusion*: manage as pancreatic ascites/fistula.

   viii. *Hemosuccus pancreaticus*: hemorrhage resulting from pseudocyst erosion into peripancreatic vessel. Tx w/ endovascular embolization of involved vessel, possibly followed by surgical exploration and packing.

2. *Chronic pancreatitis*

    a. Most commonly from recurrent alcoholic pancreatitis, resulting in pain and potentially exocrine a/o endocrine insufficiency.

    b. *Surgical tx can be divided into 2 broad approaches*: ductal drainage (theorizing that problem is ductal hypertension) or resection (theorizing that nerve proliferation or sensitization is responsible for pain *or* if duct is too small to drain).

        i. *Resection procedures* (have generally fallen out of favor)

           • *Whipple*: sometimes performed for benign, inflammatory mass in head w/ nondilated duct. Entails pancreaticoduodenectomy followed by jejunostomy/gastrostomy + gastrojejunostomy + choledochojejunostomy.

           • *Subtotal pancreatectomy*: generally less than 80% (if remove 95%, leaving thin rim along duodenum and CBD, termed Child's resection).

        ii. *Drainage procedures*

           • *Partington-Rochelle* (modification of Puestow, *vide infra*): side-to-side pancreaticojejunostomy w/out resection of pancreatic tail or spleen.

        iii. *Combination procedures* (procedures of choice for vast majority, good results up to 95% reported): Puestow, Beger, Frey

B. Developmental anomalies

1. *Pancreas divisum*:

    a. *Etiology/presentation*: failure of fusion of dorsal and ventral ducts (ventral duct [duct of Wirsung) assoc. w/ CBD and migrates inferiorly to dorsal duct [duct of Santorini] to drain via major papilla). Result is the normally smaller duct of Santorini draining the pancreatic body through minor papilla instead of the duct of Wirsung through the ampulla of Vater; it should be noted that variations of this anomaly are common (up to 5–10%). Usu. asymptomatic, but may result in pain/pancreatitis.

    b. *Dx*: made via ERCP/MRCP, but all efforts must be made to r/o other possible causes of pancreatitis.

    c. *Tx*:

        i. *Endoscopic*: balloon dilatation or papillotomy may be used in minimally symptomatic pts.

        ii. *Operative*: surgery is indicated for pts w/ pancreatitis (or in pts w/ pain in whom stenting is technically not possible).

2. *Annular pancreas*: see "double bubble" on x-ray, as w/ duodenal atresia or malrotation. Perform duodenojejunostomy w/out resecting pancreas.

C. W/u of pancreatic lesions

1. *Solid*—consider as malignant until proven otherwise:

    a. *CT w/ 3-mm cuts should be obtained*: adenocarcinomas are often slightly hypodense, but this is not diagnostic.

        i. *CT criteria for unresectability include*: evidence of distant/extrapancreatic spread; obliteration of fatty plane between mass and superior mesenteric vein; encasement of SMA.

        ii. *Pts w/ unresectable dz need bx for palliative tx (chemo, XRT); this is best obtained by EUS. Pathologic dx is not required preop, however*. In pts w/ strong possibility of having an inflammatory mass instead of cancer, endoscopic FNA may be considered, but carries a 10% risk of being false-negative due to sampling error.

    b. Endoscopic U/S a/o ERCP useful to identify lesions < 2 cm. Endoscopically placed stents may also be used to provide symptomatic relief, tx cholangitis, or help correct hepatic dysfunction preop, but should be plastic, not metal, if surgery is planned.

    c. In pts w/ tumors > 2 cm that appear resectable on CT, laparoscopy sometimes used to confirm resectability before proceeding w/ open operation (assuming one would not need to perform open biliary a/o gastric bypass regardless of findings).

2. *Cystic*: pseudocyst >> neoplasms > congenital.

    a. *Hx*: pancreatitis (esp. alcoholic, chronic) or trauma suggests pseudocyst.

    b. *CT characteristics*: septations suggest neoplasm.

c. *ERCP/MRCP*: pancreatic duct communication suggests pseudocyst or intraductal papillary mucinous neoplasm.

d. *Aspirate*: high amylase suggests pseudocyst whereas mucin or high CEA a/o CA 19-9 suggest neoplasm.

e. *Bx*: epithelial cells in cyst wall exclude pseudocyst.

CHAPTER 15

HERNIAS

I. INGUINAL HERNIAS

A. In men, indirect hernias 2× more common than direct. Direct hernias even less common in females; females have femoral hernias more commonly than men (but still relatively uncommon).

1. Indirect and femoral hernias both 2× more common on the right. (Right testis descends more slowly on right, and sigmoid colon may tamponade left femoral canal.)

2. Infant females may have fallopian tube/ovary in inguinal ring. 1% of pediatric female inguinal hernias assoc. w/ testicular feminization; obtain buccal smear for chromatin testing in female infants w/ inguinal hernia. If no chromatin found, leave gonad in canal to generate estrogen until puberty, then take out to prevent malignant degeneration.

3. Young males (up to 3 yo) should undergo contralateral groin exploration esp. if presenting hernia is on left.

B. Anatomy

1. *Conjoined tendon*: fusion of fibers from internal oblique and transversus abdominis aponeuroses. Inserts on pubic tubercle, pectineal ligament, and superior pubic ramus.

2. *Genital nerve*: motor to cremaster muscle *and* sensory to lateral scrotum/labia (not leg). Arises from L1 to L2. Lies on iliopubic tract, accompanying cremaster vessels, generally divided w/ impunity. Runs along spermatic cord, often in inferoposterior aspect of cord along w/ external spermatic vessels. In males can be divided w/ impunity; females may experience undesirable hypesthesia of labia majora, however.

3. *Hesselbach's triangle*: although not exactly the same boundaries as initially described in 1814, circumscribes area through which *most* direct hernias protrude. Superolateral = inferior epigastric vessels; medial = lateral border of rectus sheath; inferior/base = inguinal ligament.

4. *Iliopectineal arch*: medial thickening of iliopsoas muscle deep to inguinal ligament; external oblique aponeurosis and fibers of inguinal ligament insert into it and also serve as lateral attachment of iliopubic tract.

5. *Ilioinguinal nerve*: mixes w/ fibers of iliohypogastric nerve to provide sensation to groin, penile base/scrotum, medial upper thigh. Arise from T12 and L1. Found superficial and superior to spermatic cord in 60%, but may be behind or in cremasteric muscle.

6. *Iliopubic tract*: transverse aponeurotica at upper border of femoral sheath; aponeurotic band extending from iliopectineal arch to superior pubic ramus. Passes medially, contributing to inferior border of internal ring, then crosses femoral vessels to form anterior margin of femoral sheath. Attaches to pectineal ligament and is often confused w/ inguinal ligament. More simply, a ridge-like thickening of aponeurotic tissue along superior rim of inferior pubic ramus immediately deep/posterior to inguinal ligament, essentially where transversalis fascia attaches to the ramus.

7. *Inguinal ligament* (Poupart's ligament): thickened inferior aspect of external oblique aponeurosis. Extends from AS iliac spine to pubic ramus; middle $1/3$ has a free (shelving) edge, lateral $2/3$ attached to iliopsoas fascia.

8. *Lacunar ligament* (Gimbernat's ligament): inferiormost portion of inguinal ligament, which recurves to attach to pectineal ligament.

9. *Pectineal ligament* (Cooper's ligament): formed from tendinous fibers of internal oblique, transversus, and pectineus muscle. More simply, a somewhat broad ridge of thickened ligamentous tissue found immediately posterior to iliopubic tract (which itself is immediately posterior to the inguinal ligament), in the medial portion of the groin. Division of the transversalis fascia is mandatory to view this structure.

10. *Reflected inguinal ligament* (Colles' ligament): thick band formed mostly by fibers of lacunar ligament and fibers of internal oblique, transversus abdominis, and pectineus muscle; formed by aponeurotic fibers from inferior aspect of external ring. Fixed to periosteum of superior pubic ramus.

11. *Semiarculate line of Douglas*: in lower ¼ of abdominal wall, aponeuroses of internal oblique and transversus abdominus pass anterior to muscle, which is bounded posteriorly by transversalis muscle only.

12. *Shelving edge of inguinal ligament*.

C. **Hernia nomenclature and types**

1. *Incarcerated hernia*—irreducible.

2. *Taxis*—manipulation of the hernia resulting in reduction.

3. *Strangulated hernia*—vascularity of viscus is compromised.

4. *Richter's hernia*—contents of the sac consist of only a portion of the intestinal wall of the intestine; esp. precarious in that strangulation can occur w/out obstruction.

5. *Sliding hernia*—internal retroperitoneal organ (cecum, sigmoid colon for indirect, bladder for direct) forms part of the wall of the hernia sac.

6. *Indirect hernia*—dilated persistent processus vaginalis, emerges lateral to inferior epigastric vessels, and lies along anteromedial aspect of cord. Properitoneal fat may be found w/in, inappropriately called "cord lipoma." If remains completely open and contains testicle, is termed communicating hydrocele. *Note:* 80% of newborns and 50% of 1-yr-olds have patent processus vaginalis; only 20% of adults remain patent.

7. *Direct hernia*—protrusion through inguinal floor, via Hesselbach's triangle (*almost* always medial to inferior epigastric vessels, which are the last branch of external iliacs).

8. *Femoral hernia*—herniation between femoral vein/sheath laterally and lacunar ligament medially; limited anteriorly by inguinal ligament and posteriorly by Cooper's ligament. Often contains node(s) of Cloquet/Rosenmüller.

9. *Pantaloon hernia*—defect w/ herniation both medial and lateral to epigastric vessels.

10. *Littre's hernia*—any inguinal hernia which contains a Meckel's diverticulum.

D. **Repairs**

1. *Lichtenstein's tension-free repair:* sew mesh to Cooper's ligament, then tack down to conjoined tendon above and shelving edge of inguinal ligament below, reinforcing transversalis fascia floor (for direct hernias), and can tighten "legs" of mesh to reconstruct internal ring (for indirect hernias). Open procedure of choice for almost all inguinal hernias.

2. *Others:* Marcy, Bassini, Shouldice, McVay-Lotheissen. In last one, transverse aponeurotic arch is sutured to Cooper's ligament medially and to femoral sheath laterally; requires excision of medial portion of iliopubic tract. The nonmesh procedure of choice for femoral hernias.

3. *Laparoscopic:*

   a. Results in fewer recurrences compared to open suture, but not mesh repairs.

   b. Takes longer, possibly fewer infections, possibly earlier return to work.

   c. *Two approaches:*

      i. Transabdominal preperitoneal (TAPP)

      ii. Totally extraperitoneal (TEP)

4. *Open preperitoneal* (Nyhus): esp. good for strangulated hernias as can provide direct access to peritoneal contents for bowel resection w/out additional incision. Also useful for femoral and recurrent hernias.

E. **Complications**

1. *General*

   a. *Neuralgia:* pain, paresthesias, a/o numbness result from partial nerve division or entrapment in mesh or scar tissue, but most largely subside w/in 2 mo. Completely transecting nerve can avoid this for nerves at risk, yielding only a variable degree of numbness.

   b. *Injury to vas deferens:* may present as painful spermatic granuloma; tx by granuloma excision and repair of vas.

   c. *Recurrence:* most repairs report 1–10% recurrence rate.

   d. *Ischemic orchitis/testicular atrophy:* most often from venous, not arterial, insufficiency. Initially presents as swollen, firm cord, epididymis, and testis, most often 2–5 d postop; symptoms may last several mo. Decrease risk by not dissecting medial to pubis and not dissecting distal hernia sac (except in sliding hernias).

2. *Laparoscopic*

   a. *Triangle of doom:* defined by vas deferens medially, spermatic vessels laterally, and external iliac vessels inferiorly. Contains external iliac artery/vein, deep circumflex iliac vein, genital branch of genitofemoral nerve, as (covered by fascia) femoral nerve. Stapling in this area can cause significant bleeding a/o neuralgia.

    b. *Triangle of pain*: defined by spermatic vessels medially, iliopubic tract laterally, and inferior edge of skin incision. Contains lateral femoral cutaneous nerve and anterior femoral cutaneous nerve. Stapling in this area can cause neuralgia.

    c. *Circle of death* ("corona mortis"): vascular ring formed by anastamosis of aberrant branch of obturator artery w/ a branch of internal iliac artery. Injury can lead to considerable bleeding.

II. NON-INGUINAL HERNIAS (*note*: paraesophageal hernia discussed in Chapter 6)

A. Epigastric hernia: risk factors include obesity and pregnancy. Differentiate from diastasis recti, as the latter does not present risk of significant complication.

B. Ventral hernia

  1. Mesh repair standard of care either open or laparoscopic.

  2. Ramirez (1990) first described component release (ext oblique and posterior rectus fascia) for abdominal closure; can get up to 20 cm at waist. [Ramirez OM et al., *Plast Reconstr Surg*, 1990;86(3):519-26.]

C. Spigelian hernia: Spigelian fascia lies between aponeurotic edge of transversus abdominus and lateral border of rectus sheath. Majority are w/in 6 cm of level of iliac crest. Often difficult to appreciate on abdominal exam; CT generally procures dx. Repair through incision directly over hernia or through preperitoneal or laparoscopic means.

D. Petit's hernia: like Grynfeltt's hernia, is a lumbar hernia. Petit's is inferior and represents an upright triangle bounded by latissimus dorsi, iliac crest, and external oblique muscle; it is covered only by superficial fascia. Repair requires prosthesis or myoaponeurotic flap.

E. Grynfeltt's hernia: like Petit's hernia, a lumbar hernia. Grynfeltt's is superior and represents an inverted triangle defined by 12th rib, internal oblique muscle, and sacrospinalis muscle; it is covered by latissimus dorsi. Repair requires prosthesis or myoaponeurotic flap.

F. Parastomal hernia: for first-time hernias, moving site of stoma and mesh repair of hernia is preferred. For recurrent hernias, mesh repair is recommended. [Rubin MS, et al., *Arch Surg* 1994;129(4):413–8.]

G. Obturator hernia: most common variant of pelvic hernias, and is generally seen in elderly, cachectic females, often strangulated upon presentation. Compression of obturator nerve may result (50%) in hip, knee, and medial thigh pain, esp. w/ internal rotation of thigh (Howship-Romberg sign). Mass may be palpable in upper medial thigh, or on pelvic/rectal exam. Exploration through lower midline incision useful to assess bowel and repair hernia. Can often be repaired w/out mesh.

H. Umbilical hernia: black > white children. F > M adults. Risk factors include multiple pregnancies and ascites; latter condition may result in rupture requiring emergent portal decompression. Strangulation of colon, omentum not uncommon. Infants w/ defects 2 cm or smaller may be observed while defects larger than 2 cm or any defect in a child older than 3 yo should be repaired. The Mayo "vest-over-pants" imbrication remains the standard for small hernias; prosthetic repair for larger defects is appropriate.

CHAPTER 16

SPLEEN

I. ANATOMY

A. Tethered by gastrosplenic, gastrocolic, splenorenal, and phrenosplenic ligaments, must take down superior, lateral, and inferior ligaments to mobilize. Splenic artery branches off celiac axis, and divides into 6 segmental end branches. Accessory spleens in ~ 25%, from failure of anlagen to fuse—most often in hilum, splenic ligaments, omentum, mesentery, and rarely along left ureter or left gonad. Histologically arranged into inner white pulp (w/ lymphatic follicles and immunologic function), marginal zone (filters material from white zone), and outer red pulp (w/ sinuses; serves phagocytic function).

II. TRAUMA: see Chapter 7.

III. NONTRAUMA INDICATIONS FOR SPLENECTOMY (splenectomy, splenorrhaphy details in Chapter 7.)

A. ITP: splenectomy reserved for the 75% of adults who fail steroid +/– IVIgG, +/– Rho(d) immunoglobulin tx; > 85% get good response to surgery. Thrombocytopenia and intracranial bleed are indications for emergent splenectomy. Nuclear medicine scans such as SPECT imaging useful to identify accessory spleens in refractory cases.

B. TTP: if pt fails plasmapheresis and FFP +/– steroids +/– aspirin (~ 30–50%).

C. Gaucher's dz: deficent β-glucosidase leads to glycosylceramide accumulation in RES. Can cause hypersplenism or mechanical sx from splenomegaly. *Partial* splenectomy recommended (over total splenectomy) to lessen risk of malignancy and accelerated bone dz.

D. Felty syndrome: constellation of rheumatoid arthritis, autoimmune neutropenia (often w/ recurrent infections), and splenomegaly. Splenectomy can improve neutropenia.

E. Pyruvate kinase deficiency, thalassemias, and elliptocytosis: splenectomy can help w/ hemolytic anemia if significant.

F. Spherocytosis: from RBC lack of spectrin; splenectomy only useful tx. Eval for cholelithiasis (55%), do concomitant cholecystectomy as appropriate.

G. Splenic vein thrombosis (often from pancreatitis): can lead to "left-sided ("sinister") portal hypertension" manifesting w/ isolated gastric varices. Splenectomy, not shunt, is indicated.

H. Part of total gastrectomy or other surgery.

I. Sarcoidosis: granulomatous dz of spleen may lead to anemia, which is improved w/ splenectomy.

K. Hairy cell leukemia: tx first w/ interferon a/o cladribine, reserving splenectomy for failures (primarily palliative at that point—very rare).

L. Giant hemangiomas: rarely may lead to platelet entrapment and Kasabach-Merritt syndrome as in the liver.

M. Infections: formerly, splenic abscesses warranted splenectomy, but majority can be handled w/ percutaneous drainage and abx.

IV. CONSEQUENCES OF SPLENECTOMY

A. Howell-Jolly bodies: nuclear remnants in RBC.

B. Heinz bodies: denatured hgb remnants (think Heinz ketchup = red = hgb).

C. Pappenheimer bodies: iron granules.

D. Leukocytosis.

E. Thrombocytosis: conventionally, aspirin given if > 1,000,000, although little data to support.

F. Loss of tuftsin (helps PMNs phagocytose) and properdin (helps initiate alternate complement pathway) and major site of IgM synthesis. Leads to OPSS (below).

G. Risk of "overwhelming postsplenectomy sepsis."

   1. Avoid splenectomy if pt less than 4 yo if possible.

   2. Mortality > 50% in children, decreases w/ age.

   3. Typically occurs in first 2 yr postop, but can occur > 5 yr later.

4. *Streptococcus pneumoniae* (50–90%), *H. influenzae*, *N. meningitidis* should all be vaccinated against; last not as commonly indicated though. *E. coli*, β-hemolytic strep, and *Pseudomonas* are other potential pathogens. (Encapsulated bacteria require opsonization for optimal elimination.) Increased risk for severe malaria, babesiosis.

5. Risk greater if splenectomy for heme/onc dz than trauma or if pt less than 4 yo.

6. Prodrome of F, C, ST, D, V → hypotension, DIC, death.

7. No data to support prophylactic abx in adults.

    a. *Children < 5 yo*: amoxicillin 20 mg/kg PO q d or penicillin VK 125 mg PO two times per day (*alt*: TMP-SMX, clarithromycin).

    b. *Children > 5 yo*: penicillin VK 250 mg PO two times per day × 1 yr postsplectomy (*alt*: TMP-SMX, clarithromycin).

    c. *All children*: self-tx w/ ampicillin-clavulanate for febrile illness while awaiting eval by physician.

H. Most common complication is LLL atelectasis, followed by subphrenic abscess. Placement of drain in splenic fossa unnecessary (unless pancreatic injury/leak), and contributes to risk of subphrenic abscess.

CHAPTER 17

BREAST

(See Chapter 10 for breast cancer.)

I. ANATOMY AND VASCULATURE OF BREAST AND AXILLA

A. Vascular and lymphatic

1. *Vascular:* 60% blood supply from subclavians via internal mammary perforators. 30% blood supply from axillary artery via lateral thoracic artery → external mammary artery. 10% from aorta via posterior intercostals. Batson's plexus refers to anastamotic network connecting intercostal veins w/ vertebral veins, thought to be important for vertebral metastases.

2. *Lymphatic drainage:* majority to level I—lateral to pectoralis minor (includes axillary, which drains arm; ext mammary, which drains breast; and subscapular). Level II refers to nodes deep to pectoralis minor (aka "Rotter's nodes"). Level III medial to pectoralis minor.

B. Nerve: long thoracic n. (innervates serratus anterior) 1–3 cm anterior to thoracodorsal n. (innervates latissimus). Transverse intercostobrachial n. crosses axilla transversely to provide sensory function to medial arm. Lateral pectoral nerve runs under and medial to pectoralis minor to innervate pectorals.

C. Anatomic anomalies: 2–6% women w/ polymastia (typically in axilla) or polythelia (typically inferior to primary nipple). < 10% women w/ benign nipple inversion.

II. BENIGN DISEASE

A. Mastodynia: 66% of women. Do H&P; if abn, manage accordingly. If WNL, do mammogram; tx lesions accordingly. If no lesion, 5–10% will respond to medical tx; primrose oil (gamma-linoleic acid) or Danazol (FDA-approved).

B. Nipple discharge: may be physiologic, from meds, or pituitary tumors. Pathology usu. papilloma. More worrisome if spontaneous (doesn't require squeezing/induction), bloody, unilateral from 1 duct, assoc. w/ mass, or if age > 60 yo.

C. Breast abscess: abx and aspiration likely to be successful unless > 20 cc volume, > 5 cm diameter, or > 1 wk delay dx, in which case I&D probably required. [Ervilmaz R et al., *Breast*, 2005 Oct ;14(5):375–9; Schwarz RJ et al., *Am J Surg*, 182(2):11–9.]

D. Fibroadenomas: most common lump if < 30 yo. R/o cystosarcoma phylloides. Observe, or if sx (or > 2–3 cm), excise. No increased cancer risk.

E. Fibrocystic dz: 50% United States females meet clinical definition, 70% meet histologic criteria. 58% premenopausal females have microcysts, 21% have macrocysts. Of female w/ cysts, 54% will refill, and 10% refill after aspiration. Intraop, classically have appearance of "blue domed cysts." Appropriate to cytology and excise if atypical pathology or if persistently symptomatic.

F. Breast lumps: if cystic, aspirate, f/u w/ mammogram; if nonbloody (which does NOT require cytology) or if disappears, just observe (some would add if strong fam hx, bx too). If mass recurs × 2, or aspirate is bloody, or if persists, or if get positive cytology, or if initial size was > 5 cm, bx. If is solid, but clinically benign *and* mammogram/sonogram (–) *and* CNBx/FNA benign, then observe (triple test—neg predict value 100%). If solid but indeterminate or mammo suspicious and CNBx or FNA malignant or benign, bx.

G. Mondor's dz: superficial thrombophlebitis of the breast. *Tx:* NSAIDs, warm compresses.

H. Benign lesions and breast CA risk

1. *No increased risk*:

   a. Apocrine metaplasia.

   b. Duct ectasia.

   c. Mild epithelial hyperplasia of unusual type.

2. *1–4× increased risk*:

   a. Moderate (3–5+ cell layers above BM—normally only 2)—florid (> 70% luminal filling) hyperplasia.

   b. Sclerosing adenosis.

      c. Papilloma.

      d. Radial scar/complex sclerosing lesion.

      e. H/o fibroadenoma (some say no risk w/ fibroadenomas, though).

   3. *4–5× increased risk*:

      a. Hyperplasia w/ atypia (indication for tamoxifen).

   4. *8–10× increased risk*:

      a. Lobular or ductal carcinoma in situ.

III. DIAGNOSTIC MODALITIES

  A. Mammogram: indications include screening, palpable mass (> 25 yo), mastodynia (> 35 yo), bloody nipple d/c, skin/nipple retraction.

   1. < 35 yo only get for dx. 35–40 baseline mammogram. 40–50 q 1–2 yr. 50–74 annual (highest yield). > 75 controversial.

   2. *BI-RADS*: 0—incomplete, do complete w/u. 1—no findings, regular f/u. 2—benign findings, regular f/u. 3—probably benign findings, 6-mo f/u (1–2% bx +). 4—indeterminate finding, bx (core or open, 20–30% +). 5—highly suspicious finding, excise (85% CA).

  B. U/S: useful to eval cystic vs solid, for palpable masses a/o mammo abn or screening in young females w/ dense breasts; also consider for high-risk pts.

  C. FNA: 10-cc syringe w/ 22-g needle. False neg 1–35%, False pos 1–18%.

  D. Core needle bx: for histo of masses. False neg 5%. Rare false pos. Can do mastectomy based on results. Stereotactic core needle bx another option.

  E. Mammotome: get 8× volume as w/ core needle bx; can do w/ U/S or stereotactically.

  F. Open bx: for atypical ductal hyperplasia or BI-RADS 5 lesions.

CHAPTER 18

PEDIATRIC

I. VITALS, FLUIDS, AND OTHER PEDIATRIC BASICS
   A. See Table 18.1.

TABLE 18.1. Normal Vital Signs

Age	Wt (kg)	Heart Rate	Systolic BP	Resp. Rate
0–1 mo	2–4	120–180	60–70	30–60
2–12 mo	4–10	80–160	70–100	20–50
12–24 mo	10–13	80–140	75–110	20–40
2–6 yo	13–25	80–120	80–110	20–30
6–12 yo	20–40	70–110	85–120	20–30
> 13 yo	> 40–60	55–105	90–120	12–20

Modified with permission from Cline DM, et al. *Emergency Medicine, Fifth Edition*. New York, NY: The McGraw-Hill Companies, Inc., 2000, page 754.

   B. **Fluid management**
      1. *Per h*: 4 mL/kg for 1st 10 kg (40 mL) *PLUS* 2 mL/kg for 2nd 10 kg (20 mL) *PLUS* 1 mL/kg thereafter.
      2. *Per 24 h*: 100 mL/kg for 1st 10 kg (1000 mL) *PLUS* 50 mL/kg for 2nd 10 kg (500 mL) *PLUS* 20 mL/kg thereafter.
   C. **Nutrition** (*note*: infants should gain ~ 30 g/d)
      1. *Calories*:
         a. *< 1 yo*: 100–120 kcal/kg/d
         b. *1–3 yo*: 100 kcal/kg/d
         c. *4–6 yo*: 90 kcal/kg/d
         d. *7–10 yo*: 70 kcal/kg/d
      2. *Protein*:
         a. *< 1 yo*: ~ 3 g/kg/d
         b. *9 yo*: ~ 2 g/kg/d
         c. *18 yo*: ~ 1 g/kg/d
      3. *Carbohydrate*: neonate: min. 5 mg/kg/min, increase up to 10 mg/kg/min
      4. *Fat*: begin 0.5 g/kg/d, increase up to 3 g/kg/d
   D. See Table 18.2.

II. HEAD AND NECK
   A. **Thyroglossal duct cyst** (see Chapter 23 on head and neck)
   B. **Branchial cleft cyst** (see Chapter 23 on head and neck)
   C. **Cystic hygroma** (see Chapter 23 on head and neck)
   D. **Tracheoesophageal fistula** (see Chapter 6 on thoracic)

III. HEART (see Chapter 5)

IV. PULMONARY
   A. **Diaphragmatic hernia**: 80% left, 20% right. Exceedingly rarely bilateral. Results from failure of pleuroperitoneal canal to close. ~ 60% survival, largely limited by pulmonary hypoplasia and pulmonary hypertension.
      1. Usu. presents w/ respiratory insufficiency and cyanosis, which may not be immediately apparent postpartum; up to 20% may deteriorate more than 24 h after birth. Dx may be made w/

TABLE 18.2.   Resuscitation

Broselow-Luten	Wt (kg)	Fluids	Equipment
Grey	3–5	3 Kg: Bolus: 60 crystalloid; 30 colloid Maint: $D_5W+\frac{1}{4}$ NS+20 mEq KCl at 12 mL/h 4 Kg: Bolus: 80 crystalloid; 40 colloid Maint: $D_5W+\frac{1}{4}$ NS+20 mEq KCl at 16 mL/h 5 Kg: Bolus: 100 crystalloid; 50 colloid Maint: $D_5W+\frac{1}{4}$ NS+20 mEq KCl at 20 mL/h	Use Pink/Red zone equipment, except Foley (5 Fr) and BP cuff neonatal/inf.
Pink	6–7	Bolus: 130 crystalloid; 65 colloid Maint: $D_5W + \frac{1}{4}$ NS + 20 mEq KCl at 28 mL/h	Laryngoscope: 1 straight ETT: 3.5 uncuffed, insert to 10–10.5 cm Chest tube: 10–12 Fr Foley: 8 Fr NGT: 5–8 Fr Vasc: 22–24 Ga Intraoss: 18–15 Ga BP cuff: inf/child
Red	8–9	Bolus: 170 crystalloid; 85 colloid Maint: $D_5W + \frac{1}{4}$ NS + 20 mEq KCl at 35 mL/h	Same as Pink (above).
Purple	10–11	Bolus: 210 crystalloid; 105 colloid Maint: $D_5W + \frac{1}{4}$ NS + 20 mEq KCl at 40 mL/h	Laryngoscope: 1 straight ETT: 4.0 uncuffed, insert to 11–12 cm Chest tube: 16–20 Fr Foley: 8–10 Fr NGT: 8–10 Fr Vasc: 20–24 Ga Intraoss: 15 Ga BP cuff: child
Yellow	12–14	Bolus: 260 crystalloid; 130 colloid Maint: $D_5W + \frac{1}{4}$ NS + 20 mEq KCl at 45 mL/h	Laryngoscope: 2 straight ETT: 4.5 uncuffed, insert to 13.5 cm Chest tube: 20–24 Fr Foley: 10 Fr NGT: 10 Fr Vasc: 18–22 Ga Intraoss: 15 Ga BP cuff: child
White	15–18	Bolus: 325 crystalloid; 165 colloid Maint: $D_5W + \frac{1}{4}$ NS + 20 mEq KCl at 55 mL/h	Laryngoscope: 2 straight ETT: 5.0 uncuffed, insert to 14–15 cm Chest tube: 20–24 Fr Foley: 10–12 Fr NGT: 10 Fr Vasc: 18–22 Ga Intraoss: 15 Ga BP cuff: child
Blue	19–23	Bolus: 420 crystalloid; 210 colloid Maint: $D_5W + \frac{1}{4}$ NS + 20 mEq KCl at 65 mL/h	Laryngoscope: 2 straight or curved ETT: 5.5 uncuffed, insert to 16.5 cm Chest tube: 24–32 Fr Foley: 10–12 Fr NGT: 12–14 Fr Vasc: 18–20 Ga Intraoss: 15 Ga BP cuff: child

Broselow-Luten	Wt (kg)	Fluids	Equipment
Orange	24–29	Bolus: 530 crystalloid; 270 colloid Maint: D_5W + ¼ NS + 20 mEq KCl at 70 mL/h	Laryngoscope: 2 straight or curved ETT: 6.0 cuffed, insert to 17–18 cm Chest tube: 28–32 Fr Foley: 12 Fr NGT: 14–18 Fr Vasc: 18–20 Ga Intraoss: 15 Ga BP cuff: child
Green	30–36	Bolus: 660 crystalloid; 330 colloid Maint: D_5W + ¼ NS + 20 mEq KCl at 75 mL/h	Laryngoscope: 3 straight or curved ETT: 6.5 cuffed, insert to 18.5–19.5 cm Chest tube: 32–38 Fr Foley: 12 Fr NGT: 18 Fr Vasc: 16–20 Ga Intraoss: 15 Ga BP cuff: sm. ad.

Above information adapted from *Broselow™ Pediatric Emergency Tape*, © Copyright Vital Signs, Inc., 2002 Ed. A, Armstrong Medical Industries, Inc., Lincolnshire, Illinois.

prenatal U/S or postnatal CXR w/ gastric air bubble or intestinal air in the chest. Mediastinal shift or polyhydramnios (from gastric obstruction) may also be seen.

2. *Bochdalek hernia* = left posterolateral diaphragm.

3. *Morgagni hernia* = anterior central herniation.

4. Congenital diaphragmatic hernia often assoc. w/ pentalogy of Cantrell (omphalocele, anterior diaphragmatic hernia, sternal cleft, ectopia cordis, intracardiac defect [ventricular septal defect or diverticulum of left ventricle]).

5. *Tx:* fetal surgery not supported by data. Postnatal intubation and NGT placement are routine. Acute decompensation may reflect PTX, which will be contralateral to diaphragmatic defect. Ventilation w/ permissive hypercapnea may be sufficient if ECLS is not pursued.

   a. Surgery should be delayed for 24 to 72 h after dx to physiologically stabilize the pt.

   b. Repair diaphragm w/ interrupted nonabsorbable sutures is via subcostal or thoracotomy approach. Large defects may require prosthetic (Gore-tex, Permacol) patch or muscle flap closure; patch repairs assoc. w/ higher recurrence rate. Excise hernia sac if present.

B. **Pulmonary sequestration**

1. Both forms receive systemic arterial blood supply and do not connect to tracheobronchial tree.

2. *Intralobar* sequestrations most often drain into pulmonary veins and are most often on the left (~ 2/3), in medial or posterior segments of lower lobes. Blood supply most frequently from infra-diaphragmatic aorta in inferior pulmonary ligament. Resection via segmentectomy or lobectomy is usu. indicated because of risk of infection and bleeding.

3. *Extralobar* sequestrations drain into systemic (azygous) veins, are on left (~ 3/4), and are more common in males. 40% are assoc. w/ other anomalies (pectus excavatum/carinatum, diaphragmatic hernia, congenital heart defects, enteric duplication cysts, etc.). Resection not usu. indicated except in cases of diagnostic uncertainty.

C. **Congenital cystic adenomatous malformations (CCAMs)**

1. Lesion w/ proliferation of bronchial structures w/ relative paucity of alveolar tissue, and, unlike sequestrations, typically has bronchial and arterial/venous flow from pulmonary vasculature.

2. *Three types:*

   a. *Type I* (macrocystic): single or multiple cysts > 2 cm diameter, may result in shift of remaining parenchyma. ~ 50% of cases, no assoc. anomalies.

   b. *Type II*: multiple small (< 1 cm) cysts, often assoc. w/ other congenital anomalies (renal, cardiac, skeletal, etc.). Prognosis depends on assoc. anomalies.

   c. *Type III*: bulky, appears solid, but has microscopic cysts, often results in mediastinal shift, and is assoc. w/ nonimmune hydrops and poor prognosis. Nonimmune hydrops → 100% fatal.

3. Poor prognosis if involves more than 1 lobe or if type II or III. Small risk of malignant transformation. Resect all.

D. Congenital lobar emphysema

1. Due to insufficient cartilaginous support of bronchus, resulting in bronchial collapse, air trapping, and overdistention. LUL affected in ~ 50% of cases, w/ RML and RLL each about 25%.

2. May be asymptomatic, w/ incidental dx of radiolucency. Observation may be pursued, but resection indicated if sx (dyspnea, recurrent pneumonia). In neonates w/ large CLE, may mimic tension PTX—should be differentiated, as thoracotomy and resection, not chest tube (w/ potential of penetrating the lung), would be indicated.

E. Bronchogenic cysts

1. Usu. solitary, w/ $2/3$ in lungs (generally communicate w/ bronchus), and $1/3$ in mediastinum (gen. do not communicate w/ bronchus).

2. May be asymptomatic or present w/ pneumonia, cough, dyspnea, hemoptysis, etc. Tx is resection for sx as well as the (small) risk of malignant transformation.

V. GASTROINTESTINAL: type of lesion

A. Stomach

1. *Pyloric stenosis*:

   a. Classically presents in first born males (M:F = 4:1) about 1 mo of age w/ "projectile" vomiting. Caused by both hyperplasia and hypertrophy of pyloric musculature.

   b. Often results in w/ hypokalemic, hypochloremic metabolic alkalosis.

   c. Clinically, an "olive" may be palpated in RUQ; dx confirmed w/ U/S (dx = 16 mm × 4 mm).

   d. For majority of resuscitations, give bolus of NS (20 mL/kg) followed by $D_5^{1/2}$ NS w/ 20 KCl at 6 mL/kg/h. Take to OR once pt is euvolemic w/ serum bicarb less than 30 and normal K^+.

   e. Tx is open vs laparoscopic Ramstedt pyloromyotomy (incision longitudinally across pylorus down to mucosa, then close transversely).

B. Intestinal atresia

1. Usu. due to interruption of blood flow, commonly secondary to gastroschisis herniation; multiple in 10% of cases. Jejunoileal > duodenal (see section 7. on duodenal atresia below) > colonic > pyloric.

2. Prenatally, polyhydramnios present; maternal U/S → dilated stomach a/o duodenum.

3. Postnatally, see emesis (usu. bilious, depends on level) w/in 48 h, +/– abdominal distension (depends on level).

4. KUB → if demonstrates "double bubble," then dx is duodenal atresia. If demonstrates multiple loops of dilated bowel, need to order contrast study. Contrast enema reveals microcolon.

5. *Type I* = intact bowel and mesentery w/ septum. *Type II* = ends connected via fibrous cord and intact mesentery. *Type IIIa* = ends in discontinuity w/ wedged gap of mesentery. *Type IIIb* = terminal ileum wrapped in spiral fashion around ileocolic vessel → "apple peel" or "Christmas tree" lesion (results from loss of majority of SMA w/ gut supplied by ileocolic and right colic arteries via anastamoses from IMA). *Type IV* = "string of sausages."

6. *Tx of jejunoileal atresia*:

   a. Obtain BE preop, as up to 15% of pts have multiple atretic segments. *Note*: 10% of pts w/ jejunoileal atresia have cystic fibrosis—diagnostic testing for this entity is appropriate.

   b. Anastomosis of atretic ends is performed. Size discrepancy between proximal and distal segments may be addressed by a resection (if limited to short length) or enteroplasty.

7. *Duodenal atresia*:

   a. Failure of recanalization by 8th wk gestation. Most always at or just distal to ampulla of Vater. Most often forms a diaphragm/web of mucosa/submucosa that is stretched into "windsock" configuration, although can result in 2 ends. Assoc. anomalies common (annular pancreas, biliary atresia, malrotation); 30% assoc. w/ trisomy 21 (r/o cardiac anomalies). *Ddx* = malrotation w/ volvulus (surgical emergency), annular pancreas.

   b. *Dx*: AXR classically reveals a "double-bubble" sign (air in stomach and duodenal bulb). If air is noted elsewhere in small bowel, an upper GI study should be obtained to r/o midgut volvulus.

    c. *Tx*: Duodenal web is *not removed* via duodenotomy, because of risk of injury to major ampulla. Duodenoduodenostomy or duodenojejunostomy is performed via open or laparoscopy approach.

C. Pancreas

1. Pancreas divisum (see Chapter 14)
2. Annular pancreas (see Chapter 14)

D. Colon

1. *Hirschsprung's disease*

    a. Common etiology of neonatal intestinal obstruction. Due to absence of ganglion cells in distal segment of bowel, w/ resultant failure of relaxation in that segment.

    b. Presents w/ constipation, distention, possibly diarrhea. *Always think of this w/ failure to pass meconium w/in 48 h of birth.*

    c. Contrast enema often procured to demonstrate transition zone, but false negatives not infrequent in infants.

    d. Do transrectal bx for *absence* of ganglia cells AND acetylcholinesterase. Bx must be at least 1 cm proximal to dentate line.

    e. Initially manage w/ rectal irrigation or temporary colostomy.

    f. Definitive management is pull-through procedure in first 3 wk of life (primary surgery) or, if following colostomy, around 6 mo of age.

    g. Hirschsprung's pts are at lifelong risk of high morbidity/mortality enterocolitis.

E. Anorectal

1. *Imperforate anus*

    a. Slightly more common in males, mechanism unknown. Sometimes assoc. w/ VACTERL (esp. tetrology of Fallot, VSD), Down syndrome, duodenal atresia, a/o Hirschsprung's dz.

    b. Original classification based on relation of rectal end to the levators. Newer dichotomy is based on tx (need for colostomy).

      i. *Need for protective colostomy*: rectourethral, rectovesical, or vaginal fistula; cloaca; anorectal agenesis (no fistula); rectal or vestibular atresia. Note, these infants usu. have a "flat" bottom.

      ii. *No need for protective colostomy*: cutaneous fistula; anal stenosis; anal membrane.

    c. *Dx*:

      i. Clinical. Look for perineal fistula; if present, observe up to 48 h for meconium; if (+), then pt has a "low" lesion. Invertograms have been supplanted by prone, cross-table film.

      ii. Eval for VACTERL w/ NGT, echocardiogram, abdominal/renal U/S, plain films of vertebrae, +/− lumbar MRI.

    d. *Tx*:

      i. Maintain NPO w/ parenteral nutrition until operation.

      ii. If need protective colostomy (see entry 1bi. above), perform colostomy (and urinary diversion if indicated [rare]).

        • Postop, irrigate mucous fistula to remove meconium and perform distal colostogram to define anatomy. PSARP is generally performed between 2 and 12 mo of age.

      iii. If rectocutaneous fistula (i.e., no need for protective colostomy), perform primary posterior sagittal anoplasty (PSARP) w/in first few wks of life.

F. Intussusception

1. Usu. in age group 4 mo to 3 yo (peak = 8 mo). In children of this age range, usu. at ileocecal junction w/ no identifiable lead point, but significant mesenteric/gut lymphadenopathy. Tends to follow viral URI/gastroenteritis.

2. Typically presents w/ crampy, intense abdominal pain w/ emesis in an otherwise healthy child, causing child to flex hips/knees during episodes of pain, and punctuated by periods of relative calm.

3. "Currant jelly" stool that reflects ischemic bowel producing mucus admixed w/ clotted blood is frequently reported. A palpable mass in the abdomen may be noted, a/o relative lack of fullness in RLQ—"Dance's sign."

4. *Radiology*: all → 3-way KUB: if air/stool throughout colon, unlikely dx—suspicious if lack of air in RLQ. Often followed by air contrast enema. If low index of suspicion → *U/S*: "target" sign of intussuscepted bowel on transverse view and "pseudokidney" on longitudinal view. If low index of suspicion → *CT*: "target" or "bullseye" w/ mass in RLQ and SBO proximally. If high index of suspicion → contrast, saline, or *air enema* (can do under fluoro) can be diagnostic as well as therapeutic (80% effective), but should be bypassed if pt is unstable or has peritonitis (go to OR). Manage 1st recurrence w/ repeat enema, but if recurs twice, should go to OR. If intussusception is known to not involve colon (involves small bowel only), A-C enema not likely to be therapeutic, and therefore not indicated.

5. *Operation*:
   a. *Indications*: peritonitis, failure of enema to reduce, high index of suspicion of nonviable gut, complete SBO, lack of colonic involvement, and multiple recurrences.
   b. *Procedure*: laparoscopy may be used for incomplete reduction, but generally a transverse incision in right abdomen is made to access the bowel, which is milked from distal to proximal for reduction (push, don't pull). Adhesions, if any, are lysed, and the appendix is removed. Bowel is resected if reduction can't be achieved, if lead point is identified, or if intestine is nonviable.

6. *Prognosis*: recurrence is ~ 5% after either enema reduction or operative intervention.

7. *Caveat*: in older children, the risk of the lead point being a malignancy increases.

G. Malrotation

1. GI tract develops outside coelomic cavity from gestational wk 4–10, then begins counterclockwise rotation of 2 segments around the SMA. The duodenojejunal segment first rotates 270° and then is fixed at the ligament of Treitz. The cecocolic segment then rotates. At completion, intestines are fixed to the retroperitoneum via a broad mesentery, the duodenal C-loop, and right/left colon. If the fixation is incomplete, intestines can rotate around a narrow stalk and strangulate the superior mesenteric vessels.
   a. Will always occur to some degree w/ omphalocele, gastroschisis, and congenital diaphragmatic hernia.
   b. Assoc. to lesser degree w/ intestinal atresia and Hirschsprung's dz.

2. *Three specific anomalies*:
   a. *Nonrotation*: most common variant. Neither segment rotates appropriately, but are closely apposed, sharing a mesentery w/ a narrow base that is prone to volvulus. Duodenum courses "vertically" (cephalad–caudad) along right side of abdomen.
   b. *Duodenojejunal anomalies*: frequently manifest as duodenal obstruction from Ladd's bands extending down to colon, across duodenum. Comparatively broad mesenteric base.
   c. *Cecocolic anomalies*: Cecum and proximal colon are medially situated. Prone to volvulus as w/ nonrotation due to narrow mesenteric base.

3. *Dx*:
   a. *Clinical*: most severe presentation is w/ bilious emesis from volvulus. Hematemesis, melena, a/o sepsis may ensue as bowel becomes compromised and the child becomes increasingly ill.
   b. *Roentgenographic*:
      i. *Plain films*: may demonstrate gas pattern consistent w/ obstruction, or relatively gasless abdomen due to intraluminal transudate.
      ii. *UGI*: demonstrates obstruction (if present) and malrotation (incomplete duodenojejunal rotation). Normally, LOT to left, but will be on right w/ malrotation.
      iii. *BE*: less useful than UGI, as cecal position relatively variable in children, and may be normal in some children w/ malrotation.
      iv. *U/S*: can demonstrate absence of usual position of SMV to the right of SMA.

4. *Tx*:
   a. *Incidental malrotation*
      i. *Ladd procedure* [Ladd WE. *NEJM* 1932;206:277–83.]
         • *Eviscerate*: via supraumbilical midline incision.

- *Lyse Ladd's bands*: divide these peritoneal bands as they compress 2nd/3rd portion of duodenum.
- *Widen mesenteric base*: move small bowel to lie along right gutter and colon to the left (ileocecal valve will be oriented opposite direction as usual).
- *Verify duodenal patency*: perform additional dissection as necessary to properly orient and decompress duodenum. Also, r/o atresia/stenosis or tx if present.
- *Appendectomy*: to avoid future diagnostic quandaries.

  b. *Malrotation w/ volvulus*

    i. Resuscitate w/ IVF, NGT/OGT then to OR emergently.

    ii. Operative steps same as above, except that immediately after evisceration (before lysing Ladd's bands), detorse bowel by counterclockwise rotation. Examine bowel for areas of viability/ischemia/necrosis. Condition of bowel may warrant second look 24 h later, or immediate resection +/– primary anastamosis.

  5. *Prognosis*:

    a. Recurrent volvulus in 5–10% of pts after Ladd procedure, and ~ 5% risk of adhesive obstructive dz.

H. Meconium ileus variants: *note*, the below diagnoses are variably assoc. w/ cystic fibrosis, which is diagnosed w/ pilocarpine iontophoresis sweat test. Positive = chloride concentration > 60 mEq/L, but less reliable in infants. Testing for mutated *CFTR* gene required for definitive dx.

  1. *Meconium plug*: most affected pts are normal, but is assoc. w/ CF as well as Hirshprung's, maternal diabetes, hypothyroidism, preterm delivery. Usu. presents as distal intestinal obstruction; water-soluble contrast enema diagnostic and therapeutic.

  2. *Meconium ileus (simple)*: virtually pathognomonic for CF in white children in North America. Terminal ileum dilated w/ inspissated meconium. Typically, KUB shows dilated small bowel w/ meconium mass and small bowel gas often interpreted as "soap bubble" or "ground glass" appearance. Water-soluble contrast enema effective tx in 75%. Failure of enema is indication for operation, as is 3rd occurrence (2 recurrences). In OR, evacuate meconium via enterotomy in dilated ileum. Irrigate proximally and distally w/ saline or 4% *N*-acetylcysteine through a red rubber catheter. Meconium can be milked into colon or out through enterotomy. Enterotomy may be closed, partly diverted w/ Bishop-Koop or Santulli ostomy, or end small bowel enterocutaneous ostomy. Rarely, a T tube may be placed for postop irrigation.

  3. *Meconium ileus (complicated)*: refers to meconium ileus w/ perforation, resulting in peritonitis. May present w/ obstruction or calcified cyst if occurred prenatally, or superinfection, ascites, or dense adhesions.

I. Foreign body ingestion / aspiration

  1. *Ingestion*:

    a. *3 most common places to lodge in the esophagus*: cricopharyngeus (most common), mid-esophagus (region of left mainstem bronchus), diaphragmatic hiatus.

      i. Evaluate w/ CXR and retrieve w/ rigid or flexible esophagoscope.

    b. 95% of ingested foreign bodies safely pass once distal to the esophagus, usu. w/in 48 h. Those who have blunt objects w/out projections beyond the esophagus may be sent home w/ appropriate precautions including instructions to return if no passage w/in 5 d. Surgery is reserved for no passage after 5 d, or significant N/V/pain/bleeding. Emetics and cathartics are contraindicated.

    c. Long, blunt, slender objects (tools, pencils, etc.) pass less frequently, and should more frequently be followed in the hospital w/ serial x-rays.

    d. Ingestion of sharp objects (glass, needles, etc.) mandates hospitalization for serial abdominal exams and daily KUBs. As long as object continues distal travel w/out peritonitis or significant bleeding, observation is reasonable and usu. successful.

    e. Battery ingestion poses a significant risk of alkali burn or mercury poisoning and requires emergent removal. Remove them endoscopically if in the stomach. If distal (i.e., duodenum), q 6 h films must document rapid transit if the pt is to avoid celiotomy.

  2. *Aspiration*

    a. Right mainstem bronchus most common due to relatively shallow angle w/ trachea compared w/ left.

      b. CXR often demonstrates hyperinflation; less often the foreign body will be demonstrated.

      c. Rigid bronchoscopy for definitive dx and removal.

J. **Necrotizing enterocolitis (NEC)**

  1. Most common neonatal GI emergency. Primary risk factor is prematurity.

  2. 80% of cases occur during first postnatal mo, but rarely in the first several days. Typically involves distal ileum and right colon, but may affect entire GI tract. 80–90% are successfully treated w/ supportive care alone (nonsurgically).

  3. Frequently presents w/ nonspecific sx such as bradycardia, dyspnea, irritability, labile temperatures, poor feeding, a/o hematochezia/melena. This may progress to sepsis and DIC.

  4. Classic roentgenographic finding is pneumatosis intestinalis, although portal gas, free air, and ascites may also be seen.

  5. *Tx*:

      a. Begin w/ NGT, fluid/blood products resuscitation, broad-spectrum IV abx for 3 wk.

      b. *Operation*:

         i. *Absolute indication*: perforation.

         ii. *Relative indication*: worsening clinical picture (i.e., progressive sepsis, worsening neutropenia/thrombocytopenia/acidosis/sepsis), palpable abdominal mass, abdominal wall cellulitis, radiographic fixed loop of intestines.

      c. Resect nonviable bowel and create enterostomies as needed. In severely ill, unstable pts, bedside placement of peritoneal drains under local anesthesia may be sufficient.

      d. Mortality 10–50% of operative candidates. Primary long-term sequelae include short gut syndrome and strictures.

VI. <u>**GASTROINTESTINAL DIFFERENTIAL DIAGNOSIS**</u>: type of symptoms

  A. **Vomiting**

    1. *Malrotation*

      a. Etiology of bilious emesis in newborn until proven otherwise.

      b. May see "double bubble."

      c. Ladd's procedure

         i. Divide Ladd's bands.

         ii. Counterclockwise rotation of gut.

         iii. Place small bowel on right, large bowel on left.

         iv. Appendectomy.

    2. *Duodenal atresia*

      a. Assoc. w/ Down syndrome.

      b. May see "double bubble" on AXR (r/o malrotation!).

    3. *Annular pancreas*

    4. *Pyloric stenosis*

    5. *Intussusception*

      a. Most common cause of intestinal obstruction to age 2 yo.

      b. 95% of pediatric cases w/ no identifiable mass to act as lead point.

      c. Ileal "intussusceptum" into colonic "intussuscipiens" most common.

      d. Most resolve w/ air or barium enema.

      e. If require laparotomy, push mass out from distal bowel rather than pull out proximal bowel.

  B. **Abdominal distension**

    1. Intestinal obstruction

    2. Pneumoperitoneum

    3. Pseudocyst (assoc. w/ CF, meconium ileus)

    4. Mesenteric cysts or intestinal duplication

    5. Hydrocolpos/hematocolpos

     6. Instestinal inflation (TEF, or secondary to CPAP)

     7. Hydrops (Rh dz w/ anasarca and hepatosplenomegaly)

C. Scaphoid abd ddx

     1. CDH

     2. Esophageal atresia

     3. Duodenal atresia

D. Diarrhea

     1. Intussusception

E. Constipation

     1. Meconium ileus

     2. Hirschsprung's dz

     3. Intestinal neuronal dysplasia

F. Blood in stool

     1. Intussusception

     2. NEC

     3. Volvulus

G. Respiratory distress

     1. Esophageal atresia +/− TEF

     2. Congenital diaphragmatic hernia

     3. CCAM

     4. CLE

     5. PTX

     6. Congenital heart dz

VII. ABDOMINAL WALL

A. Umbilical hernia

     1. Caused by incomplete contraction of umbilical ring.

     2. More often in African Americans, premature babies, twins, mucopolysaccharide storage disorders (esp. Hurler's syndrome).

     3. Majority spontaneously close by 2 yo. Surgical repair indicated after age 5 or if > 2-cm diameter after age 2.

B. Omphalocele

     1. Proposed etiology is failure of lateral/cranial/caudal mesoderm ingrowth and fusion during gestational wk 4–7.

     2. Assoc. w/ pentalogy of Cantrell (diaphragmatic hernia, ectopia cordis, sternal cleft, etc.), bladder extrophy, cloacal extrophy, imperforate anus, and meningomyelocele. 10–30% chromosomal anomalies (i.e., 12, 13, 18, 21). 35–81% w/ major congenital anomaly(ies), most frequently cardiac ($^1/_5$, such as TOF, ASD, VSD). In addition to VACTERL, also assoc. w/ Beckwith-Wiedemann (visceromegaly, neonatal hypoglycemia, macroglossia).

          a. *VACTERL w/u should include* echocardiogram; renal U/S; plain films of chest, pelvis, and spine; karyotype/chromosomal analysis; thorough physical exam.

     3. If not already diagnosed in utero, presents postnatally as > 4 cm umbilical defect (< 4 cm = "cord hernia") w/ eviscerated organs covered w/ amnion (minority rupture in utero or during delivery).

     4. *Tx*:

          a. Place OGT. Do not mask ventilate (intubate).

          b. Excise sac, correct malrotation (usu. present), explore abdominal contents.

          c. Primarily close abdomen if defect small enough and sufficient peritoneal domain exists.

          d. Alternatives for closure include patch, skin flaps, or silo (serially tighten, then close in delayed fashion).

    e. If pt not stable for anesthesia, consider applying Silvadene to sac to create eschar and allow for epithelialization; repair ventral hernia when able (usu. at 1 yo).

  5. *Prognosis*: usu. limited by assoc. anomalies (~ 80% long-term survival).

C. Gastroschisis

1. Thought to be related to defect from early right umbilical vein involution w/ resultant weakness to the right of umbilicus (95+% of cases are on the right). Not assoc. w/ other anomalies, other than intestinal atresia (10–15%), probably secondary to incarceration in utero, and undescended testes.

2. Presents postnatally, defect almost always just to right of umbilicus w/ eviscerated organs *not* covered by amnion. Organs covered by generally thick rind from exposure to amniotic fluid (this will resolve w/ time in the abdomen). Variable degrees of malrotation present.

3. *Tx*:

    a. Place NGT to prevent distention.

    b. Wrap eviscerated contents in bowel bags or saline-moistened gauze.

    c. Generally need to enlarge defect to facilitate reduction.

    d. Repair atresias if possible, but inflammation may preclude this, requiring revisit 6–8 wk after reduction. Correct malrotation as indicated.

    e. Tension-free closure of abdomen may require use of patch, flaps, etc.

    f. Anticipate prolonged ileus (up to 6 mo postop) w/ early institution of TPN. NEC also more common than in omphalocele pts as gastroschisis pts more frequently born premature.

4. Prognosis excellent w/ appropriate early management.

D. Eagle-Barrett (prune belly) syndrome: 1 in 50,000 live births, more common in males.

1. Triad consists of absent/deficient abdominal wall musculature, cryptorchidism, urinary tract malformations (usu. ureteral dilatation). Some pts lack 1 or more of the classical components. Pt at risk for complicated UTI due to frequent vesicoureteral reflux. Increased risk for postop respiratory complications due to compromised respiratory mechanics. Malrotation common. Orchidopexy should be performed by 2 yo; abdominoplasty may be performed concurrently.

VIII. GENITOURINARY AND ADRENAL

A. Sexual development

1. See Tables 18.3 and 18.4.

TABLE 18.3.   Tanner Score (Male)

Male	Testis	Pubic Hair	Penis	Other
Stage 1 Prepubertal	< 4 cc or 2.5 cm long	No coarse, pigmented hair	No growth	
Stage 2	4 cc, 2.5–3.2 cm long (9.5–13.5 yo)	Minimal coarse, pigmented hair at base of penis (9.9–14 yo)	Earliest increased length and width (10.5–14.5 yo)	
Stage 3	12 cc, 3.6 cm long (11.5–16.5 yo)	Coarse, dark curly hair over pubis (11.2–15 yo)	Increased length and width (10.1–14.6 yo)	Possible gynecomastia (13.2 yo avg). Voice breaks (13.5 yo avg). Muscle mass increases.
Stage 4	4.1–4.5 cm	Adult quality, but not to junction of thigh w/ perineum (12–15.8 yo)	Continued growth in length and width (11.2–15.3 yo)	Axillary hair (14 yo avg), voice changes, acne vulgaris (14.3 yo avg).
Stage 5	> 4.5 cm	Adult quality. Spread to medial thigh but not linea alba.	Mature size by 16.5 yo	No further height gain after 17 yo.

TABLE 18.4. Tanner Score (Female)

Female	Breast	Pubic Hair	Other
Stage 1 Prepubertal	Papilla elevation only	Villus hair only (not coarse)	
Stage 2	Breast buds palpable, areolae enlarge (8.9–12.9 yo)	Minimal coarse, pigmented hair, mainly on labia (9.0–13.4 yo)	With increasingly earlier puberty, these changes may appear 1–2 yr earlier.
Stage 3	Elevation of breast contour, areolae enlarge (9.9–13.9 yo)	Dark, coarse, curly hair over mons (9.6–14.1 yo)	Axillary hair (13.1 yo avg), acne vulgaris (13.2 yo avg).
Stage 4	Areolae forms secondary mound on breast (10.5–15.3 yo)	Adult quality, no spread to thigh/ perineal junction (10.4–14.8 yo)	
Stage 5	Adult breast contour, areola recedes to contour of breast	Adult quality, spread to medial thigh, but not linea alba	No further height gain after 16 yo.

B. **Congenital adrenal hyperplasia (CAH):**

1. Most common cause of female fetal virilization.

2. Shunts precursors for both cortisol and aldosterone to make sex steroids.

3. Due to deficiency of enzyme needed for cortisol synthesis, leading to excess ACTH production; 21 hydroxylase deficiency responsible for 90–95%; ¾ of these cases are "salt-wasters" as well. Remainder of CAH pts lack 11-β-hydroxylase, 3-β-hydroxydehydrogenase, or 17-hydroxylase.

4. *Prenatal* (females): Mullerian tissue (ovaries, fallopian tubes, uterus) unaffected, but have masculinized external genitalia. W/ correction of endocrine problem and reconstructive surgery, can bear children.

5. *Postnatal*:

   a. *Both*:

      i. Pts w/ 21-hydroxylase deficiency appear well immediately after birth, but after 2–3 wk decompensate due to salt loss and resulting hypovolemia (hyperkalemia also common). *Consider dx in any hypotensive infant w/ hyponatremia, hyperkalemia, and metabolic acidosis.*

      ii. Less dramatic cases may present w/ rapid somatic growth, advanced bone age, early closure of epiphyses (short stature), +/– hyperpigmentation.

   b. *Females*: virilization, hirsutism, polycystic ovaries, menstrual irregularities.

   c. *Males*: enlarged phallus, increased muscle mass, body hair by 2–3 yo; fertility may be impaired.

   d. *Note: virilizing sx in children may also be due to adrenocortical carcinoma—must consider this dx. Unlike CAH, pts usu. will have hypercortisolism.*

IX. **GASTROINTESTINAL BLEEDING:** most common cause in young children is Meckel's diverticulum. Other sources to consider include anal fissure from constipation, juvenile polyps, and other dx more commonly seen in adults such as ulcers (often due to NSAIDs), varices, etc.

X. **PEDIATRIC ONCOLOGY**

A. **Most common tumor in children is leukemia.**

B. **Most common solid tumor in children is brain cancer.**

C. **Neuroblastoma:** slightly less common than nephroblastoma (below) at ~ 1:10 million children.

1. Derived from neural crest cells, demonstrate wide range of behavior (benign/spontaneous regression to malignant).

2. Majority of cases present in infancy. *Site of primary tumor*: adrenal > other retroperitoneum > mediastinum > pelvis > neck > other. Most commonly metastasizes to bone. Median age at dx = 2 yo.

3. Etiology linked to proto-oncogene N-*myc* amplification; inversely assoc. w/ *TRK* expression.

4. *W/u*: imaging depends on site of primary tumor but should include chest CT scan as well as MIBG scan to r/o metastasis. Labs should include complete chemistry w/ BUN/Cr, LFTs, LDH, plasma/urine homovanillic acid and vanillylmandelic acid.

5. Early stage tx → excision alone. Mod/high risk → neoadjuvant chemotx + surgery + BM transplant +/− XRT.

D. Nephroblastoma (Wilm's tumor): most common extracranial solid tumor in childhood (~ 1:9 million children).

1. Derived from metanephric blastema, but often contains extrarenal tissue as well (cartilage, muscle, etc.).

2. *Assoc. syndromes:*

   a. *WAGR* (**W**ilm's tumor, **a**niridia, **G**U malformations, mental **r**etardation).

   b. *Beckwith-Wiedemann:* other tumors include hepatoblastoma, rhabdomyosarcoma, and adrenal cortical carcinoma. (See section X. on Syndromes below.)

   c. *Denys-Drash:* male pseudohermaphrodism a/o renal dz (nephritic syndrome or glomerulonephritis) and nephroblastoma.

3. Etiology linked to deletion of WTI (Wilm's tumor suppressor gene) at 11p13.

4. Most commonly present w/ abdominal mass, abdominal pain, HTN, hematuria, a/o fever at 3–4 yo.

5. *Tx*: transperitoneal nephrectomy (inspect contralateral kidney, bx LN, etc.); neoadjuvant chemotx given if tumor extends into IVC. Prognosis overall 85% long-term survival.

E. Rhabdomyosarcoma: < 5% of childhood malignancies.

1. Commonly presents in head/neck, GU tract, and extremities.

2. Most cases sporadic, although condition assoc. w/ Li-Fraumeni syndrome, neurofibromatosis-1, and Beckwith-Wiedemann syndrome.

3. *Tx*: multimodality (usu. surgery + chemo +/− XRT). 60% overall 5-yr survival.

F. Liver tumors: 2% childhood malignancies.

1. *Hepatoblastoma*: usu. between 1–3 yo. 70% overall long-term survival.

   a. Usu. unifocal.

   b. Assoc. w/ Beckwith-Wiedemann syndrome and hemihypertrophy, children w/ parents w/ FAP, fetal alcohol syndrome, Wilm's tumor, Fanconi's syndrome; trisomy 2, trisomy 20, 11p and β-catenin gene mutations frequently implicated. Tx similar to hepatocellular carcinoma (below); neoadjuvant chemotx can facilitate resection more frequently than for HCC (below).

2. *Hepatocellular carcinoma*: usu. ~ 12 yo or older, more often multicentric and aggressive than hepatoblastoma, same risk factors as in adult HCC in addition to hepatocyte growth factor gene (*Met*) mutations (see Chapter 10). 25% overall long-term survival.

G. Teratoma

1. Tumors that contain more than 1 embryonic germ cell layer, at least 1 of which is ectopic.

2. Most often present in infancy, often in sacrococcygeal area, particularly in females; those fitting this pattern are generally benign.

3. In older children, tumors are more likely to involve gonads and be malignant.

4. Surgery is the common principle for all teratomas (critical to resect coccyx in sacrococcygeal lesions), although some malignant varieties warrant multimodality intervention.

XI. SYNDROMES

A. Trisomy 21 (Down syndrome): neonatal hypotonia, protruding tongue, mental retardation, simian crease, assoc. also w/ duodenal atresia and cardiac lesions.

B. Trisomy 18 (Edward syndrome): low birth wt, delayed mental development, low-set ears, micrognathia, umbilical hernia, inguinal hernia, diastasis recti, cryptorchidism, VSD/ASD/PDA, horseshoe kidney, hydronephrosis, polycystic kidney, coloboma, pectus carinatum, microcephaly.

C. Trisomy 13 (Patau syndrome): severe mental retardation, seizures, microcephaly, microphthalmia, cleft lip/palate, hypotelorism, coloboma, simian crease, polydactyly, umbilical hernia, inguinal hernia, cryptorchidism, micrognathia, hypotonia, skeletal limb anomalies.

D. **Beckwith-Wiedemann syndrome**: macrosomia, macroglossia, visceromegaly, umbilical hernia/omphalocele, neonatal hypoglycemia, hemihypertrophy, various malignancies (hepatoblastoma, adrenocortical carcinoma, etc.).

E. **Pentology of Cantrell**: epigastric omphalocele, sternal cleft, Morgagni hernia, cardiac defect (usu. VSD or left ventricular diverticulum), ectopia cordis.

F. **VACTERL**: vertebral, anal, cardiac, tracheoesophageal, renal, radial limb.

CHAPTER 19

ORTHOPAEDIC AND HAND

I. **SPINE**

A. **C-spine trauma (see Chapter 7)**

1. If trauma pt alert, awake, no mental status changes, no neck pain or tenderness, no distracting pain, no neurologic deficit, then no x-rays needed.

2. If fails to meet above criteria, then lateral film (from occiput to upper border T1), AP (spinous processes C2 to T1), and open mouth odontoid (lateral masses C1 and entire odontoid). This is being rapidly replaced by CT c-spine in larger hospitals as the c-spine trauma series.

3. If plain radiographs normal but pt complains of significant neck pain/tenderness, consider place in collar and obtain flexion/extension c-spine films in 2 wk. Any neuro deficit or suspicion for ligamentous injury → MRI acutely.

5. If neuro deficit possibly referable to c-spine injury, immediate spine surg consult and MRI.

6. Trauma pts w/ anticipated altered mental status for > 24 h (i.e., traumatic brain injury), may be considered to have stable cervical spine if adequate 3-view radiographs (including CT as necessary) and thin-cut axial CT images through C1 and C2 are read as normal [consensus statement from Eastern Association for the Surgery of Trauma, 1998.]. MRI is becoming the gold standard to clear the c-spine in an obtunded pt in the ICU in whom an exam cannot be performed, the CT c-spine is negative, and there is a wound care issue or tissue break down from the hard collar.

7. If c-spine abnormalities discovered on any of the above imaging modalities, spine surgery should be consulted.

8. *Guidelines for radiographic "clearing" of c-spine*:

a. Proper alignment of posterior cervical (had ligamentous) vertebral body line, anterior (had ligamentous) cervical vertebral body line, posterior longitudinal ligament line, spinolaminal line, and tips of spinous processes.

b. Predental space 3 mm or less in adults, 4–5 mm or less in children.

c. No hypo-/hyperdensity in vertebral bodies suggestive of compression fx, etc.

d. No intervertebral or interspinous process angulation greater than 11°.

e. No fanning of spinous processes suggestive of posterior ligament disruption.

f. No abnormality in atlantooccipital region abnormality.

g. No step off > 3 mm between vertebral bodies

h. *Prevertebral soft tissue distance*:

i. Less than 7 mm at C2, < 5 mm at C3–4, < 23 mm at C6.

ii. In children < 2 yo, prevertebral space may appear widened if not an inspiratory film.

B. **Specific types of spinal fx**:

1. *Occipital condyle fx*: result from combined axial loading and lateral bending. Generally stable and managed w/ cervical orthosis/collar.

2. *C1 (atlas) Jefferson's fx*: C1 burst fx of ring from axial loading.

3. *C2 (axis)*:

a. *Odontoid fx*: 3 types, most initially managed w/ HALO.

b. *Hangman's fx* (traumatic spondylolisthesis of axis): C2 fx of posterior elements from hyperextension. Initial management = cervical orthosis, *except* type III (bipedicle fx w/ facet dislocation) = traction.

4. *Thoracolumbar fx*:

a. *Compression fx*: most common.

b. *Burst fx*: anterior and middle column fx +/– posterior column injury from high-energy axial loading w/ mild flexion.

   c. *Chance (flexion-distraction) fx*: involves all 3 columns; classic mechanism is MVC w/ pt wearing seat belt resulting in shearing forces to vertebra. *25% risk of assoc. intraabominal injury, most often of mesentery, small bowel, a/o pancreas; CT findings of retroperitoneal or intraabdominal fluid or other abnormalities should prompt strong consideration for surgical exploration.*

II. LOWER EXTREMITY

A. Pelvic fractures

1. *Anatomy*:
   a. *Important structures involved*: internal iliac artery (gives off anterior branch = pudendal and vesicular arteries and posterior branch = sup/inf gluteal arteries), 4th and 5th lumbar/sacral nerve roots, splanchnic nerves, sacral venous plexus (difficult to embolize).

2. *Assoc. injuries*:
   a. Always look for rectal/vaginal tears, blood at urethral meatus, lower extremity malrotation, ecchymoses about trunk and perineum, leg length discrepancy, focused neurovasc exam of lower extremities.
   b. Also assoc. w/ thoracic aorta rupture.

3. *Dx*:
   a. AP pelvis films procures dx. Inlet/outlet films +/− CT define posterior injury and stability.
   b. *Young and Burgess fx classification*:
      i. *Anteroposterior compression* (APC)
         - I = stable: diastasis of pubic symphysis < 2 cm, ant. SI ligament stretched, post. SI ligaments intact.
         - II = stable vertically, unstable external rotation: diastasis of pubic symphysis > 2 cm, anterior sacroiliac, sacrotuberous, and sacrospinous ligaments torn.
         - III = unstable vertically and rotationally: diastasis of pubic symphysis and complete disruption of all ligamentous structures of sacroiliac complex and pelvic floor.
      ii. *Lateral compression* (LC)
         - I = stable: oblique fx's of anterior pubic rami, minor sacral body/alar crush.
         - II = stable vertically, unstable internal rotation: oblique pubic rami fx's, posterior SI ligamentous rupture a/o posterior ilium/sacral fx.
         - III = stable vertically, unstable rotationally: type II + contralateral APC ("windswept pelvis").
      iii. *Vertical shear*
         - Complete osseous or ligamentous disruption of hemipelvis w/ vertical displacement. Vertically and rotationally unstable.
      iv. *Combined mechanical forces*: any combination of the above injury types.
   a. *Indications for binder for pts w/ pelvic fx*:
      i. Age > 55.
      ii. SBP < 90.
      iii. AC II, III or LC III or VS pattern.
   b. Management of hemodyn. unstable blunt trauma pt w/ both pelvic fx and intraabdominal potential injury (*assuming have rapid access to highly experienced interventional angiography team, such as a level I trauma center*):
      i. If LC I or APC I (stable fx), then address intraabdominal as source first (celiotomy, then possibly angio).
      ii. If LC II, III or APC II, III (unstable fx), consider angio first (even in hemoperitoneum). [Eastridge BJ, Starr A, Minei JP, O'Keefe GE, Scalea TM. The importance of fracture pattern in guiding therapeutic decision making in patients with hemorrhagic shock and pelvic ring disruptions. *J Trauma*, 2002 Sep;(53):446–50.]

B. Femoral shaft fx

1. Can lose 1500 cc's (3 U blood) from each femur. Treat w/ traction splint before definitive management.

    2. Assoc. w/ pelvic/acetabular fx. 5% assoc. w/ femoral neck fx.

    3. Early stabilization is critical to avoid complications (i.e., pneumonia, ARDS, etc.).

C. Tibial shaft fx:

  a. *Gustillo classification for open tibial fx's:*

    i. *Grade I:* wound < 1 cm, minimal soft tissue injury, minimal comminution.

      • Tx w/ IM nailing, union in 21–28 wk.

    ii. *Grade II:* wound > 1 cm, moderate soft tissue injury, moderate comminution.

      • Tx w/ IM nailing, union in 26–28 wk.

    iii. *Grade III*

      • Segmental fx w/ displacement

      • Diaphyseal segmental loss

      • Assoc. vascular injury requiring repair

      • Farmyard injuries/highly contaminated wounds

      • High-velocity gunshot wound

      • Crushing injury by fast-moving vehicle

      • *Grade IIIa*

        ◦ Wound > 10 cm, crushed tissue, contamination, local soft tissue coverage possible → nail, union 30–25 wk.

      • *Grade IIIb*

        ◦ Wound > 10 cm, crushed tissue, contamination, requires regional or free flap → nail, union 30–25 wk.

      • *Grade IIIc*

        ◦ Major assoc. vascular injury requiring repair for limb salvage.

        ◦ Fx classified using mangled extremity system score (MESS).

        ◦ Occasionally necessary to perform BKA. Remember the appropriate abx to give as per the start of this section above.

D. Tibial plafond (pilon) fx:

    1. Combined fx of medial malleolus and anterior/posterior distal tibia; ¼ are open fx. 75% w/ fibula injury.

    2. From vertical/axial loading. Assoc. w/ compartment syndrome, L1 fx, pelvic/acetabula fx.

    3. High incidence of complications (soft tissue coverage compromise, arthritis, etc.).

E. Calcaneal fx:

    1. If assoc. w/ fall, look for assoc. thoracolumbar fx.

    2. High risk for compartment syndrome (as are tibial fx, supracondylar humeral fx). Consider obtaining XR in trauma pts or high-energy mechanisms.

III. DISLOCATION

A. Shoulder

    1. *Anterior* most common (~ 85%). Methods of reduction include "Hippocratic" (reducer's foot in axilla, maintain traction), or have pt lie prone w/ arm hanging off bed w/ 10-lb wt. Alternately, may tie sheet around pt's arm w/ elbow flexed, then pass another sheet around chest. Apply countertraction w/ sheets around physician's and assistant's waists.

    2. *Posterior* much less common than anterior dislocation, and frequently appears normal on AP x-rays. Reduce by abducting shoulder of supine pt, then externally rotate w/ elbow bent 90°.

B. Hip

    1. *Posterior most common.* Typically presents w/ flexed, adducted, internally rotated, relatively immobile hip.

      a. Commonly w/ sciatic injury (10–20%), sometimes just peroneal component.

    2. *Anterior dislocation rare* (5%): typically presents w/ abducted, externally rotated hip.

      a. Uncommonly assoc. w/ injury to femoral vessels, femoral nerve.

    3. *Dx:* plain films (AP, Judet/oblique) views to confirm. CT postreduction to assess adequacy of reduction as well as possible fx and retained intraarticular fragments.

4. *Tx*: reduce w/in 6 h to diminish chances of avascular necrosis of femoral head. Reduce in ED if conscious sedation is available then put on traction if unstable.

C. **Knee dislocation (usu. anterior):**

1. Assoc. w/ popliteal artery injury, particularly posterior dislocation. Any pulse or ABI asymmetry (before *or* after reduction) or neurologic sx (*note*: tibial/peroneal nerve also prone to injury and may mimic vascular compromise sx) suggests vascular injury.

2. *Tx*:

   a. Knee instability w/ clinically obvious vascular insufficiency demands emergent operative exploration of popliteal artery.

      i.   Reduce and stabilize knee w/ external fixator then perform vascular repair. Fixator can be adjusted intraop to facilitate vascular surgery.

   b. If limb not acutely threatened, but sx suggestive of vascular injury, procure arteriogram.

   c. If pulse exam before and after reduction are normal, many report that routine angiography is not required; *however*, this does not evaluate for injury such as intimal flap, which could lead to late thrombosis. An ankle brachial index > 0.90 had a negative predictive value for vascular injury of 100% and < 0.90 was 100% for vascular injury [Mills WJ et al, *J Trauma*, 2004;56(6):1261-5.].

IV. SKELETAL NEOPLASMS

A. **Benign**

1. *Enchondroma*: "fluffy calcification" on x-rays typical. Multiple enchondromas = Ollier's dz (risk of malignant change ~ 30%). Ollier's + hemangiomas = Maffucci's syndrome. Risk of malignancy high.

2. *Osteochondroma*: cartilage-shaped cap of bone that grows from surface of normal bone.

3. *Osteoid osteoma*: painful lesion (esp. at night), which induces osteoblastic response. Although sx may respond dramatically w/ aspirin, excision is recommended. Most resolve or burn out after 2 yr.

4. *Osteoblastoma*: osteoblastic lesion, typically larger than osteoid osteoma. Tx = curettage.

5. *Unicameral bone cyst*: usu. in proximal humeral metaphysis (carpals, tarsals less often). Often presents w/ pathologic fx. Tx = steroid injection a/o curettage.

B. **Malignant**

1. *Chondrosarcoma*: relatively resistant to chemotx or XRT. Tx is wide surgical excision.

2. *Osteosarcoma*: "sunburst" pattern and a "Codman's triangle" on x-ray. Aggressive tx required.

3. *Ewing's sarcoma*: generally presents before 30 yo, arises in diaphyses, and grows rapidly w/ early spread to lungs. X-rays classically demonstrate diaphyseal lucency w/ periosteal "onionskin" reaction. Generally tx w/ XRT/chemotherapy before considering surgery.

4. *Giant cell tumor of bone*: 90% are "benign;" 10% metastasize to lung. Begin in metaphysis.

5. *Multiple myeloma*: most common primary malignancy of bone. Arises in diaphyses (like Ewing's) or other bones that contain marrow. Tx w/ XRT and chemotherapy.

6. *Metastatic tumors*

   a. More common (80%) than primary bone cancer; in descending order of frequency—breast, prostate, lung, kidney, thyroid (follicular), pancreas, stomach.

   b. Usu. osteolytic, but may be all or partly osteoblastic w/ breast or prostate metastases.

   c. Bone scan or skeletal survey useful to evaluate for multiple sites. Most common primary for isolated single metastasis is renal cell carcinoma.

V. HAND SURGERY

A. Always perform Allen test before invasive procedures distal to elbow. Have pt elevate hand, squeeze into a fist (~ 30 sec), then physician compresses both arteries. Pt then opens hand and physician releases 1 of the arteries and evaluates for perfusion. Test is then repeated for the other artery. Hand should reperfuse w/in ~ 6 sec. Abn in up to 15% of pts.

B. **Trauma**

1. *Hand injuries and deformities*

   a. *Boxer's (fighter's) fx*: neck fx of 4th or 5th metacarpals. Up to 50° of angulation acceptable. If involves 2nd or 3rd metacarpals, only 15° of angulation accepted. Reduce and place in ulnar gutter splint, refer to specialist.

b. *Scaphoid fx*: usu. from fall on outstretched hand; usu. pt has "snuffbox" tenderness. If initial x-rays (–), place in thumb-spica splint, and f/u w/ specialist w/in 10–14 d.

c. *Nail bed injury*: removal of nail, repair of bed w/ fine (i.e., 7-0 chromic gut) suture, and replacement of nail generally indicated; perform w/ loupe magnfication.

C. Infections

1. *Paronychia*—most common hand infection, usu. from *S. aureus*.

   a. *Dx*: erythema, swelling, tenderness adjacent to nail.

   b. *Tx*:

      i. *Early*: warm soaks, oral abx. Superficial abscess may be drained where it "points."

      ii. *Late*: may require elevation of perionychium and skin adjacent to nail fold or even removal of part of the nail if pus extends below nail plate.

      • Abx should be continued as appropriate after drainage.

   c. *Chronic*: frequently due to fungus.

2. *Felon*—subcutaneous abscess of distal pulp involving the palmar pad.

   a. Essentially an infectious compartment syndrome of the pulp. If left untreated, risk developing osteomyelitis, septic (DIP) arthritis, a/o flexor tenosynovitis.

   b. *Dx*: pain, swelling, and tenderness distal to DIP. Frequently from penetrating foreign body.

   c. *Tx*:

      i. *Early* (cellulitis only): elevation, oral abx, warm soaks.

      ii. *Fluctuant* (assume fluctuance if > 48 h of sx):

      • Many different incisions described, but safest and most effective is probably longitudinal over point of maximal tenderness.

      • Open involved septa, culture pus.

      • Examine distal phalanx w/ probe and debride soft, necrotic bone.

      • Irrigate and place wick, sterile dressing.

3. *Herpetic whitlow*: herpes simplex virus (HSV) infection of hand, often seen in healthcare workers, and may be confused w/ paronychia or felon. Important to distinguish from the latter 2 as rest, elevation, anti-inflammatory agents, +/– antivirals (i.e., acyclovir), *not surgery*, is indicated. Crucial to obtain hx, which generally reveals prodromal pain followed by clear vesicles; confirmation may be achieved w/ viral cx a/o Tzanck smear.

4. *Suppurative flexor tenosynovitis*

   a. Most often from *S. aureus* infection of tendon sheath, other organisms such as *N. gonorrhea* can be involved.

   b. *Kanavel's signs*:

      i. Fusiform swelling of finger ("sausage digit").

      ii. Finger held in partial flexion.

      iii. Tenderness over volar finger/flexor tendon sheath.

      iv. Exquisite pain w/ passive extension of finger.

   c. *Tx*:

      i. *Nonoperative*: if early (1st 24 h), mild sx, consider IV Abx, rest, elevation. If no improvement w/in 24 h → OR.

      ii. *Operative*: limited incision (e.g., over A1 and A5 pulleys) and catheter irrigation usu. adequate; uncommonly full exposure of sheath required.

CHAPTER 20

OBSTETRICS AND GYNECOLOGY

I. PREGNANCY

A. R/o in all preoperative pts 10–50 yo.

B. **Nägele's rule:** estimated date of conception = last missed period – 3 mo + 7 d.

C. At 5–6 wk, a fetal pole of 1–2 mm can be seen on transvaginal U/S, and at 6–6.5 wk, fetal heart tones detectable. Fetus generally considered viable about 24 wk (0 survival at 21 wk and 75% at 25 wk; 11% at 401–500 g and 75% at 701–800 g [Lemons JA, et al., *Pediatrics* 2001;107:E1.].

   1. *β-hCG:* detectable in maternal serum as early as 8 d postconception. Should increase at least 53% every 48 h early in pregnancy [Barnhart KT, et al., *Obstet Gynecol* 2004;104:50–5.] Peaks ~ 65 d after conception, generally decreasing in 2nd and 3rd trimesters then stabilizes at about 20,000 mIU/mL.

   2. *Ultrasonography:*
      a. *Transabdominal U/S:* can see intrauterine gestational sac w/ mean diameter of 5 mm (5 wk gestational age) or 6000–6500 mIU/mL β-hCG.
      b. *Transvaginal U/S:* should see intrauterine gestational sac by 4–5 wk, 1500–2400 mIU/mL β-hCG.
      c. Be aware of gestatational pseudosac of ectopic pregnancy.

D. **Uterus:** by 12 wk moves out of pelvis into abdomen, by 20 wk is at umbilicus, by 34–36 wk at costal margin.

E. In gravid pts in shock, consider ectopic pregnancy in 1st trimester, placental abruption (esp. after blunt trauma/MVA due to shearing between elastic myometrium and inelastic placenta), amniotic fluid embolism later in pregnancy.

F. **Physiologic changes in pregnancy:**

   1. *Cardiovascular:*
      a. Plasma volume increases 40–60% between 12–36 wk gestation. Hct 31–35% normal in late pregnancy. May lose 30% of blood volume before sx occur. CVP does not significantly change.
      b. After wk 10, CO increases by 1.0–1.5 L/min (increased volume, decreased uterine/placenta resistance). However, in late pregnancy, supine compression of IVC can decrease CO 30%.
      c. Heart rate increases by 10–15 bpm during pregnancy (max in 3rd trimester).
      d. DBP drops 5–15 mm Hg during 2nd trimester, then rise again to near-normal at term. SBP changes minimally. Left-lateral decubitus position will help if hypotensive from IVC compression while supine.
      e. *EKG:* left shift by 15° common. T wave flattening or inversion in III, AVF, and precordial leads may be normal. Ectopy increases in incidence.
      f. Hypovolemic shock results in compensatory increase in uterine resistance. Normal maternal vital signs do NOT imply adequate fetal oxygenation.

   2. *Pulmonary:* minute ventilation increases (mostly from increased – Vt); $PaCO_2$ as low as 30 not uncommon in 3rd trimester, whereas $PaCO_2$ 35–40 may herald respiratory failure. Oxygen consumption increases.

   3. *Hematologic:* WBC increases; 15K not unusual, may be as high as 25K during labor. Fibrinogen and clotting factors markedly elevated, resulting in possibly shorter PT/PTT, but unchanged bleeding time. RBC mass increases by $1/3$, but not as fast as plasma volume initially, w/ resultant hematocrit drop until end of 2nd trimester. Plt count has been shown to decrease in some studies (possibly due to increased platelet consumption in pregnancy). Prostacyclin and thromboxane A2 production increase.

   4. *Gastrointestinal:*
      a. GI motility slows due to progesterone effects. Gastric emptying prolongs during pregnancy; NGT decompression esp. important. Gastrin levels also rise, and GERD worsens due to increased acidity, decreased emptying, and cephalad migration of stomach.

    b. Gallbladder stasis predisposes to gallstone formation.

    c. More water than usual is absorbed, often resulting in constipation.

    d. Albumin drops to 2.2–2.8. Alkaline phosphatase rises from placenta.

- **G. Abnormal outcomes**:

    1. *Ectopic pregnancy*: 1% of all pregnancies; 99% are tubal. ↑ risk: low SE status, h/o difficulty conceiving, IUD users, prior ectopic pregnancies or PID. *Always consider in ddx for abdominal pain in reproductive age females.* Tx: surgical emergency if symptomatic → open/lap salpingectomy if ruptured, linear salpingostomy if unruptured; follow β-hCG until normalizes if salpingostomy performed. *Early, minimal sx cases*: consider methotrexate, in-house serial β-hCG and clinical exams (outpt if min sx, stable, reliable pt).

    2. *Molar pregnancy*: (hydatidiform mole, invasive mole, and choriocarcinoma). Tumor of fetal tissue. *Risk factors*: women < 20 yo or > 40 yo, low economic status, low diet protein or folate.

        a. Assoc. w/ 1st trimester uterine bleeding, preeclampsia and hyperemesis, absence of fetal heart tones, inappropriately rapid growth of uterine size, inappropriately high β-hCG, a/o passage of vesicles.

        b. *Tx*:

            i. *Hydatidiform mole*: suction curettage, then follow exam and β-hCG to ensure both normalize by 15 wk; if they don't, then consider malignant process.

            ii. *Malignant gestational trophoblastic neoplasia*: depending on presence of metastasis (usu. lung), tx options are chemotherapeutic (methotrexate most often) +/– surgery.

II. PID: SPECTRUM OF DZ, WHICH RANGES FROM ENDOMETRITIS TO TUBO-OVARIAN ABSCESS AND PERITONITIS.

- **A.** Most often from *N. gonorrhea* a/o *C. trachomatis* (note, classic "STD organism" not recovered in up to ⅓ of cases), although anaerobic bacteria may play a significant role.

- **B.** Most consistent findings are lower abdominal pain and tenderness, cervical motion tenderness, and adnexal tenderness. Cervical discharge not infrequent.

- **C.** W/u should include CBC, specific testing for gonorrhea and chlamydia, urinalysis, β-hCG. Consider U/S if concern for TOA.

- **D. Tx**:

    1. *Primary*: cefoxitin (2 g IV q 6 h) or cefotetan (2 g IV q 6 h) and doxycycline (100 mg PO/IV two times per day).

    2. *Alternatives*:

        a. Clindamycin (900 mg IV q 8 h) and gentamicin (load 2 mg/kg IV/IM, then 1.5 mg/kg IV/IM q 8 h).

            i. If pt improves on IV medication after 24 h, may transition to oral abx for 2 wk (clindamycin 450 mg PO four times per day or doxycycline 100 mg PO two times per day).

        b. Ofloxacin 400 mg IV q 12 h and metronidazole 500 mg IV q 8 h (inpt regimen); Ofloxacin 400 mg PO two times per day and metronidzole 500 mg PO two times per day (outpt regimen—14 d).

    3. *Surgical* (or percutaneous if appropriate) intervention should be considered if no improvement after 3 d of medical tx, abscess rupture, or bleeding from erosion into vessel.

III. OVARIAN TORSION/CYST

- **A. Risk factors**: ovarian cysts, tubal ligation, ovarian malignancy.

- **B. Presentation**: presents w/ crampy, sharp abdominal pain w/ radiation to flank/groin +/– N/V.

- **C. Dx**:

    1. PEx often demonstrates abdominal tenderness and palpable mass on pelvic exam.

    2. Doppler U/S is appropriate initial study to assess structure, size, and flow.

- **D. Tx**: laparoscopy or ex lap: detorsion usu. possible, occasionally require unilateral oophorectomy and salpingectomy for ischemia.

IV. MALIGNANCY

- **A. Ovarian**

    1. *Risk factors*: age (esp. postmenopausal), BRCA 1 > 2, Lynch syndrome type II (colorectal and gastric, endometrial and ovarian), nulliparity, infertility, endometriosis. Decreased risk of ovarian CA if h/o use of OCPs, pregnancy, breastfeeding.

2. *Dx*: routine screening not recommended, but do evaluate signs and sx. Can consider screening high-risk women (family h/o ovarian CA, breast CA, BRCA mutation) w/ transvaginal U/S and CA-125 q 6 mo (CA-125 is elevated in 80% of cases, but this is a nonspecific marker).

3. *Tx*: TAH/BSO w/ surgical staging, infracolic omentectomy +/– appendectomy, pelvic and para-aortic LN sampling, tumor debulking, multiagent IV chemotherapy +/– intraperitoneal chemotherapy.

B. **Management of the incidental ovarian mass (found on U/S or physical exam):**

1. If symptomatic, will usu. require intervention (surgery, abx, medical management).

2. Simple cysts ≤ 10 cm in both pre- and postmenopausal women are usu. benign and can be followed.

3. *Postmenopausal women*: most masses except simple cysts will likely require surgical intervention esp. if U/S suspicious for malignancy (solid areas, excrescences, ascites) and elevated CA-125 (preferably by gyn oncologist).

4. *Premenopausal women*: can observe if U/S reveals benign characteristics (unilocular thin-walled cysts w/ smooth borders) and asymptomatic. Refer to gyn onc if CA-125 > 200 U/mL, ascites, FH of breast or ovarian CA, evidence of metatstatic dz. (Adnexal masses in pregnant women seem to have low risk for malignancy and can be considered for observation.)

5. If surgical evaluation of malignancy indicated, perform TAH, BSO, omentectomy, periaortic LN sampling, and peritoneal irrigation for cytology.

CHAPTER 21

UROLOGY

I. ANATOMY, AND PHYSIOLOGY

A. **Vascular**

1. Right kidney apposed to liver, right adrenal, psoas, duodenum, ascending colon. Left kidney apposed to spleen, left adrenal, pancreatic tail, descending colon.

2. Renal vein anterior to artery. Right artery passes behind IVC, and left vein passes in front of aorta (10% pass behind). Renal arteries may be singled or paired, and divide into segmental → lobar → arcuate → interlobar arteries (end arteries), which supply glomeruli via afferent arterioles.

B. **Ureter:** blood supply to ureter is segmental, from medial proximally and lateral distally; maintain adventitia during dissection to preserve feeding anastomoses. Crossover iliac vessels at pelvic brim. Renal pelvis is posterior to the renal artery.

C. **Bladder:** normal adult capacity ~ 400 mL. Ureters enter posterolaterally, ~ 5 cm apart. Median umbilical ligament (obliterated urachus) extends from dome to umbilicus.

D. **Male genitalia:**

1. *Phallus:* corpora invested in tunica albuginea, enveloped in turn by Buck's fascia. Underneath skin of penis and scrotum lies (from corona to urogenital diaphragm) Colles' fascia, continuous w/ abdominal Scarpa's fascia.

2. *Testes:* spermatic arteries from aorta anastomose w/ arteries of vas deferens, which come from internal iliac artery, making arterial supply somewhat redundant. Venous return is via pampiniform plexus, which becomes spermatic vein at level of internal ring. Right vein empties into IVC while left vein empties into left renal vein. Left adrenal vein and lumbar vein also empty into left renal vein.

    a. *Sertoli cells:* produce inhibin (Mullerian inhibiting factor); provide blood–testis barrier as well as some nutrition to spermatids en route to epididymis; also convert testosterone to estrogen.

    b. *Leydig (interstitial) cells:* produce testosterone, DHEA, and progesterone, and estradiol.

II. CONGENITAL DISORDERS

A. **Vesicoureteral reflux:** usu. due to abn. intramural ureter, occ. intrinsic ureteral abnormalities. Depending on etiology, observation, suppressive abx, or surgery may be appropriate.

B. **Cryptorchidism:** occurs in ~ 3.5% of term births (rate increases almost 10× w/ prematurity). ½ descend w/in 1 mo of birth. Tx w/in 1 yr. Most feared complication is testicular cancer (rate increased 40× over lifetime, even after placement in scrotum). Surgery recommended if hormonal tx fails (hCG a/o LHRH). Orchidopexy usu. recommended except in children > 10 yo or (more controversial) intraabdominal testis—orchiectomy reserved for such cases. Pts w/ bilateral cryptorchidism and hypospadias should get a karyotype analysis.

III. ACQUIRED DISORDERS

A. **Anatomic (nontraumatic; see Chapter 7 for management of urologic injury)**

1. *Voiding disorders*

    a. *Benign prostatic hyperplasia*

        i. Generally due to effects of dihydrotestosterone although prostatic smooth muscle tone can contribute.

        ii. *Sx:* diminished force of urinary stream, hesitancy, nocturia, urgency typically reported.

        iii. *Dx:* ddx: prostate/bladder CA, urethral stricture, prostatitis, cystitis, urolithiasis, and neurogenic bladder.

        iv. *Tx:*

          • *Medical:* alpha blockers, 5α-reductase inhibitors usu. used in combination.

          • *Surgical:* transurethral resection of prostate (TURP), open prostatectomy.

            ▪ *TUR syndrome:* ~ 2% of pts in immediate postop period, due to absorbtion of glycine or sorbitol from irrigant solution, resulting in dilutional hyponatremia. Mental status or vision changes, N/V, HTN reported. Tx w/ furosemide (occ. w/ hypertonic saline as well).

- Open prostatectomy (retropubic or suprapubic).
  - Reserved for surgical candidates w/ prostates > 100 g or w/ orthopedic issues precluding lithotomy position.

b. *Neurogenic bladder*

   i. Continence requires coordination of CNS, autonomic nervous system, detrusor, and external and internal sphincters.

   ii. *Tx*: depends on etiology, but usu. involves anticholinergics to diminish unwanted bladder contractions; alpha agonists can help augment sphincter pressure.

2. *Urolithiasis*: may present w/ flank, abdominal, or testicular pain +/− dysuria, +/− hematuria. 85% of stones are radio-opaque (exceptions = cystine, xanthine). Calcium oxalate = majority; risk factors include distal small bowel inflammation, bypass, or resection (reason = excess intraluminal fat binds calcium, which is unavailable to bind oxalate to prevent its absorption in colon). Urinary infection w/ urea-splitting organisms raises risk factor for formation of struvite stones (magnesium ammonium phosphate). Hypomagnesemia, hypocitratemia, high sodium intake are also general risk factors. Stones < 6 mm usu. pass. Acute w/u includes CT scan of abdomen and pelvis w/out any contrast, CBC, chemistry, and urinalysis. Urinary obstruction and fever might need decompression of the kidney via a ureteral stent or percutaneous nephrostomy tube, + IVF, abx. *W/u for recurrent stones*: serum (calcium, phosphorus, oxalate, cystine, etc.), stone analysis, urine analysis (pH, 24-h mineral assay).

3. *Phimosis, paraphimosis*

   a. *Phimosis*: inability to retract foreskin back over glans, tx w/ dorsal slit or circumcision.

   b. *Paraphimosis*: inability to reduce foreskin distally back over glans, may cause significant pain and swelling; gentle uniform compression often reduces edema enough to reduce foreskin. Occasionally a dorsal slit is needed.

4. *Testicular torsion*: usu. in adolescence, although significant incidence in infants w/ undescended testis. Usu. a swollen, tender, high-riding testicle. Cremasteric reflex absent. Duplex to evaluate blood flow can be useful, but if any doubt, take pt to OR for exploration and detorsion w/in 4 h of sx onset. Ddx includes torsion of appendix testis and epididymitis.

5. *Varicocele*: engorgement, dilatation of pampiniform plexus. Found in up to 10% of young males. Most commonly of the left. Presents w/ palpable "bag of worms," which may be painful; can contribute to infertility. Palpate pt upright and recumbent; failure of varicocele to decompress while recumbent, or presence of a right-sided varicole may represent obstructing renal neoplasm. Definitive tx: ligation of internal spermatic veins.

B. **Infectious**

1. *Urinary tract infection and pyelonephritis*: simple UTI—3 d of fluoroquinolone or SMP-TMX. Complicated infections such as pyelonephritis generally manifest w/ constitutional symptoms such as fever, often CVA tenderness. Usu. require hospital admission and IV abx, but can be treated on outpt basis in healthy individuals who tolerate fluids orally.

2. *Epididymo-orchitis*: assoc. w/ scrotal swelling, pain, often dysuria. Under 35 yo most often from STD. Over 35 yo, usu. from gram-negative rods. "Prehn's sign" is improvement in scrotal pain w/ elevation of scrotum. Pts w/ testicular torsion do not experience relief w/ scrotal elevation. Tx w/ oxafloxacin is effective for both.

3. *Fournier's gangrene*: synergistic necrotizing infection of scrotum/perineum, usu. seen in diabetics.

C. **Neoplastic**

1. *Testicular*

   a. *Seminoma*:

      i. *Dx*: may see increased hCG or LDH, *not AFP*.

      ii. *Tx*: sensitive to *XRT*. Tx depends on stage. Early stage dz is usu. treated w/ XRT. Late stage dz w/ platinum-based chemotherapy.

   b. *NSGCT*:

      i. *Dx*: 85% w/ increased hCG or AFP.

      ii. *Tx*: sensitive to platinum-based *chemo*; early stage dz is usu. treated w/ surgery or chemotherapy, while late stage dz is treated w/ chemotherapy followed by selective RPLND if residual masses are noted.

2. *Renal cell carcinoma* (adenocarcinoma of kidney)

a. Classic triad of pain, hematuria, and palpable flank mass in less than 10%. Fever, HTN, nonreducing left varicocele, a/o wt loss may also be present. Majority present as incidental findings on CT/MRI.

b. *Paraneoplastic syndromes common*: may see [hypercalcemia, HTN, erythrocytosis] > [Cushing's syndrome, hypoglycemia, amenorrhea, galactorrhea, hirsutism].

   i. *Stauffer's syndrome*: hepatic dysfunction (may include ↑ PT) +/− fever assoc. w/ RCC, which typically resolves w/ nephrectomy.

c. CT is imaging study of choice. MRI superior though in imaging IVC and renal vessels.

d. *Tx*:

   i. Partial nephrectomy is standard of care for all masses < 4 cm in size and for masses < 7 cm if technically feasible.

   ii. Radical nephrectomy (en block excision of kidney w/ Gerota's fascia, adrenal gland, proximal ½ of ureter and hilar LNs) reserved for large tumors that are not amenable to partial nephrectomy.

   iii. Up to 10% of cases present w/ luminal involvement of renal vein +/− IVC. IVC thrombectomy can be curative in pts who otherwise have no distant metastases. This is typically done in combination w/ a thoracic/vascular surgeon.

   iv. *Metastatic dz* (lung > bone > lymph nodes): current tx includes tyrosine kinase inhibitors or mTOR inhibitors (no cures). IL-2 can be given to very select healthy pts w/ a cure rate of < 5%.

3. *Prostate cancer*

a. The most common cancer in males. 70% arise in peripheral zone; thus often readily palpable on DRE. Most commonly adenocarcinoma.

b. *W/u*: DRE and PSA (note, DRE can elevate transiently PSA level), followed by transrectal U/S-guided needle bx. CT, MRI, bone scan may be warranted as well.

c. *Tx*:

   i. *Early* (T1, T2): radical prostatectomy *or* XRT (long-term survival > 80% w/ either). Some pts w/ very low-risk prostate cancer are offered active surveillance.

   ii. *Locally advanced* (T3, T4): surgery or XRT w/ hormone ablation.

   iii. *Metastatic*:

   • Hormonal tx (estrogens, orchiectomy, LH-RH agonist, antiandrogens) primary modality (chemotx not as effective).

   • Taxol-based chemotherapy for pts who fail hormone ablation.

   • XRT used for bone pain or other local bone complication refractory to hormonal tx.

4. *Bladder cancer*

a. 90% transitional cell. 5–10% in U/S squamous cell. < 2% adenocarcinoma.

b. Majority w/ painless gross hematuria. Frequency, urgency, dysuria, nocturia may be present, as may sx of bladder/ureteral obstruction (i.e., azotemia).

c. *Dx*: urine cytology and cystoscopic bx.

d. *Tx*: ranges from transurethral resection (TUR) +/− intravesical bacillus Calmette-Guérin to radical cystectomy, +/− adjuvant tx depending on stage.

IV. <u>ACUTE RENAL FAILURE (ARF)</u>

A. Usu. from ischemia or toxins, and lasts 7–21 d. Major cause of death in ARF pts is infection. Predictors of poor outcome include oliguria, poor nutritional markers, mechanical ventilation, acute MI or CVA or sz, and chronic immunosuppression.

B. Dx:

1. Rise in serum Cr 0.5 (or 50%) or more above baseline; reduction in calculated creatinine clearance of at least 50% from normal.

2. *Creatinine clearance*:

a. *Normal*: males 97 – 137 mL/min/1.73 m²; females 88 – 128 mL/min/1.73 m².

b. *Calculation* (requires 24-h urine): (Urine Cr × Urine volume in mL) / (Serum Cr × 1400).

    c. Increased w/ pregnancy, exercise. Decreased w/ renal insufficiency, increasing age (decreases 1 mL/min/yr > 30), certain medications (cimetidine, procainamide, various abx, quinidine).

    d. Alternately, can gauge renal function w/ GFR (unless pt is vegetarian, uses creatine supplement, is malnourished, or an amputee).

        i. *GFR (male)* = $(140 - \text{age}) \times (\text{wt in kg}) / (\text{Serum Cr} \times 72)$

        ii. *GFR (female)* = $(140 - \text{age}) \times (\text{wt in kg}) \times 0.85 / (\text{Serum Cr} \times 72)$

C. Tx:

  1. *Dietary restrictions*: avoid high-phosphorus foods, carefully monitor K^+.

D. Prophylaxis

  1. *Dye nephropathy*—for high-risk pts (diabetics, CRI, etc.).

    a. *Sodium bicarbonate*:

        i. 1 h prior to procedure give 3 cc/kg (max 330 cc) over 1 h of 3 amps (150 mEq $NaHCO_3$ / 1 L D_5W or sterile water).

        ii. Post-scan continue infusion as 1 cc/kg (max 110 cc/h) for 6 h. [Merten GJ, *JAMA*, 2004;291(19):2328–34.]

    b. *N-acetylcysteine* (Mucomyst)

        i. 600 mg PO two times per day preprocedure day and 600 mg PO two times per day on day of procedure.

        ii. Also give $^1/_2$ NS at 1 cc/kg × 12 h pre- and postprocedure [Tepel M, *N Engl J Med*, 2000;343(3):180–4.]

    c. Fenoldopam is a selective renal dopamine D-1 agonist (no effects on other dopamine or adrenergic receptors). Although its use may result in augmented renal perfusion, natriuresis, and UOP, data do not suggest any consistent renal protective effects.

CHAPTER 22

NEUROSURGERY

I. **NEUROLOGIC EXAM**
   A. **Glasgow coma scale**: see Chapter 7.
   B. **Altered mental status**: see Chapter 25.
   C. **Trauma**
      1. *Brain*
         a. *Elevated intracranial pressure*:
            i. Normally 10–15 mm Hg; maintain less than 20 mm Hg.
            ii. CPP = MAP – ICP; maintain ≥ 60.
            iii. *Cushing's triad*: hypertension, bradycardia, respiratory irregularity.
            iv. *Management*:
               • Elevate head 30–45°.
               • Avoid hypotension (consider early use of pressors instead of excessive fluids).

TABLE 22.1.   Cranial Nerves

Cranial Nerve	Innervates / Function	Deficit Manifestation
I – olfactory	Smell	Anosmia
II – optic	Vision	Altered vision (*note*: diminished perception of the color red may be early sign of nerve compression)
III – oculomotor	Opens eyelid; sup. rectus, inf. rectus, med. rectus, inf. oblique motor supply	Eyelid ptosis; palsy of respective ocular muscles
IV – trochlear	Superior oblique motor	Inability to look down and in
V – trigeminal	Facial sensation, mastic	Facial sensory loss, weakness of mastication
VI – abducens	Lateral rectus motor	Inability to look laterally
VII – facial	Taste, facial animation	Loss of taste, altered facial animation
VIII – vestibular	Hearing / balance	Neural hearing loss, vertigo
IX – glossopharyngeal	Swallowing/gag (aff); taste posterior $1/3$ tongue	Impaired gag reflex
X – vagus	Swallowing/gag (eff), vocal cord	Impaired gag reflex, dysphagia, hoarseness
XI – spinal accessory	Motor to trapezius, SCM	Weakness of "shrug" a/o turning head *contralaterally*
XII – hypoglossal	Motor to tongue	Tongue "points to" side of deficit when stuck out

TABLE 22.2. Spinal Nerves

Root Level	Sensory	Motor	Reflex
C2	Occipital area		
C3	Medial supraclavicular		
C4	Acromial area	Diaphragm / breathing	
C5	Lateral arm	Deltoid / arm abduction	
C6	Dorsum thumb	Biceps / elbow flexion	Biceps
C7	Dorsum middle finger	Triceps / elbow extension	Triceps
C8	Dorsum little finger	Flexor carpi ulnaris / wrist flexion	
T1	Medial arm	Lumbricals / finger abduction	
T2	Axilla		
T4	Level of nipple		
T10	Level of umbilicus		
L1	Infrainguinal region	Hip flexion	Cremasteric
L2	Mid. medial thigh	Iliopsoas / hip flexion	
L3	Medial knee	Quadriceps / knee extension	
L4	Anterior / medial leg, medial foot	Tibialis anterior / knee extension	Patellar tendon
L5	Dorsum foot / hallux	Dorsiflex (toe, ankle)	Medial hamstring
S1	Lateral foot / heel	Plantarflexors / knee flexion	Achilles' tendon
S2	Popliteal fossa	Rectal tone	Bulbocavernosus
S3	Medial gluteal area		
S4–5	Perianal area		Anal wink

TABLE 22.3. Peripheral Nerves

Peripheral Nerve	Origin	Sensory	Motor
Axillary	C5–C6	Deltoid region	Deltoid (arm abduction)
Musculocutaneous	C5–C6	Lateral forearm	Biceps
Radial	C6–C7	Radial dorsum of hand	Wrist and elbow extension
Median	C5–T1	Radial palm of hand	Pincer strength
Ulnar	C8–T1	Ulnar $1/3$ of hand	Finger abduction
Femoral	L1–L4	Anterior thigh / medial calf	Hip flexion / knee extension
Peroneal (deep)	L4–L5	Calf	Dorsiflextion of ankle
Tibial	S1–S2	Plantar and lateral foot	Plantarflexion of ankle

TABLE 22.4. Motor Strength (United Kingdom System)

Score	Ability
0	No contraction
1	Palpable contraction without limb movement
2	Able to move limb when gravity's effect eliminated
3	Able to move limb against gravity
4	Diminished strength
5	Normal strength

- Avoid hypercarbia (ventilate to keep pCO_2 35–40 mm Hg).
- Appropriate analgesia (i.e, fentanyl) and sedation (i.e., lorazepam 1–2 mg IV q 4 h prn); alternate, propofol gtt.
- Drainage w/ intraventricular catheter/EVD prn.
- Chemically paralyze (i.e., pancuronium 3–5 mg IV q 2–3 h prn); alternate, vecuronium gtt.
- Mannitol 0.25–1.0 g/kg, then 0.25 g/kg q 6 h; stop if serum osmol < 330 or hypotension.
- Pentobarbital 100 mg IV q 4 h (2–5 mg/kg IV q 4 h in peds); consider burst suppression w/ continuous EEG monitoring.

   b. *Sz prophylaxis*: pts at risk for early posttraumatic seizures (acute intracranial hemorrhage/ hematoma, open depressed skull fx w/ parenchymal injury, etc.) should be prophylaxed w/ loading dose of phenytoin/fosphenytoin at 20 mg/kg, then maintaining therapeutic levels for 1 wk.
   c. *Epidural hematoma*: bleed between skull and dura
      i. Assoc. w/ skull fx (usu. temporal fx and middle meningeal artery).
      ii. "Classic" (only seen in $^1/_3$) pattern is brief LOC, then "lucid interval" followed by deterioration of mental status. Ipsilateral pupil dilatation, contralateral hemiparesis follows in significant cases.
      iii. Noncontrast CT demonstrates hyperdense lenticular lesion.
      iv. Surgical evacuation indicated unless asymptomatic.
   d. *Subdural hematoma*: bleed between dura and brain
      i. Assoc. w/ tear of bridging veins over cortex.
      ii. Noncontrast CT demonstrates crescentic lesion.
      iii. Surgical evacuation indicated for symptomatic cases.
      iv. Prognosis worse than for epidural hematomas.
   e. *Diffuse axonal injury*
      i. Most common closed head injury pattern.
      ii. CT frequently normal, requiring MRI for detection (multiple hyperdense lesions on T2 images).
   f. *Cerebral contusion*
      i. Temporal lobe > frontal lobe > other locations.
      ii. Initial CT may show patchy low-density lesions +/– hyperdense hemorrhagic lesions.
      iii. May worsen w/ time, demonstrable on CT.
         - Monitor w/ serial CT scans for increase in size.
   g. *Basilar skull fx's*
      i. *Clinical findings*: rhinorrhea/otorrhea, hemotympanum, Battle's sign, raccoon's eyes, possible cranial nerve deficits.
      ii. *Dx*: CT.
      iii. *Management*: do not place NGT; otherwise generally expectant.

h. *Depressed skull fx's*

   i. *Surgery indicated*: open fx; fx depth exceeds thickness of cranial bone (usu. 8–10 mm); surgical brain injury/hemorrhage or dural laceration w/ CSF leak; less often, cosmesis.

i. *CSF leak*

   i. *Dx*:

- "Target sign" on filter paper as CSF moves further than blood.
- β-2 transferrin specific for fluid from CSF, perilymph, or vitreous humor.

   ii. *Tx*:

- Expectant management w/ elevation of head, bowel regimen, avoidance of sneezing/coughing/etc.
- Routine antibiotic prophlaxis not indicated.
- Lumbar puncture or drainage may be indicated if lasts longer than 2 d.
- Surgery indicated for persistent leaks.

j. *Physiologic sequelae of intracranial lesions*:

   i. *Syndrome of inappropriate antidiuretic hormone secretion* (SIADH); ~ 5% of CHI.

- *Dx*:
  - Hyponatremia (< 134 mEq/L), hypernatriuria (> 18 mEq/L), hypoosmolar serum (< 280 mOsm/L).
- *Tx*:
  - *Mild*: water/fluid restriction.
  - *Symptomatic or severe*: water/fluid restriction, HTS, furosemide, salt tablets.
  - *Chronic*: water restriction, demeclocycline (ADH antagonist), furosemide.

   ii. *Cerebral salt wasting* (CSW)

- Common w/ aneurismal SAH.
- Serum and urine laboratory findings similar to that of SIADH.
- *Unlike pts w/ SIADH, those w/ CSW will be intravascularly volume depleted.*
- *Tx*:
  - Restore volume w/ NS (0.9%) or HTS (3%) a/o salt tablets.
  - Avoid too rapidly correcting sodium level (see Chapter 1).
  - Fludrocortisone usage reported effective, but accompanied by significant side effects such as hypokalemia, pulmonary edema, and HTN.

   iii. *Diabetes insipidus* (DI)

- More common after basilar skull fx or severe TBI.
- Generally manifests w/ polyuria UOP > 250 cc/h, w/ urine SG < 1.005 and urine osmolality of 50–150 mOsm. Serum osmolality may be normal or high. Pts often crave water, and risk hyponatremia from polydipsia.
- *Management*: depends on severity and if pt is cooperative.
  - Mild cases may be managed w/ simply drinking water.
  - *Desmopressin* (DDAVP): 2.5–20 mcg intranasally two times per day drug of choice, although certain medication such as HCTZ may help in partial ADH deficiency (not intuitive as HCTZ is diuretic; use w/ caution).
  - In noncooperative pts, give IVF as D_5½ NS + 20 mEq KCl/L at 75–100 cc/h and replace UOP cc/cc w/ ½ NS. If behind on fluid losses:
    - Desmopressin 2–4 mcg SQ/IV q d in divided doses, a/o . . .
    - Vasopressin 5 U IV/IM or SQ q 4–6 h or as a drip, begun at 0.2 U/min (titrate up prn).

   iv. *Cushing's triad* (seen in $1/3$ of pts w/ intracranial HTN): hypertension, bradycardia, respiratory irregularity. *Note*: pts > 40 yo and those w/ systemic hypotension at increased risk of having intracranial HTN w/ normal head CT scan.

v. *Cushing's ulcers*: gastric ulcers assoc. w/ severe head injury, increased ICP, and hypergastrinemia. Provide appropriate acid blocker (i.e., proton-pump inhibitor) for pts at risk.

2. *Spinal cord*

a. *Blunt spinal cord injuries* may *benefit (i.e., 1 spinal cord level) from methylprednisolone*: 30 mg/kg initial bolus, then 5.4 mg/kg/h for 23 h. Exclusion criteria include pregnancy and pediatric pts.

b. *Patterns of injury*:

i. *Complete cord lesion*: complete loss of sensory, motor, and reflex activity below level of injury.

ii. *Anterior cord syndrome*: occurring after hyperflexion injury w/ retropulsion of disk; only posterior columns are spared, manifesting w/ only position and vibratory sensation intact.

iii. *Brown-Séquard syndrome*: ipsilateral preservation of pain and temperature w/ motor function, position, and vibratory sensation preserved contralaterally. Results from spinothalamic decussation 2–4 levels above level of cord entry w/ motor fibers crossing in brain stem.

iv. *Central cord syndrome* (anterior spinal artery syndrome): presents w/ greater strength in legs than in the arms, most likely from lesion in anterior spinar artery; generally improves w/ time.

c. *Neurogenic shock*

i. Due to disruption of sympathetic pathways (T1–L2).

ii. Cervical cord lesions assoc. w/ hypotension, bradycardia. Bradycardia may be stimulated by turning, suctioning, or other events. Tx (a/o pretx) w/ vagolytics such as atropine may be useful. In general mild, intravascular fluid expansion is sufficient, but occasionally vasopressors (alpha agonists) or even pacemaker is needed.

d. *Spinal shock*

i. Refers to lack of neurologic function immediately after trauma, lasting up to 4–6 wk. Resolution may be met w/ susceptibility to autonomic hyperreflexia.

e. *Autonomic dysreflexia/hyperreflexia*

i. From loss of central inhibition, hyperreactive sympathetic reflexes result; bladder or bowel distension can lead to severe hypertension, arrhythmias, and headache. Treat by stopping source of reflex and addition of labetalol or nitroprusside for hypertension.

D. **Tumors**

1. *Meningioma*: relatively indolent tumors that arise from dura, and are often calcified. May also induce hyperostosis of nearby cortical bone. Surgical removal is curative. Relatively radioresistant.

2. *Astrocytoma*: a form of glioma, and the most common intra-axial brain tumor. Categorized as follows:

a. *Grade I* = pilocystic astrocytoma (common in children), cured w/ gross surgical resection.

b. *Grade II* = low-grade glioma generally progresses to high grade; tx = surgery; average survival 7 yr.

c. *Grade III* = anaplastic astrocytoma; tx = surgery; average survival 3 yr.

d. *Grade IV* = glioblastoma multiforme (GBM); tx = surgery + chemotx + XRT; average survival 1 yr.

CHAPTER 23

HEAD AND NECK

I. EMBRYOLOGY AND ANATOMY

A. Branchial (pharyngeal) apparatus embryology

1. Head and neck structures develop from *branchial (pharyngeal) arches*, derived from neural crest cells. Failure of regression of the clefts gives rise to fistulas (more commonly seen in children), sinuses, or cysts (more commonly seen in adults).

   a. *First branchial arch*: develops structures for mastication, innvervated by CN V.

      i. *1st BA cleft anomalies*: present anterior to external auditory canal, passing through parotid gland and facial nerve branches.

   b. *Second branchial arch*: develops structures for facial expression, innvervated by CN VII.

      i. *2nd BA cleft anomalies*: most common place for cleft anomalies; present anterior to SCM, pass through carotid bifurcation toward pharynx/tonsil, above hypoglossal nerve.

B. Nerves:

1. *Brachial plexus*: passes between anterior and medial scalene muscles.

2. *Vagus* (CN X): runs in carotid sheath, 90% posterior to carotid artery, 10% anterior to carotid artery. Provides motor function to larynx.

3. *Spinal accessory* (CN XI): in posterior triangle (innervates trapezius, SCM).

4. *Phrenic*: runs anterior to anterior scalene (superficial), innervates diaphragm.

5. *Facial*: 5 branches, responsible for taste in anterior $^2/_3$ tongue, muscles of facial expression, including orbicularis oculi (eyelid closing). Marginal mandibular br. at risk when operating along inf. mandible.

II. BENIGN

A. Congenital

1. *Thyroglossal duct cyst*: results from failure of obliteration of the tract created by the descent of the thyroid from the foramen cecum. Presents as midline neck mass. Tx is Sistrunk procedure, which removes the cyst/tract along w/ the midportion of the hyoid bone, up to the level of the base of the tongue. Important to ensure pt has normal thyroid tissue elsewhere in the neck (i.e., w/ radionuclide scan) before removing what may represent an incompletely descended thyroid.

2. *Branchial cleft cyst/fistula*: see section I. above on Embryology. *Tx*: excision.

B. Infectious

1. *Ludwig's angina*: sublingual abscess and cellulitis. A surgical emergency, tx = I&D (and possibly extracting affected teeth), although high-dose penicillin + clindamycin (or metronidazole) is appropriate. *The first priority, however, is to protect the airway; if fiberoptic nasotracheal not available (orotracheal usu. difficult), tracheostomy may be required.*

2. *Parotitis*: usu. elderly pt w/ poor oral intake and hygiene, often immunocompromised (i.e., diabetic), and frequently w/ NGT. Tenderness/induration over parotid may extend to floor of mouth or even track down toward mediastinum, threatening aiway. Treat immediately w/ broad IV abx, oral hygiene (i.e., irrigation). Failure to respond → surgically drain the gland; raise flaps, then incise abscesses through incisions parallel to facial nerve branches and pack open.

C. Other

1. *Epistaxis*

   a. Most commonly from trauma or dessication over Kiesselbach's plexus in anterior nares; posterior bleeding is less common, but more difficult to control. Consider evaluation for contributing factors (HTN, coagulopathy, leukemia, etc.).

   b. *Tx*:

      i. *Anterior bleed*: gently compress nares between fingers for 5 min. Refractory cases should be tx'd w/ packing w/ petrolatum gauze.

      ii. *Posterior bleed*: place posterior gauze pack is 1st-line tx. Refractory bleeding may cease w/ traction applied via inflated Foley catheter passed transnasally into nasopharynx.

If not, ligation or embolization of anterior ethmoidal or sphenopalatine artery may be necessary.

iii. Correct contributing factors as appropriate.

2. *Tracheoinnominate fistula*
   a. Rare complication of tracheostomy.
   b. Classically presents w/ herald bleed before subsequent catastrophe.
   c. *Initial maneuvers include*:
      i. Inflate cuff on ETT to tamponade bleeding.
      ii. *Utley maneuver*: place finger inside trachea or in pretracheal fascial plane and compress against clavicle.
   d. Definitive tx is median sternotomy to expose innominate artery, then ligate/divide innominate and cover w/ soft tissue (i.e., muscle). Affected tracheal segment should be resected and trachea reanastamosed.

III. MALIGNANCY

A. W/u of a neck mass (squamous, not adenocarcinoma)

1. *Ddx varies w/ age and duration of lesion.*
   a. *Children*: most commonly infectious, usu. viral, may persist for months, generally < 1 cm. Bx if > 2 cm, continued growth, or matted.
      i. *Viral*: usual etiology, often preceded by URI sx. Abx, drainage may be indicated.
      ii. *Mycobacterial* (MAIS): LNs enlarged, but not tender. Perform skin test. Excision frequently necessary.
      iii. *Cat-scratch dz*: minimal tenderness, often fluctuant nodes, (+) complement fixation, self-limited.
      iv. *Hodgkin dz*: teenage/young adult, not tender, wt loss. Dx w/ bx.
2. *H&P for possible primary neoplasm.*
3. *If cannot identify primary neoplasm*:
   a. CXR, barium swallow, CT of neck indicated.
      i. MRI may be useful for deep tumors of tongue, pharynx, and larynx.
      ii. CT useful for sinus tumors. CT/MRI of chest/abdomen may be used for staging.
   b. Panendoscopy (direct laryngoscopy, esophagoscopy, bronchoscopy, and nasopharyngoscopy).
      i. If endoscopy is negative, perform random bx of right, middle, and left nasopharynx +/− tongue base bx +/− tonsillectomy.
      ii. If all bx are negative, then open neck bx w/ frozen section is indicated.

AJCC TNM Classification for Head and Neck (Squamous Cell) Carcinoma

Primary Tumor (T)	Regional Lymph Nodes (N)–Clinical & Pathological	Distant Metastasis (M)
T1 – Tumor < 2 cm	N0 – No clinically positive node	M0 – No distant metastasis
T2 – Tumor 2–4 cm	N1 – Single clinically positive node, ipsilateral to primary tumor, ≤ 3 cm in greatest diameter	M1 – Distant metastasis
T3 – Tumors > 4 cm	N2a – Single clinically positive node, ipsilateral to primary tumor, > 3 cm, but < 6 cm N2b – Multiple clinically positive ipsilateral nodes, but none > 6 cm in greatest diameter N2c – Bilateral or contralateral clinically positive nodes, but none > 6 cm in greatest diameter	
T4 – Tumor invades adjacent structure(s)	N3 – Any node(s) > 6 cm in greatest diameter	

B. **AJCC TNM staging for head and neck (squamous cell) carcinoma**

1. *Stage I* (T1N0M0) tumors receive radiation alone or surgery alone.

   a. Radiation may be preferred for functional or cosmetic reasons in early cancers. It can also tx several primary tumors as well as clinically negative regional lymph nodes simultaneously.

   b. Side effects of radiation include xerostomia, agustia, mucositis, soft tissue/dermal fibrosis, dental caries, and necrosis of bone/soft tissue.

2. *Stage II* (T2N0M0) tumors receive radiation alone, surgery alone, or combination tx.

3. *Stages III* (T3N0M0 *or* any T1–3N1M0) and IV (T4 *or* N2 *or* M1) receive surgery (including comprehensive neck dissection) and XRT +/– chemotherapy.

   a. Surgery for cure is generally not indicated in pts w/ distant metastatic dz.

   b. Cisplatin is the most common chemotherapeutic agent, and may be combined w/ 5-FU, paclitaxel, or other agents.

4. *Neck dissections*

   a. *Radical neck dissection*: an en block dissection of lymphatics, this operation includes removal of SCM, internal jugular vein and spinal accessory nerve. Indicated for SCCA in a neck mass w/ unknown primary or in conjunction w/ excision of primary tumor.

   b. *Modified radical (functional, conservative) neck dissection*: spares SCM, internal jugular, a/o spinal accessory nerve XI (most morbidity in radical neck dissection from loss of CN XI). Indicated for elective neck dissections (dissection for N0 dz); a single LN < 3 cm, which will receive adjuvant radiation tx; differentiated thyroid CA w/ neck metastases; simultaneous bilateral neck dissections.

      i. *Type I*: preserves CN XI

      ii. *Type II*: preserves CN XI and SCM

      iii. *Type III*: preserves SCM, internal jugular vein

   c. *Selective neck dissection*: removal of less than all 5 nodal regions on 1 side of the neck.

C. **Skin cancer of head/neck region** (squamous cell carcinoma, melanoma, basal cell carcinoma, melanoma, Merkel cell, etc.), see Chapter 10.

D. **Salivary gland tumors**

1. *Parotid*

   a. *Dx*: parotid masses should generally be evaluated w/ superficial parotidectomy, taking care to preserve facial nerve branches (FNA, imaging usu. not helpful). Exceptions include pts w/ high index of suspicion for lymphoma (if FNA-proven, a simple LN bx is sufficient) and pts w/ HIV (HIV-related parotid tumors w/ CT findings of multicystic architecture may sometimes be tx'd w/ XRT).

   b. *Benign* (75%)

      i. Mixed tumor (pleomorphic adenoma)—most common.

      ii. Papillary adenocystoma lymphomatosum (benign cystadenoma lymphomatosum, Warthin's tumor).

      iii. Benign lymphoepithelial tumor (Godwin's tumor).

      iv. Oxyphil adenomas.

      v. Pleomorphic adenoma > Warthin's > other.

   c. *Malignant*

      i. Mucoepidermoid carcinoma (most common malignant tumor in parotid).

         • Low grade

         • High grade

      ii. Malignant mixed tumor.

      iii. Squamous cell—rare in parotid (usu. metastatic from face/scalp; may require total parotidectomy).

2. *Submandibular*

   a. 50% benign (mostly pleomorphic adenoma).

   b. Adenoid cystic tumor most common malignancy.

3. *Sublingual and minor salivary glands*
   a. Only 25% benign (mostly pleomorphic adenoma).
   b. Adenoid cystic tumor most common malignancy.

4. *Tx:*
   a. Benign tumors may be simply excised. For parotid, superficial parotidectomy usu. adequate (total removal of submandibular, sublingual glands appropriate). Superficial parotidectomy is generally appropriate as part of regional sentinel lymph node bx.
   b. Critical to identify facial nerve in parotidectomy.
   c. Malignancy, or suspicion thereof (unusual adherence to facial nerve, regional LAD, etc.—or known high-grade carcinoma or metastatic malignancy such as melanoma), generally requires completion of total parotidectomy +/– regional cervical lymphadenectomy; facial nerve reconstruction w/ interposition nerve graft may be performed after resection.
      i. 20% of pts after parotidectomy experience gustatory sweating (Frey syndrome) as a result of cross-innervation between auriculotemporal nerve and sympathetic nerves (the latter innervate sweat glands). Although maneuvers to prevent this (i.e., placement of AlloDerm between tissue planes) may be of benefit, significant sx may require tx w/ botulinum toxin or topical scopolamine/glycopyrrolate.
   d. Adjuvant XRT indicated for high-grade neoplasms, regional lymphatic spread, and (+) margins.

E. **Paragangliomas (chemodectomas, carotid body tumors):** generally (95%) benign tumors of neural crest origin occurring in the carotid body. Angiogram classically demonstrates "lyre sign" of splayed ECA and ICA. Bx is contraindicated. Large tumors > 3 cm may be appropriately embolized preop; larger tumors frequently also require reconstruction/replacement of carotid artery. Complications of surgery include cranial nerve (i.e., superior laryngeal n.) injury and "first bite syndrome" (pain w/ beginning to eat due to reinnervation of parotid glands by aberrant parasympathetic fibers).

CHAPTER 24

TRANSPLANT

I. POST-TRANSPLANT COMPLICATIONS

A. Rejection:

1. *Hyperacute*: in minutes, from preformed Ab, prevent w/ cross-match.
2. *Acute vascular*: minutes to hours, Ab-mediated, tx w/ plasmapheresis/IVIg.
3. *Acute cellular*: 5–7 d most common, but can happen at any time, T-cell mediated, see lymphocytic infiltration, tx w/ aggressive immunosuppression.
4. *Chronic* (gradual): years, from Ab/B-cell, see fibrosis/scarring, "vanishing bile duct syndrome" in liver, glomerular sclerosis in kidneys.
5. W/u w/ H&P, immunosuppressant drug levels (esp. calcineurin inhibitors [cyclosporine, tacrolimus]), possibly bx. May be also caused by infectious etiologies (i.e., CMV, polyoma virus in kidney, etc.).

B. Malignancy:

1. *Most common*: cervical cancer (HPV), vulvar/perineal cancer (HSV), squamous cell cancer (HPV), Kaposi sarcoma (EBV), and lymphoma (HTLV-1).
2. *Post-transplant lymphoproliferative disorder* (PTLD): related to intensity of immunosuppression, particularly of T-cells. More commonly seen w/ transplantation of critical organs (heart, lung)— 5–10% vs. only 1% in renal transplant pts. Assoc. w/ Epstein-Barr virus. B-cell lymphomas of transplant organ, GI tract, or CNS most often. Most cases present w/in 1 yr, but may present 10–15 yr later. Treat by reducing immunosuppression if possible and giving anti-CD 20 monoclonal antibodies such as rituximab; 80–90% survival w/ appropriate tx.

C. Infection:

1. *First mo*: high risk of wound infection, UTI, pneumonia.
2. *First 6 mo*: increased risk of viral opportunistic pathogens—CMV (esophagitis, GI ulceration/hemorrhage, pneumonia, renal insufficiency, malaise), *Candida*, *Pneumocystis carinii*.
   a. Prophylactic antibacterials, antivirals, antifungals given as appropriate.

II. CYTOKINES

A. IL-2: T-lymphocytes secrete, upregulate immune system via B-cell proliferation and differentiation. Blocked by cyclosporine, tacrolimus, rapamycin.

III. SPECIFIC ORGANS

A. In United States, transplant organs allocated/distributed by UNOS (*www.unos.org*), which also tracks outcomes. Brain death is not absolute prerequisite for donation; 1-yr survival for most transplant pts is ~ 90%.

B. Liver

1. *Preop*:
   a. Cross-match not that important, too close can be harmful, just ABO.
   b. EtOH most common of ESLD, but hepatitis C most common cause for transplant candidates; 100% reinfection, w/ variable clinical manifestations, most w/ good long-term results. 1-yr survival 90% for nonhepatitis pts, 80% for pts w/ hepatitis C (vs 10–15% w/out transplant).
   c. *Traditional contraindications for recipient*: HIV infection; active substance abuse; life-limiting comorbidities; uncontrolled psychiatric d/o; inability to comply with pre-/post-transplant regimens.
   d. *Other criteria for liver transplantation*:
      i. *Model of end-stage liver dz (MELD) score*:
         - *3 components*: serum creatinine, total bilirubin, INR.
         - Score each from 1 upwards (max Cr = 4); max score = 40.
         - MELD = 10 [0.957 Ln(Cr) + 0.378 Ln(Tbil) + 1.12 Ln(INR) + 0.643].
         - Average score for pt undergoing transplant in United States = 20.

    e. *Hepatorenal syndrome*: renal dysfunction seen in assoc. w/ liver failure, secondary to renal vasoconstriction (pseudo-prerenal picture not responsive to fluid). Can fully reverse w/ timely liver transplantation.

    f. *Fulminant hepatic failure*. Only ~ 5% of cases of transplant. Etiologies include acetaminophen, viral dz, etc.

2. *Intraop*:

    a. *Partial transplantation*: left lateral segment transplantation developed initially for children, but right lobe transplantation has been performed for adults as well. Major drawback is risk to donor (mortality $1/300$—10× greater than for renal donors), outcome not better than w/ cadaveric sources, but do increase total number of available organs.

C. Heart

1. *Preop*:

    a. *Survival*: > 80% at 1 yr, > 70% at 5 yr.

    b. *Contraindications for recipient*: malignancy, recent PE, infection, fixed pulmonary resistance (unresponsive to vasodilators) > 6 Wood units.

    c. *Contraindications for donor*: infection, extracranial malignancy, ventricular dysrhythmias, and death from CO poisoning w/ blood carboxyhemoglobin > 20%.

    d. ABO and size (w/in 20% body wt) most important for screening; HLA done only if high PRA.

2. *Intraop*: orthotopic placement w/ 4–6 anastomoses.

3. *Postop*:

    a. *Early*:

        i. RV dysfunction common, partly secondary to high pulmonary pressures; give inotropes and pulmonary vasodilators first several days.

        ii. Tachycardia (~ 100 bpm) secondary to loss of vagal innervation, unresponsive to digoxin and atropine; bradydysrhythmias, however, respond well to isoproterenol or pacing.

    b. Acute rejection often manifests w/ fatigue and tachydysrhythmias.

    c. Leading cause of morbidity/mortality after first yr is cardiac allograft vasculopathy (CAV)—caveat, MI in transplant heart does not sense pain/angina. Only tx is retransplantation.

    d. Other problems include susceptibility to CMV; EBV; VSV; HSV types 1, 2, and 6; and exceptionally high rate of PTLD.

D. Kidney

1. *Preop*:

    a. Renal transplantation results in 2- to 3-fold increase in life expectancy compared w/ remaining on hemodialysis for pts w/ CRI, offers more independence, and is cheaper in the long run. 1-yr survival 90% (deceased donor) to 95% (living donor) postop.

    b. *Contraindications for donor*: HIV, sepsis, non-CNS malignancy. Age > 65, HTN may be appropriate to bx.

    c. *Contraindications for recipient*: cardiopulmonary insufficiency, morbid obesity, PAD, cerebrovasc dz, tobacco abuse, hepatic insufficiency.

    d. Living donors are typically 18–55 yo, in good health, w/ 2 normal, functioning kidneys. Outcomes are better w/ living donors, even if totally mismatched HLA.

        i. Oblique incision made to harvest usu. left kidney (longer vein); laparoscopic approach also done.

    e. *Prelude to transplant*: vascular access and dialysis.

        i. *Indication*:

            • *Nondiabetic*: Cr 6–7 mg/dL, GFR 10–15 cc/min.

            • *Diabetic*: Cr 4–5 mg/dL, GFR 15–25 cc/min.

        ii. Wait 2+ wk before using PTFE graft and 4–6 wk before using native fistula.

2. *Intraop*:

    a. Extraperitoneal approach through LLQ or RLQ oblique incision.

    b. Ligate lymphatics overlying iliac vessels to prevent postop lymphocele.

    c. Usu. arterial and venous end-to-side anastamoses to EIA & V.

    d. Donor ureter usu. sewn to recipient bladder, but recipient ureter can be sewn to donor renal pelvis.

    e. Frequently, mannitol a/o furosemide given before unclamping vessels.

3. *Postop*:

    a. *Oliguria, rising creatinine*:

       i. *Immediately postop*:

- Most often secondary to ATN a/o delayed graft function (~ $1/3$ of cases), usu. from reperfusion injury; much less common in living donor cases. Usu. self-limted.
- Consider duplex scan or radioisotope renal perfusion scan.
- Gradual tapering over time suggests rejection whereas sudden anuria often represents thromboses and requires emergent reexploration. Arterial injuries and majority of venous thromboses require surgery; rarely anticoagulation may be used for venous problem.
- *Urine leak*: manifest as fluid collection a/o rising creatinine. Generally from ureteral ischemia, and may be initially treated w/ stenting and percutaneous drainage, although surgical reconstruction may become necessary.

       ii. *Wks to months later may mean*:

- *Immunosuppression toxicity* (nephritis not seen on bx).
- *Graft rejection* (see interstitial nephritis on bx).
- *Renal vasculature thrombosis* (uncommon this far out from surgery).
- *CMV*: treatable w/ gancyclovir, rarely leads to graft loss.
- *Polyoma virus* (see interstitial nephritis on bx, doesn't respond/progresses w/ medical tx/immunosuppression). A nephrotropic slow virus not uncommon in general population, symptomatic in ~ 5% of renal transplant pts, w/ graft loss in 50% of those. Can monitor for this postop w/ urine cytology or serum PCR. Attempt to tx by *decreasing* immunosuppressrants.

    b. *Other*:

       i. *Urine leak*: see entry 3ai. above on immediately postop.

       ii. *Lymphocele*.

       iii. *Renal transplant artery stenosis* (RTAS): usu. 3–24 mo postop, manifesting w/ HTN, renal insufficiency. Usu. managed w/ percutaneous stenting.

       iv. *Tertiary hyperparathyroidism*: indication for subtotal parathyroidectomy or total parathyroidectomy w/ implantation of part of 1 gland into forearm.

E. Pancreas

1. Generally indicated for renal transplant pts (i.e., txp for diabetic nephropathy) w/ brittle DM.

2. *Technical aspects*: pancreas is situated in pelvis, w/ vessels anastomosed to iliacs. Pancreatic duct is drained into bladder (advantages—follow urine amylase for rejection, ease of bx; disadvantage—metabolic acidosis from bicarb loss, cystitis) or bowel.

3. *Postop*:

    a. > 70% of pts become insulin-independent, and pt survival at 1 yr > 90%.

    b. Rejection manifests w/ exocrine insufficiency before endocrine insufficiency.

IV. TOLERANCE AND IMMUNOSUPPRESIVE DRUGS

A. Steroids: block IL-I, blunting inflammatory response in kidney and pancreas transplants, rapid wean off of prednisone (i.e., after pod #5) has been achieved by administration of *thymoglobulin* + rapamycin (usu. in addition to mycophenolate and cyclosporine).

B. OKT3: murine Ab that reacts w/ CD-3 on T-lymphocytes, blocking generation and function of T-cells to Ag challenge. Side effects include fever, diarrhea, bronchospasm, pulmonary edema, meningeal irritation; profound cytokine release.

C. Cyclosporine (calcineurin inhibitor): nephrotoxic, hepatotoxic, HTN, gingival hypertrophy, hirsutism.

D. FK 506/tacrolimus (calcineurin inhibitor): nephrotoxic, hepatotoxic, neurotoxic, hyperglycemia, hyperkalemia.

E. **Azathioprim (antimetabolite)**: blocks purine metabolism; less bone marrow depression than mycophenolate.

F. **Mycophenolate/CellCept (antimetabolite)**: block purine metabolism; increased diarrhea than azathioprine.

G. **Rapamycin**: hyperlipidemia, thrombocytopenia.

CHAPTER 25

COMMON PROBLEMS ON CALL AND BLS/ACLS

I. **AIRWAY/BREATHING** (*note*: have low threshold for arranging urgent transport to ICU while addressing primary problem)

   A. **Hx**

      1. *Surgical*

         a. Recent neck surgery may result in a compressive hematoma and airway compromise secondary to laryngeal edema; difficult to intubate. Tx is emergency evacuation of hematoma/clot, often followed by cricothyroidotomy or tracheostomy.

         b. Tracheostomy. Check for obstruction, mechanical problems. Place ETT or tracheostomy for emergent control.

      2. *Medical*

         a. H/o anaphylaxis? Asthma? COPD?

   B. **Physical exam**

      1. *Dysphonia*: suggests problems w/ vocal cords (i.e., edema, nerve injury, etc.).

      2. *Wheezing*: suggests lower airway obstruction (i.e., asthma).

      3. *Stridor*: suggests upper airway obstruction (i.e., foreign body).

      4. *Look at trachea, jugular veins*: may be displaced (trachea) or distended (veins) due to mass, tension PTX. Vein distension also suggests pericardial tamponade.

      5. *Listen to breath sounds and percuss*: absent or decreased breath sounds and hyperresonance suggests PTX; absent or decreased breath sounds w/ dullness suggests hemothorax or empyema—any absent or decreased breath sounds in an unstable pt merits an emergent chest tube.

   C. **Other**

      1. *Pulse oximetry* ("pulse ox"):

         a. May not be accurate in cold extremities or in room w/ bright lights.

         b. *Hypoxia may be due to*:

            i. Carbon monoxide poisoning

            ii. Methemoglobinemia

            iii. Poisoning: cyanide, nitroprusside

      2. *Arterial blood gas* (ABG): always obtain for breathing sx; analyze as described in Chapter 4.

II. **CIRCULATION** (as w/ airway problems, have low threshold for transfer to ICU as problem is being addressed and make sure adequate IV access is obtained).

   A. **Tachycardia**

      1. *Hx*

         a. *Surgical* (thoracic—tamponade [?]; orthopaedic—fat embolism [?]; postop fluid overload—Afib [?])

         b. *Medical* (medications, caffeine)

      2. *Physical exam*: anxious? in pain? rate? arrhythmia? strong or thready pulse? fever?

   B. **Hypotension**

      1. *Hx*:

         a. *Surgical*: bleeding, anesthetic/narcotic, etc.

         b. *Medical*: medication, cardiac hx, etc.

      2. *Physical exam*

      3. *Etiology*

         a. Hypovolemia (flat jugular veins, dry mucosa, skin turgor?)

         b. Anaphylaxis (wheezing? angioedema? rash? etc.)

C. **Bleeding**
 1. *Hx*:
   a. *Surgical*.
   b. *Medical*: renal, liver dz, lupus, medications (including herbals).
 2. *Physical exam*
   a. Where is bleeding coming from? Surgical wound, rectal exam, IV or arteriogram puncture site, epistaxis.
 3. *Other*
   a. *Labs*: CBC (*thrombocytopenia ddx*: see Chapter 2), PT/PTT (*Elevation ddx*: see Chapter 2).

III. DISABILITY (NEUROLOGIC)

A. **Altered mental status**
 1. *Hx*
 2. *Physical exam*
 3. *Other*
   a. Pulse oximetry to evaluate for hypoxia.
   b. Capillary blood glucose (CBG) to evaluate for hypoglycemia.
   c. Thorough neuro exam, particular attention to symmetric reflexes and papillary size/response.

B. **Pain**
 1. *Hx and physical*
 2. *Headache*
 3. *Abdomen*
 4. *Extremity*

C. **Seizures**
 1. *Hx*
 2. *Ensure ABCs controlled*:
   a. Supplemental oxygen, airway control.
 3. *Pharmacologic control*: diazepam (Valium) 5 mg IV q 5–10 min prn; phenytoin and phenobarbital are backup agents.

IV. OTHER

A. **Cardiovascular**
 1. *Chest pain*
   a. *Hx* (acute, chronic, postprandial, etc.)
   b. *Character* (crushing, radiating, burning, etc.)
   c. *Etiology*:
     i. *Cardiac*: see section V. on Acute Coronary Syndrome below.
     ii. *Pulmonary embolism*: see Chapter 6.
     iii. *Pneumothorax*: place chest tube.
     iv. *GERD*: usu. by hx or response to GI meds.
 2. *Vascular insufficiency or pulse change*

B. **Pulmonary (see section I. above on airway/breathing)**

C. **Gastrointestinal**
 1. *Constipation* (may need disimpaction a/o laxatives).
 2. *Diarrhea* (*etiology*: meds, infectious [need stool WBC, Cx, etc.], postsurgical changes).
 3. *Nausea/emesis*: Zofran usu. better tolerated, less sedating than phenergan.
 4. *Singultus* (hiccups): usu. innocuous, but diaphragmatic irritation (e.g., subphrenic abscess) important.

D. **Genitourinary**
 1. *Urinary retention*: place Foley (flush Foley if one already placed).
 2. *Dysuria*: check urinalysis and UCx (cx may still be positive w/ negative urinalysis).

3. *Bloody or other unusual appearance to urine*: urology consult for hematuria (may ultimately require cytology, cx, cystoscopy, etc.).

4. *Oliguria/anuria*: place Foley if haven't done so, eval hemodynamics, UA, Chem 7 for starters.

E. **Metabolic**

1. *Hyperglycemic/hypoglycemic* → see Chapter 1.

2. *Electrolyte abnormality* → see Chapter 1.

V. <u>**ACUTE CORONARY SYNDROME**</u> (derived from American Heart Association, 2006)

A. **Support ABCs, prepare for CPR/code.**

B. **Give**: O_2 at 4 L/min (SaO_2 > 90%); ASA at 160–325 mg; NTG SL/IV; morphine IV if NTG not adequate.

C. **Obtain**: IV access; 12-lead EKG; portable CXR; electrolytes/CBC/troponin/CK-MB; targeted hx w/ focus on fibrinolytic checklist/contraindications.

D. **Results of 12-lead EKG:**

1. *ST elevation or (presumably) new LBBB*:

a. *Begin adjunctive tx*: beta blockers, heparin (LMWH or UFH), clopidogrel.

b. If < 12 h or high-risk (refractory ischemic chest pain, recurrent/persistent ST deviation, VT, sx of heart failure) → consult cardiology for PCI or fibrinolysis.

c. Otherwise, admit to monitored bed, continue ASA, heparin, and start ACEi/ARB and statin w/in 24 h.

2. *ST depression or dynamic T wave inversion*:

a. *Begin adjunctive tx*: beta blockers, heparin (LMWH or UFH), clopidogrel, NTG, glycoprotein IIb/IIIa inhib.

b. Admit to monitored bed, continue ASA, heparin, and start ACEi/ARB and statin w/in 24 h.

3. *Normal or nondiagnostic ST/T wave changes*:

a. If develops high-risk criteria (see above) or become troponin-positive, tx as sections D1. or D2. above. Immediately above as appropriate.

b. Otherwise, observe w/ serial cardiac markers, EKG/telemetry, etc., until resolves. Consider stress test before d/c.

VI. <u>**BASIC LIFE SUPPORT**</u> (derived from American Heart Association, 2010)

A. **Obstructed airway:**

1. Do not interfere if pt can speak or effectively cough.

2. *If conscious*:

a. *Adult/child*: Heimlich maneuver (or chest thrusts if obese/pregnant) until cleared or unresponsive.

b. *Infant*: place pt prone over arm w/ head lower than feet and give 5 back blows, then turn over for 5 chest thrusts in lower sternum. Repeat until cleared or unresponsive.

3. *If unconscious*:

a. *Adult*: call for EMS/defibrillator, then initiate CPR (after removing any visible object in mouth).

b. *Child/infant*: initiate CPR (after removing any visible object in mouth), then call EMS after 2 min.

B. **No movement or response → call code/help, then get defibrillator/AED.**

C. **Open airway, check breathing.**

1. *If not breathing, give 2 breaths.*

2. *If no response, check pulse.*

a. If pulse w/in 10 sec, give 1 breath q 5–6 sec and recheck pulse every 2 min.

b. If no pulse w/in 10 sec, give 30 compressions (100/min), then open airway, give 2 breaths, and resume compression/breath cycles. Continue until defibrillator arrives, other providers take over, or pulse is regained.

i. For *2-rescuer CPR in children*, the ratio of breaths to compressions is 15:2.

D. **Defibrillator arrives—rhythm possibly amenable to shock?**

1. *Yes*: give 1 shock, then resume CPR for 5 cycles.

2. *No*: resume CPR for 5 cycles and check rhythm every 5 cycles, continuing until others take over or pt moves.

VII. ADVANCED CARDIAC LIFE SUPPORT (derived from American Heart Association, 2010)

- **A. General (apneic, pulseless, unresponsive)**
    1. Call code, start CPR—ABCs, attach defibrillator/monitor rhythm.
        a. Open airway, check breathing—if not breathing, begin chest compressions, then breaths at ratio of 30:2 if by self.
    2. Check rhythm and pulse regularly, give 100% oxygen, get bedboard.
    3. *Simultaneous w/ resuscitation, attempt to rectify any underlying causes*:
        a. *H*: hypovolemia, hypoxia, hypo-/hyperkalemia, hypothermia, hydrogen ion (acidosis).
        b. *T*: trauma (hypovolemia, ICP), thrombosis (MI, PE), tamponade (pericardial), tension PTX, toxins.
- **B. Tachyarrhythmias**
    1. *VFib/pulseless VTach*
        a. CPR until defib available.
        b. Defib, biphasic (unsynch) 200 J → 200–300 J → 360 J (start w/ 360 if monophasic).
        c. Intubate, IV access, CPR prn.
        d. *Epinephrine* 1 mg IVP → 360 J **or** *Vasopressin* 40 U IVP → 360 J.
            i. May give epinephrine 1 mg IVP q 3–5 min.
        e. Immediately resume CPR, then check rhythm/shock again in 2 min (5 CPR cycles), and consider:
            i. *Amiodarone* (300 mg IVP—can repeat w/ 150 mg)→ 360 J **or**
            ii. If stable or converts can start w/ 150 mg over 10 min, then gtt 1 mg/min × 6 h, then 0.5 mg min × 18 h.
            iii. *Lidocaine* (1.0–1.5 mg/kg IVP—can repeat as ½ dose up to 3 mg/kg) → 360 J **and/or,**
            iv. *Magnesium* (1–2 g if torsades de pointes, hypomagnesemic, or refractory) → 360 J.
        f. Immediately resume CPR for 2 min (5 cycles) before checking rhythm/shocking again.
    2. *Unstable tachycardia w/ pulses* (monomorphic VT, PSVT, AFib, AFlutter)
        a. Oxygen, IV, pulse ox.
        b. Have intubation/code cart nearby.
        c. Consider premedication (midazolam, etc.).
        d. *Synchronized cardioversion*:
            i. 50 J (PSVT or AFlutter only) → 100 J → 200 J → 300 J → 360 J.
            ii. 100 J for all other rhythms.
    3. *Narrow complex SVT* (stable)
        a. Vagal maneuvers (carotid massage if no carotid dz/bruits, or valsalva).
        b. Adenosine (6 mg push, then 12 mg; may repeat 12 mg once).
        c. If rhythm converts, monitor for recurrence (tx w/ adenosine, diltiazem, or beta antagonist).
        d. If does not convert, control rate (diltiazem, beta antagonist, etc.), w/u cause.
    4. *Stable AFib, AFlutter*
        a. *< 48 h*:
            i. First control rate w/ beta blocker (esmolol) or calcium channel blocker (diltiazim).
            ii. Next control rhythm w/ amiodarone or DC CV as above; can also load w/ digoxin.
        b. *> 48 h*:
            i. Do not DC CV unless embolic precautions/anticoagulated; use antiarrhythmics w/ caution.
            ii. Ideally AC × 3 wk, then CV, then 4 more wk AC.
            iii. More rapidly, use heparin and TEE, CV w/in 24 h, then AC × 4 wk.
    5. *Stable wide complex tachycardia*
        a. 12 lead EKG.
        b. Amiodarone (150 mg IV over 10 min, repeat to max of 2.2 g per 24 h) or DC cardioversion.
        c. If AFib w/ preexcitation (i.e., WPW), avoid AV blocking (digoxing, diltiazem, adenosine).
        d. Torsades de pointes → magnesium sulfate, 1–2 g loaded IV over 5–60 min, then infused.

C. **Asystole/PEA/bradycardia**

1. *PEA/asystole* (confirm in 2 leads; note if only have defib pads, should shock, as only have 2 leads and could actually be fine VFib) *or PEA*

   a. Continue CPR (see section VI. above), intubate, 100% O_2, IV access.

   b. *Consider causes:*

      i. *Hypoxemia/respiratory arrest* → mechanical ventilation.

      ii. *Hyperkalemia* → 10% Ca chloride 10 cc IVP; 1 ampule D_{50} w/ 10 U reg insulin IVP; albuterol nebs 20–40 mg in 4 cc NS; Kayexalate 50 g w/ 200 cc 70% sorbitol PO. Consider sodium bicarbonate 50 mEq IV over 1–5 min; consider dialysis.

      iii. *Hypokalemia* → give potassium.

      iv. *Acidosis* → sodium bicarbonate 1 mEq/kg IV.

      v. *Hypothermia* → undertake active/passive rewarming.

      vi. *Overdose:*

         • *Narcotics* → naloxone (0.4–2.0 mg q 2 min up to 10 mg).

         • *Benzodiazepines* → flumazenil (0.2 mg IV over 15 sec, then 0.3 IV over 30 sec. Repeat up to total of 3 mg).

         • *Cyclic antidepressants* → sodium bicarbonate 1 mEq/kg (50 mEq fine for most adults). Can create gtt w/ 3 amps bicarb : 1 L D_5W (150 mEq); run at 100 mL/h, titrated to pH of 7.5.

         • *Digitalis* → digibind (chronic intox 3–5 vials IV 120–200 mg; acute intox dosage varies but average is 10 vials 400 mg, up to 20 vials [800 mg may be required]).

         • *Calcium channel blockers* → Ca chloride (10 cc of 10% soln) + glucagon (1–5 mg IV/ IM over 2–5 min).

         • *Beta blockers* → glucagon (1–5 mg IV/IM over 2–5 min).

   c. Epinephrine 1 mg IVP, repeat q 3–5 min *or* vasopressin, 40 U IV once.

   d. Atropine 1 mg IVP, may repeat once or twice every 3–5 min.

2. *Unstable bradycardia*

   a. Oxygen, IV access, EKG.

   b. Prepare for transcutaneous pacing (particularly if Mobitz type II 2nd-degree block or 3rd-degree block).

   c. Atropine 0.5 mg IV, may repeat up to total of 3 mg (pace if not effective).

   d. Consider dopamine IV 2–10 mcg/kg/min or epinephrine IV 2–10 mcg/min while awaiting pacer (or if pacer ineffective).

VIII. **SUSPECTED CVA/STROKE** (derived from American Heart Association, 2006)

A. **Immediately:**

1. *Assess vitals signs, SaO_2 (give O_2 if needed) and glucose (give glucose if needed).*

2. *Assure good IV access.*

3. *Perform neurologic screening assessment.*

   a. Review hx, establish time of sx onset, and perform neuro exam.

      i. Have pt smile, check for pronator drift (10 sec), and have pt say, "You can't teach a dog new tricks."

      ii. Acute asymmetry/abnormalities in any 1 of the above is sufficient for clinical dx.

4. *Activate stroke team.*

5. *Obtain emergent 12-lead EKG and noncontrast head CT.*

B. **CT scan w/ evidence of hemorrhage?**

1. *Yes* → consult neurologist/neurosurgeon; go to section B3. below.

2. *No* → check for fibrinolytic exclusions and repeat neuro exam.

   a. **Absolute contraindications**: h/o intracranial hemorrhage; anatomic cerebral vascular lesion such as AVM; intracranial malignancy; ischemic CVA w/in 3 mo (except ischemic CVA w/in 3 h); suspected aortic dissection; significant closed head or facial trauma w/in 3 mo.

    b. *Relative contraindications*: h/o poorly controlled HTN or acute uncontrolled HTN (SBP > 180, DBP > 110); > 10 min of CPR or major surgery w/in 3 wk; noncompressible vascular punctures; pregnancy; active peptic ulcer; current use of anticoagulants; prior allergic rxn to streptokinase (if that agent is used).

    c. *If no contraindication*, consider tPA (no anticoagulants or ASA × 24 h), go to section B3. below. *Note*: must administer tPA w/in 3 h of sx onset.

    d. If either of above questions are positive, give aspirin and go to section B3. below.

3. *For all*: begin stroke pathway, admit to stroke unit if possible, monitor tx BP/glucose, monitor neuro status, and re-image if acute deterioration.

CHAPTER 26

SAMPLE COMMON OPERATIONS

I. **APPENDECTOMY**

   A. Consider laparoscopic if obese, female of reproductive age, or anticipate heavy contamination.

   B. **(Open)**

   1. Transverse incision either at McBurney point or about 1–2 cm cephalad of point of maximal tenderness.

   2. Score external oblique in direction of fibers, then divide; appendiceal retractors or small Richardson retractors are useful. Next, using Pean clamps in alternating orientation w/ assistant, divide internal oblique and transversus abdominis muscles bluntly (muscle-splitting technique) until encounter peritoneum.

   3. Pick up peritoneum w/ DeBakey forceps along w/ assistant, release, regrasp, then sharply incise peritoneum before exploring w/ finger. Spread wound w/ appendiceal retractors. Palpate w/ index finger for indurated appendix, being careful to pause and feel for pulsation (ensure not iliac artery) before attempting to bring to wound. Alternately, can use Raytec traction on cecum to trace down to appendix by following taenia. Babcock clamps placed around base of appendix help maintain traction.

   4. Place Pean clamp at base of appendix for several sec, then move 1 cm distal. Ligate at crimped section w/ 2-0 chromic gut. Divide appendix at proximal edge of clamp w/ #15 blade, then touch tip of blade to exposed luminal mucosa and apply electrocautery to knife to cauterize mucosa (to prevent mucocele).

   5. Close peritoneum w/ 3-0 Vicryl (controversial), then posterior and anterior fascia w/ 1-0 PDS. If appendix ruptured, consider leaving skin open for delayed primary repair or to heal by secondary intent.

   C. **Laparoscopic**

   1. Tuck left arm. Place Foley. Trendelenburg w/ right side up if desired.

   2. 12-mm trocar at umbilicus for camera (initially) and stapler (later). 5-mm working ports in the LLQ and suprapubic position.

   3. Maryland dissector to open space between appendiceal base and mesoappendix.

   4. Change to 5-mm camera in LLQ and fire linear stapler w/ tissue load across the base of the appendix, then use vascular load for the mesoappendix.

   5. Place appendix in an endoscopic retrieval bag through the 12-mm umbilical port.

II. **LAPAROSCOPIC CHOLECYSTECTOMY:** multiple port options available. W/ a 5-mm clip applier, the procedure can easily be done w/ a 10- to 12-mm port at umbilicus and three 5-mm ports in the subxiphoid and right subcostal positions.

   A. **Four ports:** (1) infraumbilical, (2) epigastric ($^1/_3$ distance from xiphoid to umbilicus), (3) right subcostal midclavicular, (4) right subcostal lateral. Surgeon on left, works through subxiphoid and midsubcostal ports.

   B. Retract fundus superiorly and take down adhesions from gallbladder (GB) body bluntly; grab adhesions close to GB wall to stay in relatively avascular plane. Proceed w/ dissection from lateral to medial to expose GB neck.

   C. Retract Hartmann's pouch laterally and inferiorly to expose triangle of Calot.

   D. Identify cystic artery and cystic duct before dividing any structures. Use the Maryland dissector to bluntly create the window behind the artery and between the artery and the duct. The node of calot often lies in the space between the artery and the duct. It can be pulled down (gently), but will sometimes bleed a bit. The infundibulum/Hartmann's pouch often needs to be flipped medially as the posterolateral dissection helps delineate the cystic structures. Stay close to the GB to avoid CBD injury. Once the cystic duct and artery are identified, clips can be applied.

   E. *If planning to perform cholangiography,* place clip at junction of cystic duct and infundibulum. Cut anterior cystic duct w/ scissors. Pass cholangiogram catheter through #14 angiocatheter lumen. Clip catheter in place. Shoot IOC to demonstrate dye passage into duodenum and intrahepatic biliary tree. Remove clip securing catheter and catheter. Apply 2 clips to distal cystic duct and divide.

F. If no cholangiogram, place 2 clips on pt's side and 1 clip on GB side of the cystic duct and the cystic artery and then divide.

G. Short cystic duct:

1. Flipping GB neck medially helpful to identify junction of cystic duct and GB.
2. Primary dissection is posterolateral, then medially.
3. Using a silk tie around Hartmann's pouch instead of clip preserves length for ductotomy.

H. Significant adhesions to liver, GB:

1. Take down by sharp dissection w/ electrocautery on low power setting.
2. Be cognizant of location of duodenum and use traction/countertraction to dissect.
   a. Hydrodissection may be a useful adjunct to separating duodenum from adjacent structures.
3. Developing window at GB neck may be easier than first dividing cystic artery.

I. Midline intraabdominal adhesions:

1. Use open (Hasson) technique to achieve pneumoperitoneum.
2. Bluntly open window w/ laparoscope to allow directly visualize port placement. Subxiphoid port placed right of midline.

J. GB bed dissection:

1. After division of cystic duct and artery, begin dissection close to GB, away from hilar structures. Check w/ Maryland for posterior branch of the cystic artery. Can use cautery to remove the serosal attachments of the GB to the liver. Reposition GB as necessary to expose lateral/medial aspects of GB attachments. Inspect GB bed for hemostasis before removal of GB.

III. HERNIORRHAPHY, INGUINAL [Norton et al. (eds). 2001. *Surgery: Basic Science and Clinical Evidence*, chapter 25. New York: Springer-Verlag; Fitzgibbons et al. (eds). 2002. *Nyhus and Condon's Hernia*, 5th ed, chapters 13 and 14 (pp. 139–158). Philadelphia: Lippincott Williams & Wilkins; Rutledge RH. 1988. Dallas Cooper's ligament repair: A 25-year experience with a single technique for all groin hernias in adults. *Surgery* 103:1–10.]

A. Anterior approach

1. *Exposure*:
   a. Make oblique incision 2 fingerbreadths cephalad and parallel to inguinal ligament beginning halfway from ASIS to pubis and ending at level of pubis. Alternately, make equilateral triangle from midpubis to edge and apex equal length cepalad then connect w/ a more horizontal, Langer's line to a point slightly more inferior and medial than described above.
   b. Place self-retaining retractor after getting to level of external oblique fascia.
   c. Locate external ring just cephalad and lateral to pubis. Make superficial stab incision in external oblique fascia (w/ blade up) at lateral extent of incision in line w/ fibers going to external ring. W/ tips up and closed, run Metzenbaum scissors under external oblique fascia to external ring, w/draw, and then w/ jaws locked in semi-open position and lifting up, divide fascia down through ring by gently pushing scissors. Repeat 180° for a few cm.
   d. Grasp each edge of divided external oblique fascia w/ hemostat and pull gently apart to reveal cord underneath. Attempt to identify the ilioinguinal nerve, which is usu. just under the cephalad leaf of divided fascia. Once found, remove hemostat from closest edge of fascia, and retract nerve out of harm's way over fascial edge, then replace hemostat. If interferes w/ dissection, division of nerve is acceptable. Separate upper leaf from underlying muscle/fascia superiorly 3 cm, inferiorly down to shelving edge, and medially 2 cm beyond lateral pubis pubic tubercle.
   e. W/ fingers, Kuttner dissector, a/o moist Raytec sponge, isolate and lift up the spermatic cord at the level of the pubic tubercle, then pass Penrose drain around it. Clamp Penrose outstretched so as to expose cord fully.
   f. Divide appropriate amount of cremasteric fibers (Bovie, pulling w/ DeBakey forceps, etc.) longitudinally at the level of the internal ring, to expose indirect sac, which if present, is usu. along the anteromedial aspect of the cord. Begin dissection medially if possible.
   g. Open sac at its apex and reduce the contents. If sac spans entire canal, divide sac, leaving distal remnant open; don't dissect beyond pubic tubercle. Some recommend "fillet" of the distal sac to reduce chances of hydrocele. Close proximal w/ purse-string at base w/ 2-0 silk, then

return to peritoneal cavity. If direct sac is found, reduce into peritoneal cavity, and superficially imbricate trasversalis fascia over it to keep out of way for subsequent definitive repair. (*Note*: increasingly, authorities note that simply returning sac into abdomen w/out division does not lead to increased recurrence and causes less pain. Evaluate femoral ring through Bogros' space through an opening in canal floor.

h. Repair hernia w/ method of choice (see section IV. below). *If performing Lichtenstein, be sure to skeletonize the floor and pubis w/ good view of shelving edge and pubis (trim out cremasteric and fat) before moving on.*

i. After completing repair, close external oblique fascia w/ running 3-0 Vicryl. Approximate Scarpa's fascia w/ interrupted sutures of the same, and finally close skin w/ running 4-0 Monocryl (preferred) or Vicryl.

IV. LICHTENSTEIN

A. **Instruments**: #10 blade; #15 blade; Metzenbaum scissors; Weitlander retractors; small and medium Richardson retractors; ½-inch Penrose drain; DeBakey forceps; 2-0 Prolene on SH × 2; 8 × 16 cm polypropylene mesh; 3-0 Vicryl × 1; 4-0 Vicryl × 1; Adson forceps w/ teeth.

B. **Incidental**:

1. 8 × 16 cm polypropylene mesh is cut to conform to shape of medial end of canal and narrowed to dimensions of canal (at same time, measure length of slit needed). Create slit in lateral half of mesh dividing mesh into narrow (inferior) $1/3$ and wider (superior) $2/3$ tails. Position cord between the 2 tails.

2. Suture rounded corner to fascia sheath over inferior pubic bone, overlapping the rectus sheath by 2 cm (do not suture to periosteum). Run suture laterally w/ lower edge of mesh to shelving edge of inguinal ligament until lateral to internal ring (occasionally pull up shelving edge to make sure it is not just rolled over external oblique or superficial inguinal ligament). *Note*: If femoral hernia present, suture mesh to Cooper's ligament, up to lateral aspect of femoral vein, then transition to inguinal ligament. Similarly, anchor suture above cord, and run along transversus abdominus/conjoined tendon until at level of internal ring. Periodically pull on mesh to flatten it out so that excess redundancy doesn't exist (some slight wrinkling OK). Alternately, use double-armed 2-0 Prolene at pubis, then run 1 arm inferiolaterally, the other superolaterally. Some surgeons prefer interrupted 2-0 Ethibond instead. Retraction is key while suturing in the mesh: best results obtained w/ small or medium Richardson retractor toed in while held from medial part of exposure, w/ lip under the cord, lifting it up to expose pubis underneath. After finished medially, follow around edges of wound. Periodically identify the edges of the external oblique; if confused, trace back laterally to where the fascial incision begins.

3. Take upper/wider tail, and cross over the lower tail (both inferior edges now touching), and recreate internal ring by suturing w/ 2-0 Prolene the tails just lateral to the cord, or simultaneously recreate the shutter valve mechanism of the anatomic transversalis sling by suturing the inferior edges of both pieces of mesh to inguinal ligament just lateral to cord.

4. Trim excess lateral mesh, leaving 5 cm lateral to internal ring and tucked flat beneath external oblique aponeurosis. Close external oblique aponeurosis w/ absorbable suture (3-0 Vicryl), followed by Scarpa's (3-0 Vicryl), and skin (4-0 Monocryl/Steri-strips/Telfa/Tegaderm/staples, etc.).

V. AMPUTATION

A. **Below knee amputation**

1. *Indications*: Guillotine amputation should be performed for acutely infected/gangrenous distal lower extremity, followed by 4–5 d of IV abx to clear residual bacteria in skin/lymphatics. "Formal" or "revision" BKA should then be performed. In trauma pts w/ mangled foot, BKA may be performed as a single-stage operation.

2. *Incidental*: 80% rate of healing if Doppler signal in popliteal artery.

a. Anterior incision 11 cm below tibial tubercle (so that can transect tibia at 10 cm w/ 1 cm distal overlying skin), carry around anterior $2/3$ diameter of calf.

b. Bovie through anterior compartment, divide neurovascular structures (see section 3. on anatomy below). Divide fibula either at same level or 1 cm proximal to anticipated level of tibial transection w/ Gigli or power saw. Divide tibia w/ Gigli or power saw, creating anterior bevel. Divide remaining neurovascular structures.

c. Posterior incision parallel to long axis. Can either carry all the way to end of wound or make the length equal to the diameter of the calf at the level of proximal skin incision.

  d. Regardless of length, prepare posterior myocutaneous flap by bluntly dissecting superficial from deep posterior muscles, then bring up flap and trim to appropriate length. Alternately, can use "cake knife" to create tapered flap w/ fascia all the way to end. No need to fashion bulky muscular "pad" to lie over stump.

3. *Anatomy*:

  a. Anterior compartment contains anterior tibial artery/vein and deep peroneal nerve along posterior fascia.

  b. Deep posterior compartment contains posterior tibial artery/vein and tibial nerve along posterior fascia and peroneal artery/vein along medial aspect of fibula.

  c. Lateral compartment: no neurovascular structures.

  d. Superficial posterior compartment: no neurovascular structures; contains gastrocnemius, soleus complex.

VI CAROTID TEA

A. Indications: symptomatic carotid stenosis of ≥ 50%. Asymptomatic dz ≥ 60% (more controversial).

B. Instruments: #10 blade, Weitlaner, Rummel tourniquet, Dacron patch, umbilical tapes, Argyle shut, 6-0 Prolene, vascular needle drivers.

C. Incidental: carotid TEA can be performed through a longitudinal arteriotomy or using an eversion endarterectomy technique. The eversion technique is faster, as does not require a patch angioplasty, but is difficult to perform if shunting is desired or needed. The technique described below is through a longitudinal arteriotomy.

D. Procedure:

1. Place pt supine w/ head extended and rotated to opposite side. Incise along upper $^2/_3$ of anterior border of SCM, curving posteriorly if above level of ear lobe to avoid injury to marginal mandibular nerve.

2. Bovie through platysma, then divide, ligate facial vein to expose carotid sheath; apex of ansa cervicalis (ansa hypoglossi) often found at this point and may be divided w/ relative impunity if necessary.

3. The facial vein is generally a good landmark for the location of the carotid bifurcation. This vein will require division for adequate exposure of the carotid artery.

4. Open sheath over common carotid artery, then encircle inferiorly w/ umbilical tape (+/– and Rummel tourniquet) or vessel loop. Next approach external carotid artery, encircling first branch (superior thyroid a.) followed by separate umbilical tape (w/ Rummel) or loop around external carotid. Place a loop around the distal internal carotid in a palpably soft segment.

5. If higher exposure is required, the digastric muscle can be divided and the hypoglossal nerve mobilized. The hypoglossal nerve is fixed in place by the SCM branch of the ECA. If this small artery is divided, the hypoglossal nerve can be more easily mobilized. For higher exposure toward the skull base, the stylohyoid tendon can be divided and the stylohyoid process can be removed using a bone Rongeur. This places the glossopharyngeal nerve at great risk and should be done w/ care. If lower exposure is necessary, the omohyoid muscle can be divided. Further proximal exposure requires median sternotomy.

6. Heparinize pt (5000 U IV), then occlude internal carotid, external carotid, and common carotid (in order).

7. *Anterolateral arteriotomy from CCA across ICA lesion then made. Decision for shunt (several choices*: Argyle, Pruitt-Inahara, Javid, etc.) can be nonselective, or based on stump pressure (want at least 50 mm Hg in CCA after occlusion of all but ICA), EEG findings if neuromonitoring utilized, or mental status changes if done under awake anesthesia.

8. Endarterectomy performed, including high-pressure injection of heparinized saline at edges to identify shelves/flaps.

9. Randomized controlled trials as well as large series have demonstrated a benefit to patching (decreased restenosis), and this should be done in essentially all pts. Can use vein (saphenous vein from ankle in men, from groin in females due to risk of patch blowout), Dacron, PTFE, bovine pericardium. No differences have been found in terms of stroke, restenosis w/ different patch types.

10. *Unclamp in the following order*: ECA, CCA (allow several cardiac cycles to pass to clear the endarterectomy site), ICA.

11. Many surgeons obtain postop Duplex scan, then awaken pt in operating room to check for gross neuro deficits before extubation.

INDEX